DON'T EAT TO LIVE, EAT TO THRIVE

How to Rewire Your Mind, Heal Your Body, and Redefine the Way You Eat Forever

PHILIP ONYEAGOLU

Don't Eat to Live, Eat to Thrive

ISBN Information

Paperback: 979-8-9998029-9-6

Cover Designed by: America Publishers

TABLE OF CONTENTS

FOREWORD

To you, the reader —

for your courage to pick up this book,
to question what you've been told,
and to dare to imagine a different way of living.
May these pages be a mirror and a map —
reminding you of the strength already within you,
and guiding you gently back to wholeness.

And to Dr. Mutsa Nyamfukdza —

whose wisdom, patience, and insight have
been a compass throughout this journey.
You reminded me that science must always serve
the soul, and that food is not just fuel —
it is love, medicine, and possibility.

This book is for the seekers, the healers,
and the thrivers-in-the-making.

Yes. There is.

PREFACE:

THIS IS NOT A DIET BOOK

If you've ever picked up a so-called "Diet" book, you know the deal promises of a smaller body, a quick transformation, a lovely "before-and-after" photo without the ugly in-between. Maybe you tried to follow it to the latter You counted calories, gave up bread, drank chalky shakes, and did dumb, hard treadmill workouts.

And here you are. Still searching.

Because here is the thing: diets don't work. They never have. What you need is not another list of forbidden foods or another rigid plan that leads to you feeling like a failure. What you need is a new point of view, a new sense of self, a food story that fits your life.

This is not a deprivation book; it is about fullness. It is about creating a life in which food is your friend and not your foe, where eating is not just a ritual for trying to survive, but one for thriving. Where your health is sustained by joy and not bogged down by shame.

And yes, there is science here, but not the type of science glossed over in jargon and charts. You will see solid evidence, with simple explanations that you can follow up on, woven into stories to ensure you remember them. You will have processes that you can use immediately, even tricks, and attitudes to release yourself from the exhausting struggle between your ears.

So, if you are ready not just to live, but actually thrive, read on.

INTRODUCTION:

WAKE UP HUNGRY

Just take a moment to imagine it: You wake up in the morning, and instead of an awful, beeping, blaring alarm, the first thing you notice is your stomach gently growling—not from emptiness, but from a sense of aliveness. Your body feels energized and alert. Your mind is clear, your muscles relaxed. You're hungry—not just for breakfast, but for everything the day has to offer

But, let's be honest - most mornings don't feel that way for most of us.

Most of the timc, it looks like this: You wake up feeling groggy, and you hit snooze again, and again, and again. It hurts to get out of bed, and your body already aches. You don't feel hunger – you might feel tired – maybe bloated, or more likely just numb. You drink your coffee, not for pleasure; it's for caffeine; without it, you cannot function. You either eat breakfast, or skip it altogether, or are in a rush with guilt.

This isn't really "normal" – it's just common. And maybe the most depressing part? You have been told this is all okay – that you are just "getting older" as feeling bleary gets a little worse. That you are just like any other "menopausal woman" as your weight has slowly crept up, your brain fog is from being "busy", and your craving for sugar at 10 PM was just your "personality".

None of that is true.

You have been hijacked – and it is NOT your fault.

Your biology, not by your choices, has been literally rewired for decades because entire industries thrive off your cravings, your tiredness, your endless cycle of dieting & disappointment. Your body is not broken or faulty – it has just been misled.

But here is the absolute and exciting truth: You can take it back.

This book is your wake-up call – literally. I want you to feel hunger – not just in the morning, but hunger for life, vitality, and thriving.

PART I

REAWAKENING THE BODY'S INTELLIGENCE

CHAPTER 1:

THE THRIVE BLUEPRINT:
HOW TO BREAK FREE FROM SURVIVAL MODE
AND CRACK THE CRAVINGS CODE

THE 10 PM WALL

The microwave says 10:07 PM.

David leans against the kitchen counter, and he is exhausted from the inside out; it is the kind of exhaustion that makes your limbs feel achy simply by existing. He had promised himself again that tonight would be different. No more late-night snacks. *No more caving in*

In the soft glow of the fridge light, with the refrigerator's compressor humming to fill the silence, he can almost hear the chips calling his name. His stomach doesn't growl; in fact, it feels heavy from dinner. But the craving is penetrating and relentless; it's not hunger, but something painful, something lodged in his brain that feels urgent, insistent, and impossible to ignore.

The bag of chips crinkles like it knows it has already won. The bottle of soda is sweating on the shelf above, with the condensation causing it to glimmer. His handshakes just slightly as he reaches in.

Why is this happening? he thinks. Why now, when I don't even want food? Why am I completely at the mercy of my impulses when I should be relaxing for bed?

What he doesn't know—what so many of us don't—is that this moment is not about having weak willpower or a lack of discipline. No, it is about programming. His body and its brain are moving along a script so powerful that it overrides facts, objectives, and even respect for itself.

This is **survival mode** at work.

And survival mode, if left unchecked, becomes the silent architect of your life.

THE AFTERNOON CRASH

If you want to figure out how David ended up in the kitchen at 10 PM, you have to go back to the previous night.

It is now 3:14 PM, and David is bent over his laptop in the office. His inbox resembles a minefield, and his eyelids are drooping and heavy. The edges of the screen have become fuzzy, and his focus has collapsed into a thick fog.

What does he do? He gets another cup of coffee, this time with two sugars. And because the vending machine is shining like a lighthouse beacon in the breakroom, he also takes a candy bar. Just a quick fix, he tells himself. A boost. Something to get him through the rest of the afternoon.

For twenty minutes, it works. His brain perks up, his pulse quickens, the fog thins. But just as quickly, he crashes again, like a puppet whose strings have been cut. By the time he gets home, exhaustion has hardened into irritability. Dinner feels like another task, not nourishment.

And so the cycle spins forward, almost predictably, until it deposits him right back in the kitchen at 10 PM, chasing energy that never lasts.

This is not laziness. This is not a lack of self-control. This is biology.

DEFINING SURVIVAL MODE

Before we go any further, let's call this what it is.

Survival mode is your body's emergency operating system. It is the mode your brain shifts into when there are conditions of resource scarcity, constant stress, and unstable conditions.

It serves a purpose to protect you. In true emergencies, famine, danger, life-or-death situations — survival mode is lifesaving. It's designed to keep you alert, ready to scan for threats. It prioritizes your immediate energy needs, not your long-term repair. It tells you, Get sugar, Get fat, Get that quick fuel NOW.

But here's the twist: In the modern world, survival mode is rarely switched off.

Stress at work, screens glowing at midnight, ultra-processed food engineered to hijack your brain — all these cues signal to your body that life continues to exist as an ongoing emergency.

WHEN SURVIVAL MODE IS PERPETUALLY SWITCHED ON:

Cortisol, the stress hormone, will be elevated.

Ghrelin, the hunger hormone, will follow unpredictable patterns.

Your brain's "reward" chemical, dopamine, will become addicted to quick hits of sugar, salt, and fat.

Sleep will suffer, recovery will be delayed, and your body will begin to break down at the seams.

The outcome? You wake up foggy, drag throughout the day, and crave food at the exact moment you should be sleeping.

Does that sound familiar? That is survival mode whispering in your ear, programming your cravings, writing your story without your consent.

THE INVISIBLE PROGRAMMING

Now pause for a moment. What if David's 10 PM kitchen scene, and your cravings, your crashes, were never about you?

What if the enemy isn't discipline, but design?

Think of it like this: You are not broken. You're operating on a program. And that program has been shaped by late nights, stress hormones, and let's be real, food companies that fully understand how to work with your biology. When you have cravings, it is not a failure on your part. Those cravings are a code.

- A code written by your hormones.

- A code exploited by processed food engineering.

- A code reinforced by stress and poor recovery.

In survival mode, this cravings code becomes the default operating system. It decides what you reach for, when you eat, and even how you feel about yourself afterward, but here is the good news. Every code can be rewritten.

That is what this chapter and this book are about: moving out of survival and into a Thrive Blueprint, where your cravings no longer control you—because you've cracked the code, and now you live by another one: energy, clarity, and joy.

CONNECTION

Maybe you've never found yourself in David's exact situation, but let's be real — does any of this sound familiar?

- The parent who eats their kids' leftover chicken nuggets at 9 PM because they're too drained to cook.

- The professional who skips lunch, then raids the pantry after work like a starving animal.

- The student who survives on energy drinks, chips, and adrenaline until the paper is finished at 2 AM.

- The night-shift worker who feels upside-down, never knowing when hunger will strike, just knowing that it always does, and it always wants sugar.

Suppose you've nodded your head at one of the above scenarios or stories, welcome. You are not alone. You are not weak.

You are human, and you live in a world that is designed for you to be in survival mode.

Well, here's the cliffhanger:

If cravings aren't a mere potency of weak will power - if they are actually wired straight into our biology, then what the hell is a craving? And how do we crack that cravings code before it's too late?

To crack the cravings code, we need to get into some craving science: dopamine loops, hunger hormones, and a billion-dollar food industry that knows your brain better than you do.

Once you understand how cravings are constructed, you'll never approach a 10 PM kitchen raid the same way again.

And that's exactly where we are going.

PART 2 - THE CRAVINGS CODE - WHY IT HAPPENS

The Puppet Strings

Think about when you walk into a grocery store after work.

You only went in for eggs and spinach. But twenty minutes later, you're ok with a cart full of chips, ice cream, and a pint of soda you didn't even want until it caught your eye, shimmering under the fluorescent lights.

What happened?

Food companies, neuroscientists, and flavor chemists are manipulating your cravings in the same way as a puppeteer pulls a marionette's strings. You tell yourself you're choosing, but when you grabbed that cart, your dopamine system, your brain's "I want more" circuit, was fired long beforehand.

That's The Cravings Code. A biological program taken over by food engineering, compounded by stress hormones, and misperceived as a willpower failure.

If you've ever wondered why you're fine with a pizza at 10 PM but not a broccoli, why you can stop at one apple but not one cookie, or why your body screams for sugar when you're fatigued, you are about to discover the pattern behind these behaviors.

And once you see the pattern, you can change it.

DOPAMINE - THE HIJACKED REWARD SYSTEM

Dopamine, not hunger, is at the heart of cravings.

Dopamine's often referred to as the pleasure molecule, but that isn't correct. It's not pleasure- it's anticipation. Dopamine hits in anticipation, not when you eat the cookie, but when you think about it, when you see it, when you smell it in the oven.

Anticipation drives you to act. To seek. To want.

In prehistoric times, dopamine was a compass; it drove us to calorie-dense food in times of famine. Sweet meant ripe fruit, fat meant survival fuel, salt meant vital minerals.

Now, the compass is hacked.

The engineering goal of modern processed food is to hit what scientists call the bliss point- the right ratio of sugar, salt, and fat that maximizes dopamine release without ever fully satisfying you.

- Eat a cookie? Dopamine says: *That was good. Eat another.*

- Drink a soda? Dopamine whispers: *Don't stop now.*

- Bite into a cheeseburger? Dopamine screams: *More, more, more.*

Your biology is not at fault here; it is behaving precisely as it was supposed to behave - the difference is who is in control of the biology - a billion-dollar food laboratory or Mother Nature?

Science focus: In 2013, Dr. Michael Moss's book *Salt Sugar Fat* revealed how major food companies hire "flavor architects" to dial in bliss points so precise that they can predict your likelihood of overeating. One executive was quoted as saying:

"We don't want to make food addictive, but we want it to be so compelling you can't resist it."

Sounds familiar, does it not? Dopamine has been weaponized.

GHRELIN & LEPTIN - THE HUNGER HORMONES

Dopamine identifies the "why we want," while the hunger hormones explain the "when".

You have two important hormones in play:

Ghrelin → the "hunger hormone". Ghrelin rises before meals, directs you to eat, and drops off after meals.

Leptin → the "satiety hormone". Leptin tells your brain that you are full and to stop eating.

In a healthy system, ghrelin and leptin dance together in harmony. But in survival mode, that dance is disrupted.

Late nights, stress, and ultra-processed food shift ghrelin rhythms earlier, making you hungrier later at night than you are in the morning. Meanwhile, a habit of high-sugar foods may blunt leptin signaling, causing you not to realize you are full even if you are overeating.

Not surprisingly, you eat too much and at the worst possible time, and you do not feel satisfied.

Study highlight: Research in the journal *Nature Medicine* (2004) found that people with chronically high sugar intake can develop leptin resistance — their brain no longer "hears" the fullness signal. This leads to overeating, weight gain, and increased risk of metabolic disease.

CORTISOL & STRESS EATING

Now let's add one more layer of complication: cortisol, the stress hormone.

When we are under stress — work, financial, or emotional, cortisol is elevated. Cortisol's role is to mobilize energy (sugar and fats) for immediate activity, or at the very least, bring the body into the mode of "fight or flight".

When there is no fight or flight, just 'our overflowing email inbox,' cortisol has nowhere to go. Instead, it triggers cravings for high-calorie foods, especially sugar.

Why sugar? Because it raises blood glucose quickly and therefore gives immediate relief for the stressed brain. For the stressed brain, it feels like survival.

However, lurking just around the corner are the negatives: that relief won't last long; the crash brings greater stress as well as new cravings, and you are stuck in a cycle of cravings without an obvious exit.

Mini-case study: Sarah is 42 years old and an attorney. She described her evenings as being a "stress-snack marathon". After 12 hours of high-stakes cases, she would crash in front of a bag of chips and wine on the couch. She was not hungry; she was tired, anxious, and loaded with all the cortisol. Her cravings were not a lack of willpower; it was cortisol telling her: We need to refuel, but not like this.

SLEEP, SCREENS & CIRCADIAN HIJACK

Let's throw some logs on the fire of cravings fueled by stress.

When you are looking at your phone at 1 am, the blue light delays melatonin and sleep. Less sleep means more ghrelin, less leptin, and now more cortisol—3 strikes against cravings.

- Sleep-deprived? Ghrelin says: *Eat more.*

- Leptin says: *I can't hear you, so you'll never feel full.*

- Cortisol says: *Grab sugar now.*

The next day, you wake groggy, skip breakfast, crash by mid-afternoon, and raid the pantry by night.

Study highlight: A 2004 University of Chicago study found that just two nights of restricted sleep (4–5 hours) increased ghrelin levels by 28% and decreased leptin by 18%, resulting in a 24% increase in hunger — primarily for high-carb, high-sugar foods.

Your cravings are not random. They are predictable outputs of dysfunctional circadian rhythms.

FOOD INDUSTRY ENGINEERING

Let's pull back the curtain.

Have you ever noticed how you can't stop at one potato chip? That's not an accident. Chips are designed to have the perfect crunch, dissolve quickly in the mouth (a phenomenon called **vanishing caloric density**), and hit the bliss point of salt and fat.

Soda? Carbonation plus sugar plus acidity equals a dopamine superhit.

Cookies? Sugar plus refined flour plus fat equals rapid blood sugar spikes and dopamine fireworks.

This is not food. This is **engineering**.

Insider story: Howard Moskowitz, a food scientist, famously tested dozens of variations of pasta sauce for Prego until he found the "magic formula" that triggered the highest consumer satisfaction. This same approach has been applied to nearly every processed food on the market — optimize the bliss point, maximize repeat consumption.

So, when David opens the chips at 10 pm, he is failing. He is colliding with one of the most powerful forces on the planet and an industry that thrives on keeping people in survival mode.

WILLPOWER IS NOT ENOUGH

Here is the ugly truth that most diets will never tell you: you cannot out-willpower biology.

If your cravings are actually code — driven by dopamine, hormones, stress, sleep disruption, and deliberate food product design, then trying to battle cravings using only willpower is no different than walking into a gunfight with a knife.

Willpower is a limited resource. Cravings, however, are a 24/7 program.

The only way out is to reprogram the code.

To understand the levers of biology and reset those levers to work for you.

To stop only existing and start thriving.

And that's where the Thrive Blueprint comes in.

So far, we've uncovered the problem; cravings are not weakness; cravings are biological hijacks that are layered on top of an entire world that is designed to keep you in survival mode.

But what if you could flip that switch?

What if instead of being a prisoner to cravings, you could see cravings for what they are: signals, compasses that point you toward what your body truly needs?

That is the promise of the next part: the Blueprint Introduction, the introduction of the four pillars that free you from survival mode and will allow you to crack the cravings code for good.

(REPROGRAMMING CRAVINGS AT THEIR ROOTS)

THE MOMENT OF TRUTH — YOU ARE NOT BROKEN

Here's the most important truth: cravings are not your fault.

They are the predictable results of biology meeting modern life.

But biology can be hacked and, just as easily, biology can be retrained. Your Brain is Plastic. It rewires itself based on repetition, environment, and signals. Your hormones are rhythmic; they actually reset to the normal rhythm if you align your behaviors!

Have you ever said, " I am never going to stop craving sugar?" Science says otherwise.

Neuroimaging studies provide us with evidence that dopamine receptors begin to calibrate back to baseline after two weeks of consistent nutrition reset. Ghrelin cycles slow back down. Cortisol normalizes. Sleep deepens. Cravings fade.

This is not self-discipline.

This is reprogramming for your body and brain back to baseline.

Let us break down reprogramming cravings into concrete, scientific actions.

ACTION STEP #1: PROTEIN AT YOUR FIRST MEAL

WHY IT WORKS:

Protein increases satiety by increasing peptide YY and GLP-1, the hormones that tell your brain you are done eating.

Protein blunts blood sugar spikes that create rollercoasters in brain chemistry that lead to cravings.

Studies (American Journal of Clinical Nutrition, 2014) show that a high-protein breakfast (30-35g) reduces cravings in the evening by 60%.

HOW TO IMPLEMENT:

To get protein at breakfast, swap your cereal or toast for eggs, Greek yogurt, or a protein smoothie.

You should be able to get 30g of protein into your first meal.

ACTION STEP #2: THE CRAVING PAUSE

Wait 15-minutes

WHY IT WORKS:

Cravings feel urgent because dopamine anticipates the reward. But research in *Appetite* (2011) shows that cravings often peak and fade within **15–20 minutes** if not acted on.

How do you maximize this:

When the craving arises, hit PAUSE.

Drink a glass of water, go for a brief walk, or stretch.

Ask yourself: "Am I really hungry, or am I looking for a little relief?"

Typically, by the time you return from your PAUSE, the craving has passed.

ACTION STEP 3: THE DOPAMINE SWAP

WHY THIS WORKS:

Dopamine is not exclusively food. It can be from novel experience, bodily movement, or small wins. You're going to work to reposition the loop by more deliberately replacing food-sourced dopamine highs with other stimuli.

HOW TO DO THIS:

- Keep a craving substitution list:
    - o 5 pushups
    - o Step outside for fresh air
    - o Listen to a favorite song
    - o Text a friend
- Each time you redirect, you weaken the old pathway and strengthen a new one. Neuroscience calls this "competitive rewiring."

ACTION STEP 4: BLOOD SUGAR ANCHORS

WHY THIS WORKS:

Unstable blood sugar is arguably the most significant trigger of cravings. Stable blood sugar allows ghrelin and leptin to sync together to stabilize the cortisol baseline instead of an "emergency" spike.

HOW TO DO THIS:

- Pair every carb with **protein or fat** (e.g., apple + almond butter).
- Avoid naked carbs (bread, chips, soda).
- Prioritize **slow carbs** (beans, lentils, sweet potatoes) over fast ones (white bread, candy).

Study highlight: In *Diabetes Care* (2009), participants who paired carbs with protein experienced 55% lower post-meal glucose spikes and significantly fewer cravings.

ACTION STEP 5: SLEEP RESET RITUAL

WHY THIS WORKS:

One bad night of sleep = up to 30% more craving the next day (University of Chicago, 2004).

Sleep is the ultimate craving moderator because it optimizes ghrelin, leptin, and cortisol.

HOW TO DO THIS:

- Screens off 60 minutes before bed.

- Cool, dark, quiet room.

- Anchor sleep/wake within a 30-minute window daily.

- If needed: magnesium glycinate, chamomile tea, or a wind-down ritual (stretch, journal, read).

ACTION STEP 6: EMOTIONAL SUBSTITUTION

WHY THIS WORKS:

Many cravings are not biological, but emotional (stress, loneliness, boredom).

In a study published in Frontiers in Psychology (2015), the practice of "emotional labeling" led to a decrease in "emotional eating" of an average of 40%.

HOW TO APPLY IT:

- When craving hits, pause and ask: "What am I really feeling right now?"

- Label it (stress, tired, anxious).

- Choose a non-food outlet aligned with that emotion:
  - o Stress → breathwork or quick walk
  - o Tired → 20-min nap
  - o Lonely → call/text someone

ACTION STEP 7: ENVIRONMENT RESET

WHY THIS WORKS:

Habits are context-specific. If you can remove the cue (i.e., chips on the counter), then you can prevent the craving loop from building strength. This is cue extinction in behavioral psychology.

HOW TO APPLY IT:

- Remove trigger foods from visible places (or your home entirely if possible).

- Keep fruit, nuts, and water visible.

- Redesign your kitchen as a **thriving environment**.

QUICK-REFERENCE CHART: REPROGRAMMING CRAVINGS AT THEIR ROOT

THE CRAVINGS CODE MAP

WHY CRAVINGS HAPPEN (THE CODE)

Dopamine Loops
Processed foods frigger "anticipation dopamine" Brain rewires for quick hits, not real fuel

Hormonal Signals
Ghrelin (hunger hormone) spikes at habitual times Leptin resistance dulls satiety cues

Food Engineering
"Bliss point" blends salt + sugar + fat = hijack Designed to override natural stop signals

Sleep & Stress
Cortisol surges = sugar/ starch cravings One poor night of sleep = 30% higher appetite

Emotional Eating
Cravings as coping (boredom, stress, loneliness) Food – quick comfort → reinforced loop

HOW TO REPROGRAM CRAVINGS

Protein First
30g in first meal to blunt cravings

15-Minute Pause
Delay + distract, cravings fade

Dopamine Swap
Music, movoment, connection > food

Blood Sugar Anchors
Pair carbs with protein/fat

Sleep Reset
7–9 hrs, wind-down ritual

Emotional Labeling
What om I "really" feeling?

Environment Reset
Remove trigger foods, show thrive foods

> Cravings aren't willpower failures. They're codes - and you can rewrite them.

Cravings are not a life sentence.

They are cues. They are learned loops. And they are reversible.

When you sync up your biology with the rhythms of nature, nourish your body with real food the way Mother Nature intended, and deliberately promote rewiring, cravings will lose their power over you.

The trick is not to resist harder. The trick is to plan smarter.

Now that you have unlocked the cravings code and you have your reset toolkit, you are ready to move into the Blueprint — the thriving system that will make sure you never again feel defined by survival mode.

PART 3: THE BLUEPRINT INTRODUCTION — THE 4 PILLARS

FROM CHAOS TO COMPASS

Imagine a city without a power grid.

Traffic lights blink at random. Neighborhoods fall dark while others flare with unstable surges. Refrigerators fail, food spoils, and the people adapt with short-term fixes: flashlights, diesel generators, and late-night takeout.

That's what survival mode feels like in the human body.

Your "grid" — the system that regulates energy, hunger, and recovery — flickers. You patch with caffeine jolts, sugar hits, and late-night snacks. The system never stabilizes. Each patch sets up the next crash.

Now imagine restoring the grid. Lights synchronize, traffic flows, and food stays fresh. It isn't flashy. It isn't glamorous. But it changes everything.

The Thrive Blueprint rests on four circuit breakers: Food, Movement, Recovery, and Rhythm. There are no diets. No hacks.

These are just a foundation, and cravings lose their grip. Rebuild them, and your biology re-learns how to thrive.

PILLAR 1 - FOOD - POISON OR MEDICINE

LISA'S CRASH

Lisa, a nurse on 12-hour shifts, dreaded her afternoons. By 3 PM, she'd be shaky, craving candy bars and soda from the vending machine. By 10 PM after her shift, she was back at the drive-thru.

This isn't a lack of discipline - she lacked a strong foundation. When she shifted what she had eaten earlier, cravings evaporated. Her secret wasn't eating *less*. It was eating *smarter*.

THE SCIENCE OF FOOD AND CRAVINGS

- **The Blood Sugar Rollercoaster**
  Refined carbs spike glucose → insulin surge → energy crash → cortisol/adrenaline release → cravings.

  o 🔖 Study: Ludwig DS, JAMA (2002) showed high-glycemic meals triggered sharper hunger rebound than low-glycemic meals of equal calories.

- **Protein as Anchor**
  Protein boosts satiety hormones (GLP-1, peptide YY), lowers ghrelin, and stabilizes appetite.

  o 🔖 Leidy HJ, *Obesity* (2013): high-protein breakfast reduced late-night snacking in overweight teens.

- **Food as Medicine or Poison**
  Ultra-processed foods hijack dopamine, inflame the gut, and teach the microbiome to crave junk. Anti-inflammatory foods restore hunger signals.

QUICK REFERENCE BOX — FOOD PROTOCOLS

BEGINNER:

Add 20-30g of protein to your first meal.

Replace one processed snack per day with a whole-food choice.

INTERMEDIATE:

Use the Protein + Fiber + Color formula for your meals.

Begin your day with water + a pinch of mineral salt.

ADVANCED:

Play around with your eating window (finish dinner by 7 pm).

Document your "trigger foods" that activate cravings, and begin phasing them out.

PILLAR TWO: MOVEMENT — ENERGY CREATES ENERGY

SARAH'S WALKS

Sarah worked in corporate law and thought that working out had to be 90 minutes long at the gym. If she could not make that time commitment, she wasn't going to work out at all.

Then, she started trying 10-minute walks after meals. Within a week, she noticed her afternoon slump had improved. After a month, her evening cravings were no longer a concern. Instead of being viewed as punishment, movement became a form of medicine.

THE SCIENCE OF MOVEMENT AND CRAVINGS

- **Glucose Disposal**
  Walking after meals lowers blood sugar spikes by 30%.

  o 🏷 Colberg SR, *Diabetes Care* (2016).

- **Dopamine & Endorphins**
  Exercise restores dopamine receptor sensitivity — undoing the hijack caused by processed food.

- **Circadian Anchor**
  Morning movement + light resets your body clock, which stabilizes hunger.

QUICK-REFERENCE BOX - MOVEMENT PROTOCOLS

BEGINNER:

Walk 5-10 minutes after meals.

Get up every 60-90 mins.

INTERMEDIATE:

Add 2-3 "movement snacks" (push-ups, squats, stairs).

Strength train 2x/week.

ADVANCED:

Some type of HIIT 1-2x/week for resilience.

Train outside; benefit from natural light and daylight exposure.

PILLAR THREE: RECOVERY - THE SILENT SUPERPOWER

MIGUEL'S SLEEP DEBT

Miguel didn't value sleep. He was a dad with two children, with work and scrolling taking priority over quality sleep. He didn't recognize the connection between poor sleep and eating until he began tracking his cravings: after every short night, he would snack relentlessly. But as he focused on getting 7.5 - 8 hours, his hunger levels normalized.

THE SCIENCE OF RECOVERY

- Sleep & Hunger Hormones

    o Poor sleep = +28% ghrelin, −18% leptin.

    o Spiegel K, *Lancet* (2004): short sleep added 300–400 extra calories daily.

- **Cortisol & Comfort Food**
  High stress = high cortisol = stronger pull toward sugar and fat.

- **Parasympathetic Recovery**
  Breathwork, journaling, yoga → activate "rest and digest" mode → cravings decline.

QUICK-REFERENCE BOX - RECOVERY PROTOCOLS

BEGINNER:

- Shut down screens 30 min before bed.
- Dim lights at night.

INTERMEDIATE:

- Journal or gratitude ritual before sleep.
- Sleep-wake consistency ±30 min.

ADVANCED:

- Track HRV and improve through breathing practices.
- Use naps strategically (20–30 min, early afternoon)

PILLAR FOUR: RHYTHM — ALIGNING WITH NATURE'S CLOCK

JAMAL'S LATE-NIGHT EATS

Jamal coded late into the night. Midnight was his binge window — popcorn, ice cream, then no hunger the next morning. By shifting his light exposure and meal timing, his hunger rhythm reset. His cravings followed.

THE SCIENCE OF RHYTHM

- **Ghrelin Timing**
  Habitual eating time shifts ghrelin cycles. Late meals = late hunger cues.

  o Garaulet M, PNAS (2013): late eaters lost less weight despite equal calories.

- **Light & Clock Genes**
  Morning light synchronizes the circadian master clock: metabolism, hunger, and sleep cascade in sync.

- **Meal Timing**
  Early meals improve insulin sensitivity and curb night cravings.

  o Sutton EF, *Cell Metabolism* (2018).

QUICK-REFERENCE BOX — RHYTHM PROTOCOLS

BEGINNER:

- Get sunlight within 1 hr of waking.
- Set a "last bite" alarm in the evening.

INTERMEDIATE:

- Anchor meals at consistent times.
- Cut caffeine after 2 PM.

ADVANCED:

- Align workouts with daylight.

- Experiment with intermittent fasting (12:12 or 14:10).

THE FOUR PILLARS TOGETHER

Imagine standing in the center of a square: each wall represents a pillar. If one falls, similar losses will be felt in each of the other three. But when all four stand tall, cravings lose their power. You stop fighting food. You stop "resisting." You begin thriving.

QUICK-REFERENCE BOX — THE FOUR PILLARS OF THRIVE

- **Food:** Protein-first, nutrient-dense, hydrated.

- **Movement:** Walk after meals, joyful flow, strength snacks.

- **Recovery:** Sleep ritual, stress dissolve, naps.

- **Rhythm:** Morning light, consistent meals, early cutoff.

Bottom Line: Build the foundation. When the pillars are steady, cravings crumble on their own.

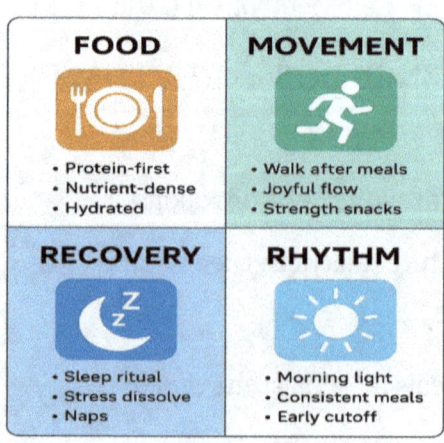

THE FOUR PILLARS OF THRIVE

FOOD	MOVEMENT
• Protein-first • Nutrient-dense • Hydrated	• Walk after meals • Joyful flow • Strength snacks
RECOVERY	**RHYTHM**
• Sleep ritual • Stress dissolve • Naps	• Morning light • Consistent meals • Early cutoff

PART 4 — THE ACTION STARTER: DAY ONE STEPS

THE THRESHOLD MOMENT

The journey of a thousand miles begins not with a giant leap, but with a first step. Imagine standing in your kitchen tomorrow morning. Nothing around you has changed yet — the cupboards still carry their stories, the cravings still whisper their promises — but something inside you is different. You've chosen to move from *survival mode* into *thrive mode.*

This chapter is not about waiting for the right moment. It is about knocking over the first domino that will release a chain reaction in the direction of health.

And it starts with small strategic Day One actions and evidence-based keystone habits that change more than what you are doing: they can also reprogram your biology.

WHY IS DAY ONE IMPORTANT?

Neuroscience tells us that the human brain craves momentum. When you take one aligned action, you are creating a "success spiral," as psychologists call it — a self-reinforcing feedback loop that makes the next decision easier.

Day One actions aren't about perfection. They are about an interruption of patterns — giving you enough time out of the survival mode cycle for your body and brain to get an experience of what a thrive mode feels like.

Think of these actions as reset buttons: small enough for immediate success, powerful enough to change your cravings, hormones, and mindset in a few hours.

DAY ONE STEP 1: PROTEIN-RICH FIRST MEAL

Action: Eat 20-30g of protein with some fibre and healthy fats within the first 90 minutes of waking.

SCIENCE:

- Protein slows the blood sugar rise that drives mid-morning crashes and cravings.

- It triggers the release of **GLP-1 and peptide YY** — satiety hormones that naturally suppress overeating.

- A 2013 study in the *American Journal of Clinical Nutrition* found that people who ate a high-protein breakfast had 60% fewer evening cravings compared to those who skipped or ate high-carb breakfasts.

Narrative: David, the late-night snacker we met earlier, tried this shift: eggs with spinach, avocado, and smoked salmon. By 10 PM, the haunting pull toward his freezer's ice cream stash was weaker than it had been in years.

QUICK REFERENCE BOX:

Day One Reset - Meal 1

- Eat eggs, Greek yogurt, or a protein shake.

- Add fiber + fat (avocado, nuts, greens) to lunch and dinner.

- Drink 8 ounces of water before your first coffee of the day.

DAY ONE STEP 2: 10 MINUTE WALK

Action: After dinner, take a 10-minute walk outside.

SCIENCE:

- Walking after meals improves **insulin sensitivity** by up to 30%, flattening glucose spikes that fuel night cravings.

- Light movement lowers cortisol, helping signal to the body it's time to wind down, not ramp up.

- A 2016 *Diabetes Care* study showed that even 10 minutes of walking post-dinner significantly reduced blood glucose compared to sitting.

Narrative: Picture yourself walking around your block at dusk. Streetlights glow. The craving clock (9–10 PM) ticks forward — but you've already shifted your biology. Muscles have absorbed the glucose surge, and the craving machinery never fully powers on.

QUICK REFERENCE BOX:

Day One Reset - Movement Anchor

- 10 minutes, as an initial version of walking after dinner

- Ideally outdoors for circadian (time of day) cues.

- Mindful walking can be used to cue both as an anchor (breathe, observe, release).

DAY ONE STEP 3: THE SCREENS-OFF RITUAL

Action: Create a **30-minute buffer zone before bed**: lights dimmed, no screens, one grounding ritual (stretching, journaling, reading).

SCIENCE:

- Evening blue light suppresses **melatonin**, delaying sleep onset and disrupting circadian alignment.

- Sleep deprivation boosts **ghrelin** and reduces **leptin**, making you hungrier (and more snack-prone) the next day.

- A 2017 study in *Sleep Health* found that reducing nighttime screen exposure improved both sleep quality and morning hunger cues within one week.

Narrative: For parents, this ritual might mean reading aloud to your child. For professionals, it might be jotting tomorrow's three top priorities on a sticky note and closing the laptop. Small signals that say: *the day is done, cravings are closed.*

QUICK-REFERENCE BOX:

Day One Reset — Recovery Ritual

- Screens off at least 30 min before bed.

- Choose: journal, stretching, reading, gratitude.

- Dim lights to cue the release of melatonin.

DAY ONE STEP 4: THE HYDRATION CUE

Action: Drink a full glass of water upon waking — *before* caffeine.

SCIENCE:

- Overnight dehydration often disguises itself as morning "false hunger."

- A 2013 study in *Appetite* confirmed that mild dehydration reduces alertness and increases subjective fatigue (which often drives sugar cravings).

- Hydration supports the **cortisol awakening response**, smoothing the transition into alertness.

QUICK-REFERENCE BOX:

Day One Reset — Hydration Anchor

- 12–16 oz water within 10 minutes of waking.

- Optional: add lemon or electrolytes.

- Delay caffeine until after water intake.

DAY ONE STEP 5: THE COMPASS CHECK IN

Action: Before your first meal, pause for 30 seconds and ask: *Am I truly hungry, or am I chasing stimulation?*

SCIENCE:

- Mindful check-ins activate the **prefrontal cortex**, the part of the brain that regulates impulse control and overrides craving loops.

- Over time, this reconditions dopamine pathways — associating reward not with processed food, but with self-mastery.

Narrative: David began jotting "Hungry / Not Hungry / Craving" on a sticky note each morning. Within two weeks, he noticed patterns: cravings clustered after poor sleep, true hunger followed hydration and movement. The notebook became his personal compass.

QUICK-REFERENCE BOX:

Day One Reset — Compass Check

- Pause 30 seconds before a meal.

- Ask: Hunger or craving?

- Optional: jot it down to track patterns.

PUTTING IT ALL TOGETHER: THE DAY ONE BLUEPRINT

If you did nothing else tomorrow other than these five steps, your biology would already be tilted toward thrive mode:

- A protein-powered breakfast blunts cravings.

- A 10-minute evening walk stabilizes glucose.

- A screens-off ritual repairs sleep.

- Morning hydration clears false hunger.

- A Compass check rewires the craving loop.

STYLED QUICK-REFERENCE RECAP: DAY ONE BLUEPRINT

1. **Protein Breakfast** — 20–30 g protein + fiber/fat.

2. **10-Min Evening Walk** — stabilize glucose, reduce cravings.

3. **Screens-Off Ritual** — 30-min buffer for recovery.

4. **Hydration Anchor** — water before coffee.

5. **Compass Check** — pause to distinguish hunger vs. craving.

These steps are your first taste of **control over cravings**. You've interrupted survival mode's circuitry. Tomorrow morning, you'll wake not in fog but with clarity.

But the real shift comes when you realize these aren't hacks — they are the opening moves in a larger **Blueprint for Thriving**.

This is where we will turn next.

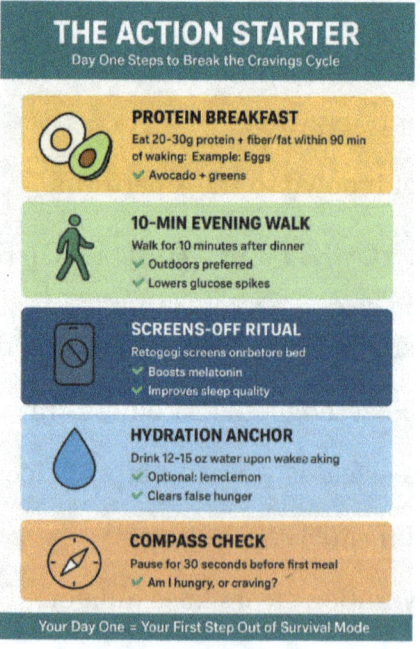

There's a moment, often subtle and quiet, when survival mode begins to loosen its grip. You feel it not as fireworks but as a soft, steady shift. It's that first night you fall asleep without your phone glowing in your hand. It's waking up clear-headed instead of foggy. It's reaching for an apple, not because you forced yourself to, but because, shockingly, it actually *sounds good.*

And in that moment, you realize thriving isn't a fantasy. It's a frequency you can tune into.

We started this chapter with David, the guy who slumped over at 3 PM, with nothing but caffeine fueling him, and whose cravings collided at 10 PM like a runaway train. That story wasn't about David alone. It was about millions of us caught in the same cycle: hustling, numbing, distracting, craving, and collapsing. That is survival mode.

Survival mode is not our natural state - thriving is. Your biology, your brain, and your circadian rhythm are developmentally designed for clarity, vibrancy, and equilibration. The only reason survival mode feels normal is because the modern world keeps us there: hyper-engineered foods, screens peering incessantly at us 24/7, broken rhythms, and endless stress.

What we've done in this chapter is expose cravings like never before. You've viewed the science - the dopamine loops, ghrelin spikes, and the "bliss point" game of engineered entrapment. You've also viewed that cravings are not a weakness. Cravings are signals. They are signals from a hijacked system.

And here is the radical truth:

If cravings can be programmed, cravings can be *reprogrammed.*

That's what the Thrive Blueprint is based upon. The Four Pillars - Food, Movement, Recovery, Rhythm - are not precognitive and irrelevant thoughts. They are your freedom levers. They are the blueprints of thriving.

And with even the smallest actions of "Day One" - protein at breakfast, a 10-minute evening walk, a screens-off ritual, you are already beginning to reprogram the code.

Now, imagine this with me for a moment.

You wake tomorrow. No foggy haze. No unseen weight sitting on your chest. Your body is present, your mind is clear. You don't reach for caffeine to awaken you - you are sipping your coffee (or tea, or water) because you choose to. You can't wait to sit down to breakfast, not with guilt or confusion, but with hunger - the clear, unconflicted kind that reminds you your body is present and ready to nourish.

That you exist. Not far away. Not someday. But here, now, waiting just beyond the cravings loop.

This is where we pivot. Chapter 2 is where the map opens wider. If Chapter 1 helped you crack the code - revealing the intricacies of cravings, and why they exist, and how to escape them - Chapter 2 is about rewiring your rhythms at their root. It gives us the opportunity to start aligning our body clock, our hormones, and our lifestyle to live in a state of thriving as the baseline and not an uphill battle.

Because here's the truth you deserve to carry forward:

You are not broken. You are not weak. You are not stuck.

You are a human being whose biology is brilliant, adaptive, and resilient. You've been wired for thriving since birth. Survival mode has been the interference—loud, distracting, insistent. But now, you've got the blueprint to quiet the noise.

So, take a deep breath. You've already started.

And as we step into the next chapter, ask yourself:

What would thriving look like for me—not in theory, but in my mornings, my meals, my movement, my rest?

Because the moment you can picture it, you're already closer than you think.

Cravings may have been your captor. But cravings, reprogrammed, can also be your compass. And tomorrow morning—the very next sunrise—could be the first time you wake not just to live but to *thrive*.

CHAPTER 2:

RHYTHM RESET:
ALIGNING YOUR BODY'S HIDDEN CLOCK

The alarm goes off. You roll over, hit the snooze button, and groan.

It's 6:30 AM, but your body feels like it's 2:00 AM. Your brain is mushy, your limbs barely lift, and the thought of breakfast feels absurd. You climb out of bed and go through the motions of taking a shower, grabbing a coffee, and telling yourself, "Tomorrow, I'll go to bed earlier. Tomorrow, I'll feel better."

But tomorrow arrives, and nothing changes.

Here is the secret no one tells you:

It's not just your sleep. It's not just your food. It's your clock.

Right now, inside your body, there is a master rhythm—an ancient, precise timekeeper—that governs when you feel alert, when you feel tired, when you get hungry, and even how you burn fat or store it. This is your **circadian rhythm**, the internal 24-hour clock written into your biology.

And here's the kicker: when that rhythm is aligned, everything feels easier. Hunger shows up at the right time. Cravings fade. Energy flows. Sleep restores. Mood stabilizes. Your body hums in harmony with its natural design.

But when this rhythm has been broken or misaligned, that is when survival mode takes over. That is when 10 PM cravings catch you off guard, right when you feel your willpower slipping. That is when mornings are like wading through mud. That is when your biology loses the capacity to thrive.

We call this chapter Rhythm Reset because it's not about willpower; it is about allowing yourself to connect back to the internal clockwork that already knows how to replenish, energize, and thrive- if you allow it.

So before we go any further, pause and ask yourself this:

What if the exhaustion, the cravings, the weight gain, the fog—it wasn't "you failing"... but your rhythm falling out of sync?

This chapter will teach you how to reset that rhythm - step by step, scientifically, and practically - so that thriving isn't something you need to fight for, but something your body remembers.

PART 1 — THE HIDDEN CLOCK: WHY CIRCADIAN RHYTHM RULES EVERYTHING

So, imagine this.

Two houses on the same quiet street. From the street, they look the same: white paint, tended lawn, porch light on. Inside? A different story.

The first house has a rhythm and hum. Lights come on when they should, coffee brewing in the kitchen, clothes tumbling in the washer, thermostat keeping the rooms warm, and at night, they turn off in unison. It isn't a château, but it runs like clockwork.

The second house? Chaos. Washer banging away at midnight; coffee being made way too late in the day, pouring out the last half stale; lights burnt out, blinking; and the thermostat literally ignores the weather. Nothing is actually broken, but it all feels off.

The truth is, your body is one of those houses.

The difference between thriving and dragging through survival mode often isn't the "quality of the house" (your DNA, your body type, your age)—it's whether your **internal timing system**, your circadian rhythm, is running in sync or out of sync.

And for many of us? We are living in the second house.

THE ANCIENT CLOCK INSIDE YOU

Every single one of your cells contains a clock. Yes—*every cell*. From your liver to your muscles, from your gut to your brain, there are microscopic oscillators ticking away, programmed to do their work on time.

But there's one master conductor: the **suprachiasmatic nucleus (SCN)**, a cluster of about 20,000 neurons in your brain's hypothalamus. Think of it as the maestro of an orchestra. The SCN keeps the beat, syncing your organs, your hormones, your metabolism, and even your mood.

- Your **liver clock** wants to process food during the day, not at 11 PM.

- Your **muscle clock** peaks for performance in the late afternoon.

- Your **melatonin clock** rises with darkness, telling your body when to sleep.

- Your **cortisol clock** spikes in the morning, giving you energy to start the day.

When everything is aligned, you live in harmony with your design. But when light, food, and stress scramble these signals, it's like the orchestra falls out of tune. Your body is still playing music—but it sounds like noise.

WHY CIRCADIAN RHYTHM RULES EVERYTHING

Let's strip away the noise of diets, hacks, and quick fixes. At its foundation:

- **Energy** → dictated by circadian cortisol and mitochondrial clocks.

- **Hunger** → driven by ghrelin and leptin pulses on a daily schedule.

- **Mood** → linked to serotonin and dopamine rhythms.

- **Repair** → optimized during deep sleep phases set by your internal clock.

- **Immunity** → strengthened or weakened depending on rhythm alignment.

A 2017 Nobel Prize in Medicine was awarded to scientists who proved this: circadian clocks regulate nearly every process in your body. Ignore the clock, and you invite chaos. Respect it, and you unlock health at its deepest level.

MINI-STORIES OF RHYTHM IN ACTION

THE NIGHT OWL NURSE

Maria, a nurse, works rotating shifts. On nights, she snacks on crackers and soda at 2 AM, sleeps fitfully during the day, and often feels wired-tired. She wonders why her digestion feels off and her cravings spike. Her rhythm isn't broken—it's just **misaligned.**

THE JET-LAGGED ENTREPRENEUR

David, a frequent flyer, crisscrosses time zones weekly. He eats dinner at 10 PM in London, breakfast at 6 AM in New York, and wonders why his weight won't budge despite working out. His hunger signals are scrambled because his **clocks can't agree on the time.**

THE PARENT ON AUTOPILOT

Jason, a father of two, collapses at night after late Netflix binges, then drags himself awake with coffee. He thinks he just needs more discipline. In truth, his circadian rhythm is like that second house—lights flickering, washer running at the wrong hour.

THE SCIENCE OF MISALIGNMENT

When you live against your circadian rhythm, here's what happens:

1. **Hormones rebel.** Ghrelin (hunger hormone) spikes at night, while leptin (satiety hormone) misfires. This is why chips at 10 PM feel irresistible.

2. **Metabolism stalls.** Your liver is "asleep" at night, meaning late-night calories are more likely to be stored as fat.

3. **Sleep fragments.** Melatonin can't rise properly when blue light floods your eyes at midnight, leaving you restless.

4. **Mood crashes.** Dopamine and serotonin get desynchronized, leading to irritability, anxiety, or flatness.

It's not a weakness. It's biology.

QUICK-REFERENCE BOX: SIGNS YOUR RHYTHM IS OUT OF SYNC

CHECK YOUR COMPASS:

- You crave sugar or salty snacks late at night.

- You wake up groggy, no matter how many hours you sleep.

- Your hunger patterns feel unpredictable.

- Afternoon crashes leave you dependent on caffeine.

- You gain weight even on fewer calories.

- You feel moody, foggy, or "wired but tired."

If you nodded to 3 or more, your house isn't broken—it's just running off time.

ACTION STEPS: RESETTING THE HIDDEN CLOCK (DAY ONE MOVES)

You don't have to overhaul your life overnight. Start with **three simple levers** that directly realign the master clock:

1. **Light as Your Anchor**

    a. Get 5-10 minutes of natural morning light within an hour of waking.

    b. Dim screens and overhead lights 90 minutes before bed.

    c. Why? Light is the most powerful signal to your SCN.

2. **Food Timing Reset**

    a. Eat your first real meal within 2 hours of waking (protein + fiber).

    b. Close your eating window 2-3 hours before bed.

    c. Why? Food timing resets peripheral clocks in your gut and liver.

3. **Movement Pulse**

    a. A 10-15 minute walk after meals lowers blood sugar and tells your body: *daytime mode, not storage mode.*

    b. Why? Movement is a cue for energy availability and circadian alignment.

Think of this: what if *everything*—your cravings, your sleep, your weight, your mood—wasn't just about what you eat or how much you move, but *when* you do it?

The Thrive Blueprint begins with rhythm. Align the clock, and suddenly the house hums, the cravings quiet, and your biology remembers how to thrive.

But before we move on, we need to decode something deeper—the invisible script running your desires, the cravings code itself.

PART 2 — THE HUNGER CLOCK: WHEN BIOLOGY MEETS RHYTHM

Before we continue, let's stop for a moment and state something so simple, but true:

Hunger is not random.

It definitely feels random when it appears at 10 PM with a tiny voice suggesting cookies, or disappears at 8 AM after not eating for 12 hours. But hunger is not random. It has a clock. When the clock is aligned, your body hums along with the natural appetite cycles. When the clock is off, cravings are in the driver's seat.

THE RHYTHM OF HUNGER: GHRELIN AND LEPTIN IN ACTION

Two hormones play lead roles here:

- **Ghrelin** → your "hunger hormone." Peaks before meals, nudging you to eat. Falls after eating.

- **Leptin** → your "satiety hormone." Signals fullness, keeps you from overeating.

Here's the kicker: both ghrelin and leptin don't just respond to food. They respond to **time**.

- If you eat at 10 PM every night, ghrelin will start rising at 9:45 PM, even if your energy stores are full.

- If you stop eating by 7 PM consistently, ghrelin shifts earlier, peaking for breakfast instead of midnight.

A landmark study in *Obesity* (Cummings et al., 2001) found ghrelin spikes in anticipation of habitual mealtimes, even if no calories are needed. In other words, your body learns the clock you set.

This means cravings are often a **timing signal, not a true energy need**.

WHY WE LOSE MORNING HUNGER

Why do so many people not have an appetite in the morning, but then become completely ravenous at night?

It's not because their metabolism is broken. It's because their **hunger clock is delayed**.

- Eating late pushes ghrelin later.

- Blue light and screens suppress melatonin, delaying sleep, which delays cortisol's morning spike.

- Cortisol normally primes ghrelin for a breakfast appetite. But when cortisol is blunted, ghrelin stays quiet in the morning.

The result?

- No hunger at 7 AM.

- A wave of "fake hunger" at 10 PM.

It's not a lack of willpower — it's a misaligned rhythm.

MINI-STORIES: HUNGER IN REAL LIFE

◇ THE LATE-NIGHT CODER

James, a software engineer, stays up until 1 AM, eating chips "to focus." He skips breakfast because he "isn't hungry." By lunch, he's starving and overeating. His hunger clock is simply trained to expect fuel when the moon is up, not the sun.

◇ THE MORNING RUNNER

Priya, a recreational runner, keeps a consistent schedule: bed by 10, run at 6, breakfast by 7. She wakes up naturally hungry and energized. Her hunger clock is tuned like the first house from Chapter 2's opening—everything runs on time.

THE CORTISOL AWAKENING RESPONSE (CAR): THE MORNING SPARK

One of the most overlooked pieces of the hunger puzzle is cortisol.

Normally, cortisol rises sharply within 30–45 minutes of waking. This isn't "stress" cortisol — it's your body's natural *ignition switch*. It mobilizes glucose and fatty acids to give you morning energy. This rise also helps set ghrelin's rhythm, creating a signal for morning hunger.

But:

- Chronic stress, late nights, and irregular sleep blunt this cortisol rise.

- Without that spark, ghrelin stays low. You feel groggy, not hungry.

A study in *Psychoneuroendocrinology* (2013) confirmed that disrupted CAR is linked with irregular hunger cues and metabolic sluggishness.

QUICK-REFERENCE BOX: WHY HUNGER SHIFTS OFF CLOCK

THE BIG 4 CAUSES OF DELAYED HUNGER:

a. **Late-night eating** → pushes ghrelin later.

b. **Screen light at night** → delays melatonin, shifts cortisol spike.

c. **Chronic stress** → blunts cortisol awakening response.

d. **Irregular meal timing** → trains ghrelin to show up at odd hours.

REPROGRAMMING HUNGER: RESETTING THE CLOCK

The good news? Your hunger clock is highly adaptable. Just as it learned late-night snacking, it can relearn morning hunger.

Here's how:

STEP 1 — ANCHOR WITH LIGHT

- Get 5–10 minutes of sunlight within an hour of waking.

- Why: This triggers cortisol's rise, syncing ghrelin for a breakfast appetite.

STEP 2 — EAT EARLY PROTEIN

- Even if you're not starving, have 20–30 grams of protein within 2 hours of waking.

- Why: Early protein shifts ghrelin earlier the next day and stabilizes leptin signals.

STEP 3 — CLOSE THE KITCHEN EARLIER

- Stop eating 2–3 hours before bed.

- Why: Teaches ghrelin to anticipate food earlier instead of at night.

STEP 4 — CONSISTENCY OVER PERFECTION

- Hunger clocks adjust within 7–10 days of consistent timing.

- Skipping breakfast one day or snacking late one night won't ruin you, but patterns matter more than exceptions.

QUICK-REFERENCE BOX: THE HUNGER RESET PROTOCOL

DAILY ANCHORS:

- **Morning:** Light + protein.

- **Daytime:** Meals aligned with daylight.

- **Night:** Screen dimming + no food 2–3 hrs before bed.

In 1–2 weeks, you'll notice:

☑ Morning hunger returns naturally.

☑ Night cravings fade.

☑ Energy stabilizes across the day.

When you begin to recognize a hunger clock, cravings stop feeling like an enemy. They become a signal — a clue or indication of whether your rhythm is in sync or not.

And here's the reframe:

- Hunger at 8 AM? That's not just appetite. Its **alignment**.

- Hunger at 10 PM? That's not a weakness. It's **mis-timing**.

In the next part of this chapter, we will take this a step further: how to incorporate hunger and rhythm into the Blueprint itself - the daily practices that transform survival mode into thrive mode.

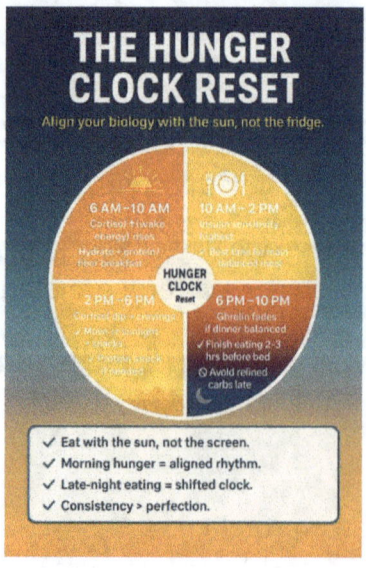

PART 3 THE THRIVE BLUEPRINT — THE 4 PILLARS

THE TURNING POINT

Envision this.

You have just recognized your hunger is no longer random - it is a signal, a rhythm, a coded communication from deep in your biology. For the first time, you're seeing your cravings not like some weakness but as some secret that is being communicated to you from your own clock inside every one of your cells.

Now, imagine you are standing on this threshold of change, and you are in a position to consider two futures:

- One where you stay locked in the old cycle, eating at midnight, waking foggy, crashing by 3 p.m., ruled by cravings.

- And another where you move in rhythm with your body's natural design, sharper mornings, steady energy, cravings dissolving like mist in sunlight.

The difference between those futures isn't willpower. It's architecture.

This is where the **Thrive Blueprint** comes in. Four pillars that turn theory into lived reality. Think of them like the frame of a house: if one pillar is weak, the structure wobbles. Together, they build a foundation strong enough to reset your hunger clock and keep it aligned — not for days, but for life.

THE FOUR PILLARS OF THE THRIVE BLUEPRINT

PILLAR 1 — LIGHT & RHYTHM

"Anchor your biology to the sun."

- **Why it matters:** Morning sunlight resets your master circadian clock, downstream clocks follow — including those that govern hunger.

- **Science Snapshot:** A 2017 trial found that just 20 minutes of morning sunlight reduced ghrelin spikes and improved appetite control later in the day.

- **Action Protocol:**

  o Morning: 5–15 minutes of outdoor light within 60 minutes of waking.

  o Evening: Dim lights 1–2 hours before bed.

  o Bonus: Use "light bookends" — morning bright, evening dim.

Quick-Reference Box: Light & Rhythm

- Morning sunlight = natural hunger reset.

- Dim evening light = melatonin protection.

- "Bookend your day with light."

PILLAR 2 — FUEL & FLOW

"Feed your body in rhythm, not reaction."

- **Why it matters:** Food timing signals your metabolism as strongly as what you eat. Eating late skews hormones, leading to a storage mode.

- **Science Snapshot:** Harvard researchers showed that shifting a main meal from 8 p.m. to 1 p.m. improved fat oxidation by 25%.

- **Action Protocol:**

  o First meal: Prioritize protein + fiber within 1–2 hours of waking.

  o Midday: Make this your largest, most balanced meal.

  o Evening: Lighter dinner, finish 2–3 hours before bed.

Quick-Reference Box: Fuel & Flow

- Protein + fiber = stable hunger signals.
- Eat more earlier, less later.
- Midday = prime fueling window.

PILLAR 3 — REST & REPAIR

"Protect the repair window — it runs the night shift."

- **Why it matters:** Sleep recalibrates ghrelin (hunger) and leptin (satiety). Skimp on sleep, and your cravings dial turns up by morning.
- **Science Snapshot:** A 2022 meta-analysis: <6 hours of sleep = 33% higher ghrelin, 26% lower leptin the next day.
- **Action Protocol:**
    - Digital sunset: Shut off stimulating screens 60 minutes before bed.
    - Sleep window: Consistent sleep + wake (±30 min).
    - Optimize: Cool, dark, quiet room → melatonin release.

QUICK-REFERENCE BOX: REST & REPAIR

- Sleep = tomorrow's first meal.
- Cool, dark, quiet = melatonin boost.
- Digital sunset = cravings control.

PILLAR 4 — MIND & STRESS

"Calm the storm that drives false hunger."

- **Why it matters:** Cortisol surges mimic hunger. Chronic stress → cravings for sugar and quick fuel.

- **Science Snapshot:** Stanford study: stressed participants ate 40% more sugary foods, independent of true hunger.

- **Action Protocol:**

  o Breath: 3–6 reset (inhale 3, exhale 6).

  o Pause: Ask, "*Am I hungry, or just stressed/thirsty?*"

  o Anchor: 5-minute mindfulness cuts stress-driven snacking by 30%.

QUICK-REFERENCE BOX: MIND & STRESS

- Stress ≠ hunger.

- Exhale longer than inhale to calm cravings.

- Check thirst before food.

NARRATIVE BRIDGE

These four pillars can be thought of like the tuning pegs on a guitar. If one peg is loose, the music will be out of tune for a long time. If all four strips are harmonized, life feels rhythmically connected; energy is steady, cravings are manageable, and hunger is in line with what's best for your health.

The Thrive Blueprint is not about fighting cravings; it is about removing the conditions that make cravings successful.

As you move through this book, each pillar will unfold slowly into practice. Daily micro-practices will be used to stack rhythm on top of rhythm, until thriving is no longer a push - but a pull; the natural state that your biology has been wanting to get back to all along.

Because thriving is not the absence of cravings.

It is the presence of rhythm.

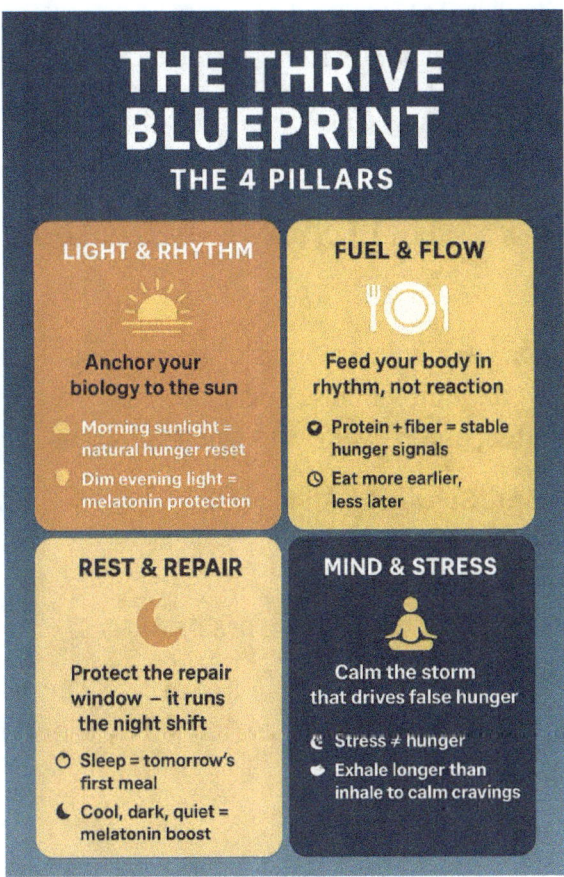

THE THRIVE BLUEPRINT

THE 4 PILLARS

LIGHT & RHYTHM

Anchor your biology to the sun

- Morning sunlight = natural hunger reset
- Dim evening light = melatonin protection

FUEL & FLOW

Feed your body in rhythm, not reaction

- Protein + fiber = stable hunger signals
- Eat more earlier, less later

REST & REPAIR

Protect the repair window – it runs the night shift

- Sleep = tomorrow's first meal
- Cool, dark, quiet = melatonin boost

MIND & STRESS

Calm the storm that drives false hunger

- Stress ≠ hunger
- Exhale longer than inhale to calm cravings

PART 4: THE ACTION STARTER

A DAY IN RHYTHM VS. A DAY IN SURVIVAL MODE

Before we discuss strategy, let's take a moment to visualize this:

You awaken to your alarm at 6:30 AM. Instead of your typical grogginess, your body feels light with your head clear. You feel a gentle hunger awakening. You hydrate and eat a balanced breakfast; by 9:00 AM, your brain is switched on, no jitteriness, no fog.

Now think of "the old way": exhausted when you wake, you skip breakfast, over-caffeinate yourself, climb the rollercoaster of cravings every hour of every day, crash mid-afternoon, and still raid the pantry at 10 PM.

These two realities hinge on the same thing: how you align your daily choices with your body's hunger clock.

This section is your Day One Blueprint: practical, actionable steps you can use today. Not a diet. Not a punishment. A rhythm.

ARCHETYPE #1: THE BUSY PROFESSIONAL

PROFILE:

Maria, 39, project manager at a tech firm. Long meetings, deadlines, and constant emails. She's used to skipping breakfast, surviving on coffee, and battling 3 PM sugar crashes.

Reset Blueprint (Circadian Aligned):

6:30 AM — Wake Window

- **Action:** Hydrate with a tall glass of water.
- **Why:** Overnight, cortisol spikes to mobilize energy. Hydration helps cortisol do its job without false hunger signals.

7:00 AM — Morning Anchor Meal

- **Action:** Protein + fiber-rich breakfast (e.g., Greek yogurt + berries + chia).
- **Why:** Ghrelin peaks here. Feeding with protein/fiber stabilizes blood sugar and reduces afternoon crashes.

10:30 AM — Focus Window

- **Action:** 5-minute walk outside + green tea.
- **Why:** Movement increases insulin sensitivity; sunlight anchors the circadian rhythm.

1:00 PM — Midday Fuel Window

- **Action:** Balanced plate (lean protein + greens + slow carbs + healthy fat).
- **Why:** This is peak insulin sensitivity — the best time for the largest meal.

3:30 PM — Cortisol Dip

- **Action:** Stretch, walk, or 5-minute breathwork. Optional protein snack (boiled egg, handful of almonds).
- **Why:** Cortisol naturally dips, creating "false cravings." Movement restores energy.

6:30 PM — Dinner

- **Action:** Light, balanced plate (protein + non-starchy veggies).
- **Why:** Keeps ghrelin stable, reduces late-night hunger.

9:00 PM — Wind-Down Ritual

- **Action:** Screen-off, herbal tea, journaling.
- **Why:** Melatonin rises only if light exposure drops. No light = better sleep = fewer cravings.

ARCHETYPE #2: THE PARENT

PROFILE:

James, 42, father of two (ages 5 and 8). His mornings start chaotic: school runs, work commute, late-night exhaustion. He often eats leftovers from the kids' plates and snacks after bedtime.

Reset Blueprint (Circadian Aligned):

6:00 AM — Wake Window

- **Action:** Hydrate + 2 mins of stretching while kids eat breakfast.
- **Why:** Hydration + light movement turns on metabolism before the chaos.

6:30 AM — Family Breakfast

- **Action:** Protein-focused breakfast (eggs + avocado + toast).
- **Why:** Eating with kids builds rhythm. Protein helps avoid sugar rollercoaster.

9:00 AM — Post-School Reset

- **Action:** Quick outdoor walk or sunlight exposure before work emails.
- **Why:** Anchors circadian clock → improves focus for work.

12:30 PM — Lunch Window

- **Action:** Balanced meal, ideally pre-prepped to avoid grabbing junk.
- **Why:** Matches peak insulin sensitivity.

3:00 PM — Cortisol Dip

- **Action:** "Snack swap" with kids (apple + nut butter vs. chips).
- **Why:** Models healthy eating while preventing his own late-night rebound cravings.

7:00 PM — Family Dinner

- **Action:** Balanced but lighter plate (lean protein + roasted veggies).
- **Why:** Kids sleep better with consistent meals; James reduces late-night hunger.

9:30 PM — Evening Anchor

- **Action:** Read with kids, dim lights, no phone.

- **Why:** Melatonin release → deep recovery → stronger morning hunger.

QUICK-REFERENCE: ACTION STARTER TIMELINE

🕐 **6–10 AM:** Hydrate + protein/fiber breakfast

🕐 **10 AM–2 PM:** Main balanced meal → fuel window

🕐 **2–6 PM:** Cortisol dip → move instead of snack

🕐 **6–10 PM:** Dinner early + light → wind-down

🕐 **10 PM–6 AM:** Sleep window → no food, deep repair

☞ This isn't a diet. It's a rhythm.

And rhythm, more than rules, is what flips your biology from *survival mode* to *thrive mode*.

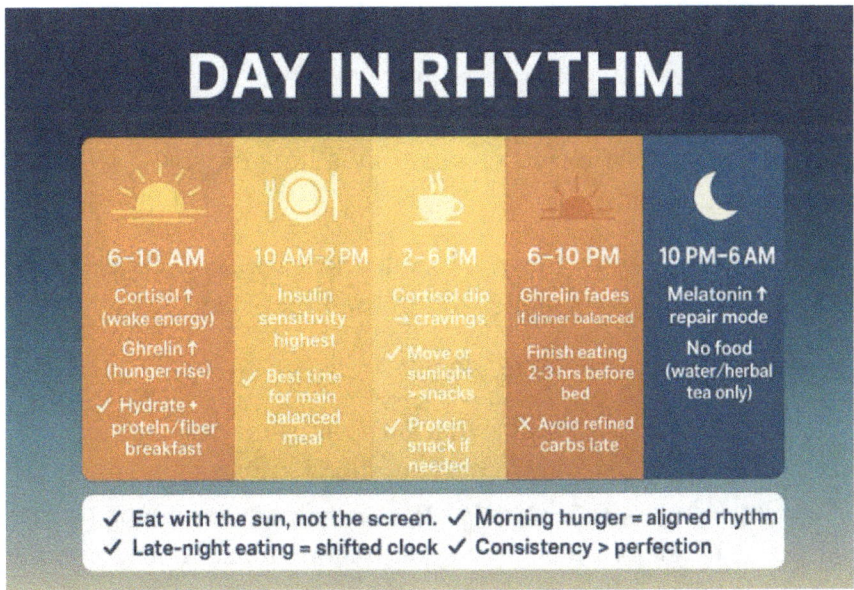

From Rhythm to Truth

The clock has always been ticking. The difference is that now, you can hear it.

Not the ticking of your watch or your phone, but the deeper rhythm your body has been whispering to you all along—a rhythm written in light and darkness, in cortisol and melatonin, in hunger and satiety.

You've seen what happens when you align with this clock: mornings no longer feel like battles, cravings lose their grip, energy steadies instead of crashing, and food begins to feel like fuel rather than a fight.

This is not about perfection; it's about partnership. When you rise with the sun, fuel in rhythm with the day, and rest in tune with the night, you stop working *against* your biology and start working *with* it. That is how thriving begins: not with a dramatic overhaul, but with a decision to let your life fall into sync with its natural beat.

But there's something else we need to talk about. Because even when you begin honoring this rhythm, there's a trap waiting just around the corner: your body will still lie to you.

It will whisper, "*I need sugar now or I won't survive.*" It will scream, "*I'm starving at 10 PM*", even when you ate dinner two hours ago. It will trick you into believing exhaustion is hunger, stress is hunger, loneliness is hunger.

And unless you know how to decode those lies, you'll keep feeding signals that were never about food in the first place.

That is where we are going next.

Chapter 3 is about pulling back the curtain on the *illusion of hunger*. It's about learning why your body sometimes sends false alarms—and how to separate true fuel needs from cravings engineered by stress, habit, or even billion-dollar food companies that have learned to hijack your biology.

You've set the foundation with rhythm. Now it's time to face the deceiver within and learn how to hear the *truth beneath the craving*.

Turn the page, and let's rewrite the way you understand hunger itself.

CHAPTER 3:

YOUR BODY IS A LIAR

THE BETRAYAL YOU DIDN'T SEE COMING

Imagine you're walking through a desert, lips cracked, skin burning. Your body screams for water. You stumble across a bottle—ice cold, glistening. You drink deeply, and relief floods you. That's how it should work: your body signals what you need, you respond, and balance is restored.

But what if I told you that in the modern world, your body no longer knows how to speak the truth?

That growling "hunger" at midnight? It's not real hunger—it's hijacked dopamine.

That 3 PM crash demanding caffeine? That's not fatigue, it's your circadian rhythm sabotaged by sugar.

That lack of appetite in the morning? That's not "just you", it's broken signaling.

Your body is lying. Not maliciously. Not because it hates you. But because it's been rewired.

HOW THE LIE BEGAN

Once upon a time, your body's signals were perfect. Hunger meant you needed food. Satiety meant you'd had enough. Cravings guided you toward nutrient salt when your body needed electrolytes, and fat when your brain required energy.

Then came the food industry.

Scientists in white coats learned to hijack your biology. They studied bliss points—the precise combination of salt, sugar, and fat that overrides satiety and keeps you eating. They tested hundreds of formulas until they discovered how to trick your brain into thinking: I *need more.*

Result? You don't crave potato chips because your body "needs" them. You crave them because they were engineered to make you crave them.

This is the lie.

STORY: THE CEREAL DECEPTION

In the 1970s, breakfast cereal companies realized something dangerous: if they could capture children's palates early, they'd own them for life. They poured millions into making cereals sweeter, crunchier, more colorful, and more addictive.

Parents thought they were giving kids "a good start to the day." Kids thought they just "liked cereal." But what really happened was this: sugar-laden flakes hijacked ghrelin, leptin, and dopamine, teaching children to crave sweet mornings.

Fast-forward thirty years: those same kids, now adults, "aren't hungry in the morning." They need coffee to survive. Their bodies lie to them because they were trained to lie since childhood.

THE SCIENCE OF LYING SIGNALS

Let's break it down:

1. DOPAMINE HIJACKING

- Dopamine is your "wanting" chemical. In nature, it motivates you to seek food, sex, and novelty.

- Ultra-processed foods—high in sugar and fat—trigger dopamine surges far beyond natural levels.

- Over time, your brain downregulates dopamine receptors. You need more stimulation to feel satisfied. This is why one cookie isn't enough—you suddenly want the whole box.

2. INSULIN CONFUSION

- Natural eating: You eat, blood sugar rises, insulin clears it, and hunger fades.

- Processed eating: Sugar spikes your blood sugar, insulin overreacts, sugar plummets, and you feel ravenous—again.

- Your body lies: *You're starving.* But you're not. You're trapped in a crash cycle.

3. LEPTIN RESISTANCE

- In a healthy system, leptin tells your brain: *Stop eating, we're full.*

- Chronic inflammation blunts this signal. You keep eating not because you're hungry, but because the "stop" button is broken.

4. CIRCADIAN RHYTHM MISFIRES

- Your body evolved to eat in daylight, fast at night.

- Blue light, late-night screens, and 24/7 access to food scramble this rhythm.

- Result: hunger at night, no appetite in the morning. Another lie.

THE EMOTIONAL FALLOUT

This betrayal has consequences far beyond the waistline.

- You blame yourself for "lacking discipline."

- You feel shame when you binge, not realizing your brain was chemically manipulated.

- You believe your cravings define you, instead of seeing them as hijacked signals.

The tragedy is not the food itself—it's the shame it creates. You begin to distrust yourself. You believe *I can't control my body.*

But the truth is: it's not that you can't control your body. It's that your body's signals can't be trusted—yet.

REFRAMING: FROM VICTIM TO DETECTIVE

Here's the shift you must make: stop seeing yourself as a victim of weak willpower, and start seeing yourself as a detective.

Your hunger, your cravings, your fatigue—they're clues. They tell you what's broken, what's misaligned. Your job isn't to suppress or ignore them. Your job is to decode them.

When you realize your body sometimes lies, you stop obeying every impulse. Instead, you step back and ask: *Is this real hunger, or hijacked hunger?*

That question alone creates space. That space is freedom.

ACTION FRAMEWORK: SPOTTING THE LIES

Here's how to start decoding your body's signals:

STEP 1: HUNGER JOURNAL

- For 7 days, write down each time you feel hungry. Note:
  - Time of day
  - What you crave (sweet, salty, protein, fresh food)
  - Energy level
  - Mood

- After a week, patterns emerge. Midnight "hunger" paired with exhaustion? Probably dopamine-driven, not real. Morning absence of hunger? Likely circadian misalignment.

STEP 2: REAL HUNGER VS. FAKE HUNGER CHECKLIST

Ask yourself:

- Would I eat plain chicken breast or boiled eggs right now?
  - If yes → real hunger.
  - If no (only pizza or cookies sound good) → fake hunger.
- How long since my last meal?
  - 3+ hours → likely real.
  - <1 hour → probably a crash.
- Am I tired, stressed, or bored?
  - Emotional cues often masquerade as hunger.

STEP 3: DELAY & DISTRACT

- When in doubt, wait 15 minutes. Drink water. Walk. Breathe.
- Real hunger persists. Fake hunger fades.

CASE STUDY: JASON'S MIDNIGHT HUNGER

Jason, 29, worked long shifts and often found himself raiding the fridge at 11 PM. He felt powerless, convinced he had "no discipline."

We ran him through the Hunger Journal. Patterns appeared: his "hunger" always struck after screens, late-night scrolling, and was always for sugar. When asked if he'd eat eggs or grilled chicken, the answer was always no.

We reframed it: *Jason, your body isn't hungry. Your dopamine is.*

He began replacing the midnight snack with a 15-minute walk around his block, followed by chamomile tea. Within two weeks, the midnight hunger was gone. By week four, he woke up hungry for the first time in years.

Jason didn't fix his willpower. He fixed the lie.

THE FIRST REPROGRAMMING EXERCISE

Tonight, before bed, try this experiment:

1. Write down what time you last ate.

2. Turn off screens 60 minutes before sleep.

3. If "hunger" strikes, test it with the boiled-egg question: Would I eat it right now?

4. If no, breathe deeply for 5 minutes, sip water or tea, and let the wave pass.

Do this for seven nights. Watch how quickly the midnight lies dissolve.

YOUR BIOLOGY FOR SALE

Think about it: every craving you feel, every hunger pang, every impulse—it's valuable real estate. The food industry spends billions each year to own it.

In 2011, a New York Times investigation revealed how food giants hired teams of neuroscientists to study the brain's reward pathways. Their goal wasn't to nourish you—it was to hook you. They weren't just selling snacks; they were buying your biology.

They perfected the "bliss point"—that precise balance of sugar, salt, and fat that maximizes dopamine release. It's the reason you can't stop at one chip or one cookie. It's not because you're weak—it's because they designed it that way.

Every colorful package, every cartoon mascot, every "limited edition flavor" is a weapon in this war. A war where the battleground is your brain and the casualty is your trust in your body's signals.

NARRATIVE: EMILY AND THE SODA MACHINE

Emily grew up in the 1990s. Every day after school, she'd put a dollar in the vending machine and watch a can of soda drop. That hiss of carbonation when she cracked it open? Heaven.

Fast forward twenty years: Emily can't go a day without soda. She tells herself it's "just caffeine," but the truth is deeper. Her brain learned long ago that soda equals reward. The sugar spikes, the caffeine boost, the dopamine hit—it rewired her pathways.

When Emily tries to quit, her body lies. It tells her she's tired. It tells her she's cranky. It tells her she "needs" soda to function. None of it is true. It's withdrawal masquerading as need.

The machine may be gone, but the programming remains.

ADDICTION PATHWAYS IN THE BRAIN

Food addiction may sound extreme, but neuroscientists agree: processed foods light up the same brain regions as drugs.

1. **Dopamine Reward Loop**

   a. Sugar triggers dopamine in the nucleus accumbens—the brain's pleasure center.

   b. The more often this happens, the fewer receptors remain. You need *more* sugar for the same high.

2. **Serotonin Depletion**

   a. Sugar provides a quick serotonin boost, a mood stabilizer.

   b. But overuse depletes serotonin, leaving you anxious, depressed, and seeking more sugar to cope.

3. **Cortisol Stress Cycle**

   a. Stress elevates cortisol, driving cravings for high-energy foods.

b. Processed food consumption then spikes cortisol even higher, creating a vicious cycle.

In short, the more you obey the lies, the more convincing they become.

SHAME: THE SILENT COMPANION

The cruelest trick isn't the craving itself—it's the shame that follows.

You eat the cookie, then hear the whisper: *See? You have no control.*

You binge on the chips, and the thought lands: *You'll never change.*

You skip breakfast again, and the voice scolds: *This is just who you are.*

But here's the truth: the shame isn't yours. It was planted in you by a culture profiting off your confusion.

Once you see the lie, you can begin dismantling the shame. Because you're not broken—you've been manipulated. And you can take it back.

ACTION FRAMEWORK: BREAKING THE CRAVING LOOP

Here's a 4-step system to rewire your response when the body lies with cravings:

STEP 1: PAUSE

When the craving hits, don't react instantly. Create a gap between the urge and the action.

STEP 2: LABEL

Name it: "This is a dopamine craving, not real hunger."

Simply labeling reduces its power.

STEP 3: REPLACE

Swap the behavior with a healthier but still rewarding action:

- Craving sugar? Eat protein + fiber (apple with almond butter, boiled eggs).

- Craving salt? Try pickles, olives, or nuts.

- Craving crunch? Raw veggies with hummus.

STEP 4: REFLECT

Afterward, note how you feel compared to when you give in. Over time, your brain learns: reward doesn't always equal processed food.

CASE STUDY: DANIEL'S AFTERNOON CRASH

Daniel, 45, felt an unstoppable pull toward the vending machine at 3 PM every workday. He convinced himself it was "hunger," but his journal revealed the truth: he had eaten lunch only two hours earlier.

We applied the Craving Loop framework. At 3 PM, instead of hitting the vending machine, Daniel paused, labeled the craving, and replaced it with a brisk 10-minute walk and a handful of nuts.

The first week was rough. His body screamed lies: *You're starving. You need sugar.* But by week three, the cravings faded. By week six, they were gone. His afternoon energy stabilized—not because he found "discipline," but because he stopped believing the lie.

THE LIE OF "ENERGY"

Here's another deception: the idea that caffeine and sugar give you energy.

They don't. They borrow it.

Caffeine blocks adenosine, the chemical that tells your brain you're tired. Sugar floods your bloodstream with glucose, spiking energy temporarily. But both demand repayment—with interest.

That crash at 3 PM? It's your debt collector. That grogginess at 10 AM? That's borrowed energy running out.

Real energy comes from mitochondria—the power plants of your cells—fueled by consistent sleep, balanced meals, and movement. The rest is smoke and mirrors.

REPROGRAMMING EXERCISE: THE "WOULD I EAT SALMON?" TEST

Next time your body tells you it's "hungry," ask: *Would I eat salmon right now?*

- If yes, it's probably real hunger.

- If no, it's likely a craving.

This isn't about salmon specifically—it's about nutrient-dense, unprocessed food. Real hunger welcomes it. Fake hunger rejects it.

Practice this for a week, and you'll be shocked at how many of your "hungers" vanish when salmon, eggs, or vegetables are the test food.

CULTURAL EXAMPLE: FRANCE VS. AMERICA

In France, children are taught to eat at set mealtimes, savoring real food. Hunger is trusted. Cravings are rare. Food is culture, not compulsion.

In America, children grow up with snacks on demand, sugary cereals, and soda at lunch. Hunger becomes mistrusted. Cravings dominate. Food is marketed, not honored.

Two bodies. Two signals. Two realities.

Which would you rather trust, your body in France, or your body in America?

THE FIRST STEP TOWARD TRUTH

You can't fix what you can't see. The first step is admitting: *My body lies sometimes.* Not because it's broken, but because it was manipulated.

Once you accept that, you gain power. You no longer obey every craving. You no longer shame yourself for every slip. You step back, investigate, and decode.

This is not a weakness. This is wisdom.

REBUILDING TRUTHFUL SIGNALS

If your body has lied for years—whispering cravings that masquerade as hunger, promising energy from sugar, scolding you with shame—how do you learn to trust it again?

You retrain it.

The human body is astonishingly adaptive. Just as it learned to crave chips and soda, it can learn to crave water, sunlight, and whole foods. The difference is this: one path is hijacked survival, the other is thriving biology.

The key? Re-establishing **signal integrity**—restoring the messages between brain, gut, and hormones to their natural state.

Here's how.

STEP 1: STABILIZE BLOOD SUGAR

Unstable blood sugar is one of the biggest reasons your body "lies." When blood glucose spikes, you feel euphoria. When it crashes, you feel panic, fatigue, and false hunger.

To stabilize:

- **Front-load protein and fat** → Breakfast with 25–30g protein reduces cravings all day.

- **Fiber with carbs** → A slice of bread with avocado is processed differently than bread alone.

- **The 3-hour rule** → Avoid grazing; give your insulin time to reset between meals.

When blood sugar is steady, hunger signals normalize. Cravings vanish.

STEP 2: REPAIR THE GUT-BRAIN AXIS

Your gut is not just a digestive organ—it's a command center. The microbiome (trillions of bacteria in your intestines) communicates directly with your brain via the vagus nerve.

- Junk food breeds **craving bacteria** (like Candida) that literally demand sugar.

- Whole foods feed **stable bacteria** (like Bifidobacteria) that regulate mood and hunger.

Think about that: when you crave sugar, it may not be *you* craving—it's the bacteria living inside you. Feed them junk, they scream. Feed them real food, and they quiet down.

To repair:

- Add fermented foods (yogurt, sauerkraut, kimchi).

- Diversify plants (aim for 30 different plant foods per week).

- Supplement with prebiotic fiber (chicory root, green bananas, Jerusalem artichokes).

Over weeks, the gut shifts. And so do your "hungers."

STEP 3: REBUILD SATIETY HORMONES

Two hormones dominate hunger truth: **ghrelin** (hunger) and **leptin** (fullness). In a hijacked body, they stop working correctly.

- **Ghrelin** rises before meals to make you seek food. But junk food consumption keeps ghrelin levels abnormally high, making you think you're always hungry.

- **Leptin** tells your brain you're full. But processed food inflammation creates "leptin resistance," so the signal never lands. You keep eating.

To restore balance:

- Sleep 7–9 hours (sleep deprivation raises ghrelin, lowers leptin).

- Eat high-volume, low-calorie foods (leafy greens, soups, broths).

- Reduce inflammatory foods (seed oils, ultra-processed snacks).

When leptin and ghrelin recalibrate, your body stops shouting lies.

CASE STUDY: MARIA'S TRUTH RESET

Maria, 39, described herself as "always hungry." She said she could eat a full dinner and still crave dessert, chips, and wine before bed.

We focused on signal restoration:

1. Protein-first breakfasts.

2. Fermented foods daily.

3. Eliminating her nightly wine (alcohol disrupts leptin).

By week 3, Maria reported something shocking: *"For the first time in years, I ate dinner and didn't want anything else."* Her body's hunger finally told the truth.

THE 21-DAY TRUTH RESET PLAN

Here's a blueprint for rewiring your hunger signals in just 21 days:

WEEK 1: THE CLEAN SLATE

- Remove added sugar completely.
- Eat three meals daily, no snacks.
- Hydrate: 16oz of water upon waking.
- Sleep target: in bed by 10:30 PM.

WEEK 2: THE GUT SHIFT

- Add one fermented food per day.
- Hit 25g fiber daily (track with a journal).
- Walk 10 minutes after each meal.

WEEK 3: THE SIGNAL STRENGTHENING

- Practice the "Would I Eat Salmon?" test with every craving.
- Journal hunger cues before and after meals (scale of 1–10).
- Reduce screen-time eating (no TV/snacking).

By the end of 21 days, most readers will notice:

- Morning hunger is sharp but calm.
- Afternoon crashes disappear.
- Cravings shrink.
- Fullness feels natural, not forced.

This isn't "discipline." It's biology restored.

EXERCISE: HUNGER JOURNALING

To help retrain signals, keep a **Hunger Journal** for 14 days:

1. Rate hunger before meals (1 = not hungry, 10 = starving).

2. Rate fullness after meals (1 = still hungry, 10 = uncomfortably stuffed).

3. Write down what triggered eating (clock, boredom, craving, social event?).

Patterns emerge. Often, you'll see that "hunger" wasn't hunger at all—it was habit or stress. With awareness, you can break the cycle.

THE EMOTIONAL LIE

It's not just biology. The body lies emotionally, too. Stress, sadness, and even joy can be mislabeled as hunger.

- Stress → Cortisol rises → body craves quick fuel.

- Sadness → Serotonin drops → sugar promises relief.

- Celebration → Brain associates food with reward → overeating feels "earned."

The truth? None of these requires food. They require **feeling**. But food becomes the translator for emotions we don't want to face.

Next time you "need" chocolate, ask: *What do I really need right now? Comfort? Rest? Connection?*

Often, the answer has nothing to do with sugar.

ACTION FRAMEWORK: EMOTIONAL REWIRING

Try this 3-step practice when emotional hunger strikes:

1. **Name the Emotion**: Write it down. (Lonely, stressed, bored).

2. **Breathe**: 5 slow breaths to regulate the nervous system.

3. **Choose a Non-Food Fix**: Call a friend, stretch, journal, or walk.

At first, it feels foreign. But soon, the brain learns: emotions are felt, not fed.

CLOSING NARRATIVE: THE WHISPER OF TRUTH

Imagine waking tomorrow and hearing your stomach growl—not in desperation, but in clarity. Imagine eating until satisfied and not feeling the pull for more. Imagine walking past the bakery and not feeling enslaved by the smell.

That is possible. Your body can tell the truth again.

But first, you must stop believing the lies.

And when you do, something extraordinary happens: hunger becomes your ally, not your enemy. Cravings lose their grip—and food shifts from a battlefield to a source of power.

That's when the paradigm flips. That's when you no longer *eat to live*—you begin to **eat to thrive.**

ACTION STEPS RECAP (CHAPTER 2)

- Recognize cravings as neurochemical manipulations, not failures.
- Stabilize blood sugar with protein, fat, and fiber.
- Heal the gut microbiome with fermented foods and plant diversity.
- Restore satiety hormones through sleep and anti-inflammatory eating.
- Use the "Would I Eat Salmon?" test to separate hunger from cravings.
- Journal hunger to reveal emotional vs. biological triggers.
- Implement the 21-Day Truth Reset Plan to retrain your signals.

PART II

**FOOD, MOOD, AND
THE INNER CHEMISTRY OF THRIVING**

CHAPTER 4:

THE ULTRA-PROCESSED FOOD PRESCRIPTION

HOW FOOD TECHNOLOGY FUELS METABOLIC DISEASE — AND HOW TO REVERSE THE TREND WITH SAVORY, PROTEIN-RICH MEALS

The fluorescent lights hum overhead in the waiting room. A row of patients shuffles forward, each clutching a plastic bag of orange pill bottles. Blood pressure meds. Diabetes meds. Cholesterol meds. Their faces are tired, their bodies heavier than they want them to be, their eyes dulled with resignation. One by one, they're called to the counter, their prescriptions refilled. It feels routine — almost normal.

But look closer.

Those bottles are not the first prescription. They are the *second*. The true prescription, the one that made the pills necessary, was written years earlier, not by a doctor, but by the food industry. By the supermarket aisle filled with neon-colored boxes at eye level. By the fast-food menu glowing late into the night. By the ultra-processed meals that became daily fuel.

This is the **Ultra-Processed Prescription.**

Unlike the piece of paper a doctor hands you, this one is invisible. You fill it every time you reach for the "quick" breakfast bar, or the microwaveable dinner, or an easily obtainable snack that professes to be "healthy." You don't notice its side effects right away, but quietly, molecule by molecule, it rewires your brain, inflames your gut, shifts your hormones, and sets you on the conveyor belt toward chronic illness.

But here's the kicker: you never signed up for it. It was designed for you - engineered to compel you to eat more, buy more, consume more. But here's the good news: just as it was written into your biochemistry, it can also be unwritten. The antidote isn't a pill; it's a plate.

The Ultra-Processed Prescription

PART 1 — THE ACCIDENTAL PRESCRIPTION

THE WAITING ROOM THAT TELLS A STORY

The waiting room is quiet except for the humming of fluorescent lights. It smells of antiseptic and paper. The chairs are filled with patients who look like they are accustomed to visiting the doctor's office. A gentleman in his fifties is slumped in his chair, the bottle of water in his hand sweating, his belly stretching the length of his shirt. Next to him sits a young woman in scrubs scrolling on her phone with heavy eyelids - a nurse who is off shift and is now a patient. Across the room, an older woman sits clutching a pharmacy bag, her knuckles swollen and stiff.

They are all waiting for the same thing - refills. Tiny plastic bottles with child-proof caps, filled with pills to manage blood pressure, blood sugar, cholesterol, or mood. When their names are called, they walk up to the counter, sign a piece of paper, and shuffle away with another month's supply of medication.

It seems routine. Ordinary. Almost inevitable.

But here's the truth: what you see in that waiting room is not a story of broken bodies; it is a story of engineered appetites. Those orange pill bottles are the second prescription. The first prescription was given out many years ago in grocery store aisles and fast-food drive-thrus. It did not come on a piece of paper. It came disguised under cellophane with delighted faces and "heart-healthy" labels, and in vibrant colors to grab our attention.

That first prescription is what brought these patients here. It's what filled their arteries with plaque, what pushed their blood sugar into chaos, what kept them up at night craving just one more bite. And it has a name: **ultra-processed food.**

THE PRESCRIPTION YOU DIDN'T KNOW YOU WERE TAKING

Here's the part most people don't realize: you don't just *eat* ultra-processed foods — you *dose* them. Just like medicine, every bite changes your biochemistry.

- A granola bar at 8 AM spikes your insulin, setting up a mid-morning crash.

- A "healthy" microwave meal at noon, filled with emulsifiers and gums, irritates your gut lining.

- A diet soda at 3 PM nudges your brain's dopamine circuits, teaching you to expect sweetness without nourishment.

- A late-night bowl of cereal rewrites your circadian clock, telling your liver to keep processing food long after it should be repairing.

You do this day in and day out, year after year, your body learns to believe the prescription. High blood sugar becomes normal. Cravings become constant. Energy crashes have become a part of everyday life. Then one day, you find yourself sitting in a waiting room, holding a different kind of prescription; pills meant to cover up what your habits have done to your body.

HOW FOOD BECAME THE INVISIBLE PRESCRIPTION PAD

The shocking reality is that none of this is accidental. Ultra-processed foods are not just "unhealthy" in the vague way we usually talk about junk food. They are engineered meticulously, scientifically, and deliberately to shape behavior and physiology.

79

Food companies employ entire teams of chemists, neuroscientists, and marketers to discover what's called the **bliss point**, the precise combination of sugar, salt, and fat that hijacks your taste buds and reward centers. Not too sweet, not too salty, not too fatty, but the *perfect* mix to make your brain say: "More. Again. Now.

This is no longer hunger. It is control.

In fact, Dr. Michael Moss, Pulitzer-winning journalist, revealed in *Salt Sugar Fat* that major food corporations have laboratories designed to test how quickly a potato chip crunch dissolves on your tongue, how cheese stretches when melted, how carbonation bubbles hit the palate, all optimized for one purpose: *to keep you hooked.*

Every time you walk into a supermarket, you're stepping into a pharmacy. But instead of healing, most of what's on those shelves is prescribing disease.

THE BODY THAT KEEPS THE SCORE

Consider David. You met him back in Chapter 1, the man dragging himself through afternoons on caffeine and collapsing into late-night binges. His story is not unusual — in fact, it's almost cliché. He wakes up groggy, skips breakfast, powers through work with coffee and snacks, grabs takeout for dinner, and crashes in front of the TV.

On paper, he's just "busy" or "stressed." In reality, he's a textbook case of what happens when the ultra-processed prescription becomes routine.

- **Energy:** Spikes and crashes all day.

- **Mood:** Irritable, anxious, distracted.

- **Sleep:** Shallow, restless, interrupted.

- **Cravings:** Insatiable, especially late at night.

- **Health markers:** creeping blood sugar, climbing waistline, and blood pressure inching higher.

David doesn't *feel* sick enough to go to the hospital. But his body is already keeping the score. Every processed snack is a dose. Every "healthy" cereal bar is another pill. His "prescription" is being filled not at the pharmacy, but at the checkout counter of his favorite convenience store.

SCIENCE BEHIND THE CURTAIN: THE MECHANICS OF THE PRESCRIPTION

This is where it gets undeniable. The science is crystal clear: ultra-processed foods don't just correlate with chronic disease, they *cause* it.

- **Study spotlight (NIH, 2019, Kevin Hall):** Researchers locked participants in a controlled metabolic ward and gave them unlimited access to either ultra-processed meals or whole-food meals. Both groups were matched for calories, sugar, fat, and salt. The result? Those eating ultra-processed diets consumed 500 more calories per day and gained weight, while the whole-food group lost weight. Why? Because processing itself — the additives, the textures, the speed of digestion — drives overeating.

- **BMJ 2019 Cohort Study:** Tracking 105,000 people, researchers found that higher intake of UPFs was linked to a 12% greater risk of cardiovascular disease and 25% higher risk of developing obesity-related cancers.

- **Gut studies (Chassaing et al., 2015):** Emulsifiers commonly added to ice cream, bread, and sauces disrupt the gut microbiome, leading to low-grade inflammation and metabolic dysfunction.

This isn't "food as fuel." This is food as pharmacology — but with a dark side. Unlike real medicine, ultra-processed foods don't heal. They harm.

THE SHOCK OF RECOGNITION

If you've ever wondered why you can't stop after just one cookie... why you crave chips at 10 PM... why you feel hungry again just an hour after eating cereal — it's not your lack of willpower. It's your biology responding to a prescription you never asked for.

Think about it:

- **Would you blame yourself for getting sleepy after taking a sedative?**

- **Would you shame yourself for feeling wired after caffeine?**

- **Then why do we blame ourselves for craving ultra-processed food, when it was designed to do exactly that?**

The guilt, the frustration, the yo-yo dieting — they're part of the trap. Because as long as you believe it's *your fault*, you'll keep reaching for another dose. And the prescription keeps working exactly as designed.

THE HIDDEN SIDE EFFECTS

Every prescription comes with side effects. Ultra-processed foods are no different. The label may not list them, but the long-term "adverse reactions" include:

- Insulin resistance.

- Chronic inflammation.

- Hormonal misalignment.

- Gut permeability ("leaky gut").

- Neurological changes in dopamine pathways.

- Altered circadian rhythms.

The side effects accumulate silently, until one day they show up as a diagnosis: diabetes, hypertension, fatty liver disease, depression.

And here's the darkest twist: once you're on the second prescription — the pills, the injections, the surgeries — the first prescription doesn't stop. People keep eating ultra-processed foods even while treating their diseases, because the cravings remain.

THE PIVOT TO HOPE

But here's the breakthrough: just like any prescription, the ultra-processed one can be **discontinued**. You can *unwrite* it.

And the antidote isn't complicated. It doesn't require elite discipline, expensive supplements, or exotic superfoods. The antidote is found in something as simple and profound as this: **protein-rich, savory meals built from whole foods.**

Why savory? Because it trains your palate away from engineered sweetness.

Why protein? Because it nourishes satiety signals, stabilizes blood sugar, and supports repair.

Why Whole Foods? Because they come without the hidden additives and engineered bliss points.

Every time you build your plate this way, you aren't just putting food into your body. You are rewriting your prescription. You are telling your body:

I choose healing over hijack.

I choose nourishment over numbness.

I choose life over labels.

The Moment of Decision

The waiting room is still full. Patients are still lining up for refills. But the questions now drift to the forefront of your mind.

What if you could step out of line? What if you could take that ultra-processed prescription, rip it to shreds in front of your healthcare provider, and write up your own - one that takes you to vitality and not disease?

THE MOMENT OF DECISION

The waiting room is still packed. Patients still line up for refills. But now there is a question in your head:

What if you could get out of line? What if you could throw out the ultra-processed prescription and write your own - one that leads not to sickness, but to health?

That's what this chapter is about. Not guilt or shame. Clarity and choice. Once you see the invisible prescription for what it is, you can choose whether to keep filling it - or whether to cancel it finally.

THE ULTRA-PROCESSED PRESCRIPTION	THE ANTIDOTE
Engineered for Bliss Point combines sugar + fat + salt at levels that hijack dopamine	**Protein + Fiber First** natural satiety signals activated, cravings reduced
Empty Calories, Hidden Chemicals preservatives, emulsifiers, and additives fuel inflammation	**Whole Food Matrix** nutrients, fiber, and phytochemicals calm inflammation and repair
Circadian Hijack late-night snacking triggered by processed food "quick hits"	**Aligned Eating Window** meals with the sun (12:12 or 16:8 rhythm) reset hunger hormones
Gut Disruption emulsifiers & additives alter microbiome diversity	**Stable Dopamine Release** savory, protein-rich meals + movement provide natural

Every bite is either a prescription for disease . . . or an antidote for thriving. Choose meals that heal, not hijack.

PART 2 — INSIDE THE PRESCRIPTION: HOW PROCESSED FOOD REWIRES YOU

THE HIDDEN LABORATORY

Before you've even crinkled open the bag, before you've even opened the pop-top on a can and heard the fizz, before your tongue even touches the first instantiation of salt-sugar-fat, there are a host of scientists already inside your head.

Not figuratively. Literally.

Behind the scenes of the bright supermarket aisles and glossy advertisements lies the hidden laboratory of the food industry. In rooms with no windows, entire departments of "food engineers" spend years perfecting a single potato chip, a single breakfast bar, a single neon-colored drink. Their tools are not pans and skillets but spectrometers, neuroimaging data, and focus groups wired to electrodes.

The goal? Not to nourish you. Not even to satisfy you.

The goal is to hit what they call the **bliss point**, the precise formula of sugar, fat, and salt that lights up your brain's reward centers more predictably than gambling, scrolling, or even sex.

That means when you walk into a convenience store, you aren't just shopping. You are entering into a behavioral experiment decade in the making.

And, for millions of people, that experiment has gone precisely to plan.

THE BLISS POINT: ENGINEERING ADDICTION

In 2015, Dr. Howard Moskowitz, a market researcher famous for coining the concept of the "bliss point", admitted in interviews that no processed food product goes to market without this equation. Every gram of sugar, every sprinkle of salt, every molecule of fat is tested in different combinations until they discover the exact ratio that causes consumers to not only like a product but also crave it repeatedly.

Here's what the bliss point actually does in your body:

- **Dopamine Hijack** → Every bite triggers a dopamine release in the nucleus accumbens, your brain's reward hub. Unlike natural foods, which have diminishing returns, engineered foods are designed for **nonlinear reward**, meaning the tenth bite feels almost as exciting as the first.

- **Satiety Interruption** → Normally, hormones like leptin (satiety) and peptide YY (fullness) signal the brain to slow eating. Processed foods disrupt these by speeding digestion, stripping fiber, and bypassing gut signaling. Your body doesn't get the "we're full" memo until it's far too late.

- **Flavor Layering** → Unlike a whole food (say, an apple) with a simple flavor profile, UPFs (ultra-processed foods) layer artificial flavors, sweeteners, and textures that **confuse sensory satiety**. Your brain keeps asking, "Maybe there's more?"

GUT DISRUPTION: THE SILENT COLLATERAL

Think of your gut microbiome as a rainforest: diverse, rich, self-regulating. Now imagine introducing daily forest fires; that's what ultra-processed foods do.

- **Emulsifiers and preservatives** strip protective gut mucus, leading to **leaky gut** and systemic inflammation (Chassaing et al., *Nature*, 2015).

- **Artificial sweeteners** like aspartame and sucralose alter microbial populations, impairing glucose tolerance (Suez et al., *Nature*, 2014).

- **Refined carbohydrates** rapidly spike blood sugar, forcing insulin surges that leave cells inflamed and resistant over time.

The result? A body in **chronic low-grade inflammation**, the soil from which nearly every modern disease sprouts: diabetes, obesity, cardiovascular disease, autoimmune flare-ups, even depression.

CIRCADIAN MISALIGNMENT: THE HIDDEN COST

It doesn't stop with the gut. Ultra-processed foods also **rewire your clock.**

Studies show that late-night eating of processed snacks suppresses melatonin, delays sleep onset, and disrupts **glucose tolerance** the following morning (Garaulet & Gómez-Abellán, *Endocrine Reviews*, 2014).

Translation: You're not just eating calories at the wrong time, you're reprogramming your circadian biology. And circadian disruption is now classified as a **probable carcinogen** by the World Health Organization.

CHRONIC INFLAMMATION: THE PRESCRIPTION YOU NEVER ASKED FOR

Doctors prescribe drugs. The food industry causes diseases.

- **Metabolic syndrome** → fueled by constant high-glycemic UPFs.

- **Cardiovascular disease** → driven by inflammatory oils and hidden trans fats.

- **Neurodegeneration** → fueled by chronic blood sugar spikes, oxidative stress, and inflammatory cytokines.

Every bite of ultra-processed food is like filling a prescription bottle you never wanted: doses of disease, one snack at a time.

The Cravings Code Within UPFs

Why can't you just stop? Why do you find yourself reaching into the bag again, even after swearing you wouldn't?

Because UPFs hijack the same wiring as addictive substances:

Because UPFs exploit the same circuitry as addictive substances:

- **Cue-triggered cravings**: Crinkling bags, soda fizz, and neon logos are designed as Pavlovian cues.

- **Dopamine tolerance**: Like drugs, repeated hits dull receptors, meaning you need more for the same reward.

- **Stress amplification**: Cortisol makes cravings for sugar/fat more intense. Guess what kind of foods are everywhere in your stressed environment?

This isn't a weakness. It's neuromarketing.

ACTION PRIMER: FIRST STEPS TO BREAK THE PRESCRIPTION

The full antidote (protein-rich, savory, whole foods) is coming in Part 4. But before that, here are **science-backed "first steps"** to begin withdrawing from the ultra-processed prescription today:

1. **The Switch Rule** → Replace one daily UPF with a whole-food equivalent (chips → roasted chickpeas, soda → sparkling water + citrus). Research shows that gradual substitution reduces withdrawal fatigue.

2. **Protein Anchor** → Begin each eating window with protein (20–30g). Protein triggers satiety hormones (GLP-1, PYY), blunting cravings for UPFs later in the day.

3. **Kill the Cue** → Don't rely on willpower. Remove branded packages from sight. Studies prove visual cues alone can trigger cravings. Keep fruit, nuts, or boiled eggs visible instead.

4. **Light Before Bite** → Get morning sunlight exposure before eating. This synchronizes circadian rhythm, reducing the evening crash-and-crave cycle.

5. **Label Decoder** → If it has more than five ingredients you can't pronounce, assume it's part of the prescription. Simplify. Whole foods don't need fine print.

PART 3 — THE CHRONIC DISEASE LINK

THE ILLUSION OF CONVENIENCE

Maria sat at her desk, the smell of crayons and dry-erase markers filling the small classroom. A pile of ungraded math tests leaned precariously to her right. She sighed, unwrapped another "healthy" granola bar, and took a bite. Oats, honey, and a drizzle of chocolate. It was quick, it was portable, and it gave her the jolt she needed to power through the next lesson. Or at least that's what she told herself.

By 2.15 PM, standing in front of thirty fidgety seventh graders, her hands were shaking a little from low blood sugar, and her brain was searching for another bar. Another coffee. Another fix.

Maria genuinely believes she is making a responsible choice with what she chooses to eat, since it is marketed as "wholesome." What she does not know is that those granola bars with added sugars, refined oils, and engineered "bliss point" are cumulatively reforming her biology. Each bite did not just temporarily fuel her; it led her closer and closer to overt metabolic dysregulation.

And she is not alone. The foods that we are convinced are going to keep us going - protein shakes, energy bars, cereal cups, "lite" snacks, flavored yogurts - are all a prescription for chronic disease. A prescription that most of us take every single day of our lives because it comes wrapped in a pseudo-health veil.

The truth? **Ultra-processed foods (UPFs) are not neutral. They are active drivers of disease.**

OBESITY & DIABETES: THE SILENT BURN OF SUGAR AND SPIKES

Visualize a faucet that cannot be turned off, and the water drips continuously into a sink. In the beginning, the sink can handle it, and the drain can keep up. And suddenly, one drip becomes a steady stream, then a torrent, and the sink is overflowing.

This is what happens when ultra-processed foods give your body almost constant glucose spikes. All those cereals, bars, sodas, and bread; all that sugar is injected into your blood in a manner that the body was not designed for. Hormonal insulin now has to work overtime. Cells stop listening. This is **insulin resistance**, the hallmark of type 2 diabetes.

Science Spotlight:

- A 2019 study in *Cell Metabolism* found that diets high in UPFs caused people to consume **500 extra calories per day**, primarily from sugar and refined starches, leading to rapid weight gain.

- Research in *The Lancet Diabetes & Endocrinology* shows insulin resistance is accelerated by frequent glucose spikes, even in "normal-weight" individuals who consume high-UPF diets.

For Maria, every granola bar meant another spike, another insulin surge, another step toward insulin resistance.

And yet, the marketing told her the opposite: "Whole grain! Heart healthy! Fuel for your day!"

But what UPFs really fuel is a **silent burn** that inflames fat tissue, dysregulates hormones, and builds the foundation for obesity and diabetes.

HEART DISEASE: THE INFLAMMATORY PATHWAYS

Ultra-processed diets don't just overload us with sugar. They lace our meals with **refined seed oils** — cheap, industrial oils extracted from soy, corn, and sunflower. Heated, refined, and deodorized until they no longer resemble food, these oils are in almost every packaged snack, sauce, and frozen dinner.

When consumed daily, they disrupt the balance of omega-6 to omega-3 fats, tipping the body toward inflammation. This inflammation doesn't stay local — it courses through arteries, irritating vessel walls, making them more prone to plaque buildup.

Science Spotlight:

- A 2021 review in *Nutrients* linked high-UPF diets to **endothelial dysfunction** — the impaired ability of blood vessels to relax and regulate blood flow.

- Inflammation triggered by UPFs raises LDL cholesterol particles, increases blood pressure, and creates the perfect storm for heart disease.

Maria's granola bar didn't just spike her blood sugar; its refined oils fueled microscopic fires in her arteries. Fires that don't show up until the day they erupt as a heart attack.

CANCER RISK: THE ADDITIVE EQUATION

Most people think of smoking when they hear the word *carcinogen*. But the additives in UPFs — preservatives, emulsifiers, and colorants- are increasingly under scrutiny.

Take **emulsifiers**, used to make ice cream creamy or keep salad dressings from separating. Studies in mice show that these compounds disrupt the gut microbiome, increasing inflammation and accelerating tumor growth. Artificial sweeteners, too, may alter gut bacteria in ways that promote glucose intolerance.

Science Spotlight:

- A large French cohort study (BMJ, 2018) found that a 10% increase in UPF consumption was linked to a 12% higher risk of overall cancer, and an 11% higher risk of breast cancer.

- The International Agency for Research on Cancer (IARC) has classified some additives found in UPFs as possible or probable carcinogens.

In Maria's classroom, the granola bar wrapper whispered words like "natural flavors" and "preservatives for freshness." Innocent enough. But beneath the surface, the **additive equation** was at work — creating an environment where cellular DNA was more likely to misfire, mutate, and multiply unchecked.

NEURODEGENERATION: THE BRAIN BETRAYED

The human brain is exquisitely sensitive to what we eat. UPFs flood it with dopamine hits that overstimulate reward pathways, while starving it of nutrients needed for repair and memory.

In the short term, this means **brain fog**. In the long term, it increases the risk for depression, anxiety, and dementia.

Science Spotlight:

- A 2022 study in JAMA *Neurology* found that high–UPF diets were associated with a **25% increased risk of dementia**.

- Research in *Molecular Psychiatry* links UPFs to depression, likely due to inflammation, gut disruption, and dopamine imbalance.

For Maria, the afternoon crash wasn't just about sugar. It was her brain, tugged back and forth between surges of artificial pleasure and plunges into fatigue. Each bar, each soda, each snack pulled her further into the cycle of reward and regret.

And the cruel irony? The foods she reached for to "keep her sharp" were eroding her sharpness.

THE PRESCRIPTION NOBODY ASKED FOR

Think about it: Maria never signed up for this prescription. She didn't walk into a doctor's office and ask for insulin resistance, arterial inflammation, increased cancer risk, or cognitive decline.

But every brightly packaged snack, every ready-to-eat dinner, every processed "health food" is a silent prescription slip. One that millions of people cash every single day without realizing the cost.

The industries behind UPFs aren't just selling convenience. They're **selling chronic illness, one bite at a time**.

And yet, the antidote exists. It doesn't come from a pharmacy, but from a plate — a plate filled with real, protein-rich, nutrient-dense, savory meals.

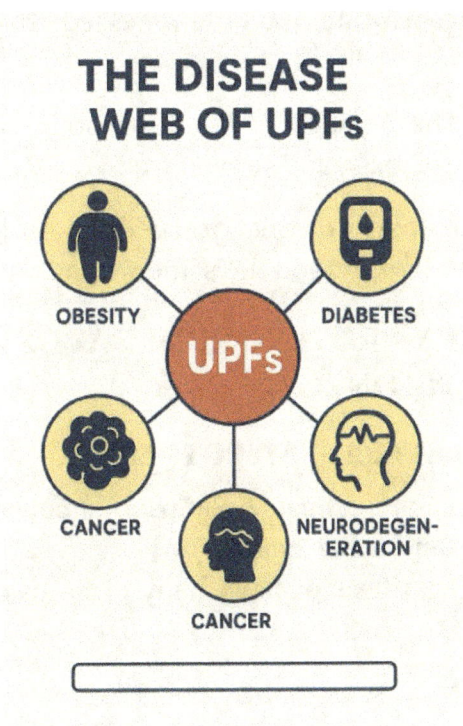

PART 4: THE ANTIDOTE

THE BREAKFAST FORK IN THE ROAD

It's now 7:30 AM.

You are standing in front of two options. On the one hand, the drive-thru window with its glowing neon signs advertising a croissant sandwich, hash browns, and a caramel latte. And on the other hand, your kitchen where eggs sizzle in a frying pan, a bowl of Greek yogurt sits ready with berries, and the coffee steams black.

Both meals deliver calories. Both fill your stomach. Both will change the trajectory of your day.

But the difference between them is seismic — not just for today's energy, but for the way your body will crave food at 3 PM, the way your brain will negotiate hunger at 9 PM, and the way your hormones will whisper instructions all week long.

One is **The Prescription** — ultra-processed, engineered to keep you hooked.

The other is **The Antidote** — whole, protein-rich, designed by nature to stabilize, satisfy, and set you free.

This is the pivot point. And once you understand how the antidote works, you'll never look at food the same way again.

SECTION 1: WHY PROTEIN-RICH, SAVORY MEALS ARE THE RESET BUTTON

THE PROTEIN LEVERAGE HYPOTHESIS

Scientists like Raubenheimer & Simpson uncovered a fascinating pattern: humans (and other animals) will keep eating until protein needs are met, regardless of how many extra calories this brings along.

- If you eat processed carbs + fats (low in protein), your body keeps the hunger switch "on," driving overconsumption.

- If you eat protein-rich meals, your brain gets the satiety signal earlier — cravings dial down, appetite normalizes, and overeating stops almost automatically.

This isn't willpower. It's biology. Protein is the *master regulator*.

Your translation – start with 25–35g of protein in your morning meal, and see your afternoon cravings substantially decrease.

THE DOPAMINE RESET

Ultra-processed foods hijack the dopamine reward system, keeping you in a cycle of "hit → crash → crave again."

But savory, protein-dense meals create *steady dopamine signals* without the roller coaster.

- Eggs with spinach don't send your brain into fireworks.

- But they *anchor dopamine tone*, giving you baseline stability.

- Over time, this recalibrates your reward pathways, making UPFs feel less magnetic.

Think of it like **volume control**: processed foods scream at your brain, but protein-rich whole foods teach it to listen at a normal volume again.

SATIETY HORMONES & GUT RESET

Protein meals activate GLP-1, PYY, and CCK — hormones that send "I'm full" signals.

UPFs bypass these, leaving you hungry despite calories.

At the same time, savory whole foods feed your *gut microbiome* the fibers, amino acids, and polyphenols it needs to thrive. Within weeks, this improves insulin sensitivity and reduces chronic inflammation.

CIRCADIAN ALIGNMENT WITH PROTEIN & SAVORY STARTS

Morning savory meals stabilize ghrelin (hunger hormone) and anchor your circadian feeding window.

Sugary breakfasts (cereal, muffins, flavored lattes) push ghrelin chaos forward, often leading to "all-day grazing."

- A protein-rich, savory first meal isn't just fuel. It's a **clock reset for hunger biology**.

SECTION 2: THE ANTIDOTE IN ACTION — PRACTICAL PLAYBOOK

STEP 1: START SAVORY, STAY STABLE

- **Aim:** 25–35g protein within 1–2 hours of waking.
- **Why:** Anchors satiety hormones, sets circadian hunger rhythm.
- **Examples:**
    o 3 eggs + sautéed greens + avocado
    o Greek yogurt (unsweetened) + hemp hearts + walnuts
    o Lentil & veggie scramble with olive oil

STEP 2: REBUILD MEALS AROUND PROTEIN FIRST

Flip the script: don't ask "what carb should I eat?" but rather:

- "What protein will I build this meal around?"
    o Lunch: chicken, salmon, or lentils as a centerpiece → then add veggies & olive oil.

o   Dinner: grass-fed beef chili, tofu stir-fry, or wild cod with roasted veg.

Protein-first = natural calorie control, no tracking required.

STEP 3: SNACK ANTIDOTE

Most UPF snacks = carb-fat-salt bombs engineered for addiction.

Replace with **protein + fiber combos**:

- Jerky + apple slices
- Hummus + cucumber
- Cheese + almonds

STEP 4: THE SAVORY FLAVOR REWIRE

Retrain your palate by emphasizing umami, herbs, and spices.

The more your tongue learns to enjoy savory depth, the less it "needs" the artificial hyper-sweetness of UPFs.

STEP 5: EVENING GUARDRAILS

- Stop eating 2–3 hrs before bed.
- Focus dinner on lean protein + colorful vegetables + healthy fats.
- Avoid eating refined carbs, as this protects sleep quality and glucose stability and reduces late-night cravings.

SECTION 3: THE LONG-TERM ANTIDOTE EFFECT

When you consistently apply this protein-rich, savory antidote, three things happen:

1. **Cravings lose their grip.** The food noise fades, and your brain regains quiet.

2. **Energy stabilizes.** No more peaks & crashes → just smooth, steady focus.

3. **Metabolic resilience builds.** Blood sugar, insulin, gut microbiome, and circadian rhythms align.

This isn't a diet. It's a **reprogramming protocol**.

QUICK-REFERENCE BOX: THE ANTIDOTE IN 5 MOVES

1. Start Savory → 25–35g protein breakfast

2. Build Meals Protein-First → anchor lunch & dinner

3. Snack Smart → protein + fiber combos

4. Rewire Flavor → herbs, spices, umami over sugar

5. Guard Evenings → finish eating 2–3 hours before bed

Think back to the fork in the road — the drive-thru croissant sandwich versus the protein-rich skillet breakfast. One path keeps you in prescription mode, forever medicating your cravings. The other path — the antidote — begins the process of reclaiming control.

Every savory, protein-centered meal is a vote for freedom. A way of saying: *I refuse to be hijacked anymore.*

And when the food noise quiets, when you wake up hungry for life, not just calories, you'll know you've begun to break the cycle.

That's the power of The Antidote.

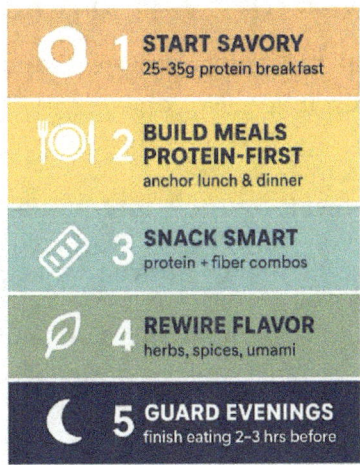

THE ANTIDOTE
IN 5 MOVES

1 START SAVORY
25-35g protein breakfast

2 BUILD MEALS PROTEIN-FIRST
anchor lunch & dinner

3 SNACK SMART
protein + fiber combos

4 REWIRE FLAVOR
herbs, spices, umami

5 GUARD EVENINGS
finish eating 2-3 hrs before

THE SUPERMARKET TRAP

Imagine walking into a supermarket for the first time on a Sunday afternoon. The automatic doors slide open with a soft swoosh, and you are immediately bombarded by sensory input. The air is filled with the baked-bread smell they inject into this environment around the bakery section—not by chance, but by skilled design. The first aisle radiates neon packaging, red and yellow purposely chosen because the actual science of food marketing tells us that red and yellow packaging works wonders on your behavior. Cereal boxes featuring cartoon characters are placed at child level. Free samples of "new protein cookies" are handed out, soft and sweet, with the promise of health layered over sugar and additives.

It feels like a choice. But it's not.

From the very first step inside, you are inside a **designed ecosystem built to make UPFs your default fuel**. If you've ever left the store with more packaged "snacks" than vegetables, it isn't because you lack willpower—it's because you walked into a carefully engineered trap.

This is survival mode packaged as convenience. And the UPF Exit Plan begins by dismantling that illusion.

STEP 1 — REFRAME THE BATTLEFIELD

Science shows that the **environment shapes up to 80% of our food decisions**. Not discipline. Not character. Not even cravings. It's environment.

- If the candy bowl is on the counter, you'll eat more candy.

- If cut fruit is in the fridge at eye level, you'll eat more fruit.

This isn't theory, it's neuroscience. A 2016 study in *Health Psychology* found that visible snacks doubled intake, regardless of hunger.

- **Action:** Before you change *what* you eat, change *what you see*. Remove UPFs from sight—stock real food in places where your eyes naturally fall. Create friction for UPFs (hide them, store them in opaque containers, or better yet—don't bring them home).

The battlefield is not your willpower. It's your kitchen.

STEP 2 — UNDERSTAND THE WITHDRAWAL CURVE

Here's what no diet book tells you: **quitting ultra-processed foods feels like withdrawal.**

Sugar, fat, and salt engineered at the "bliss point" light up the brain's dopamine system like a slot machine. When you pull back, your brain interprets it as deprivation.

- Day 1–3: Cravings intensify—irritability peaks.

- Day 4–7: Energy dips, mood swings.

- Week 2: Cravings begin to lessen.

- Week 3: Taste buds reset, subtle flavors (like roasted vegetables, savory herbs) become vivid again.

This isn't a weakness. It's **neuroadaptation.** Your dopamine baseline has been conditioned by UPFs. Breaking free requires letting your brain recalibrate.

- **Action:** Expect the curve. Don't panic. Hydrate aggressively, prioritize protein at meals (satiety hormone GLP-1 rises), and use structured meals to anchor your day.

Withdrawal isn't the end. It's the reset.

STEP 3 — ANCHOR WITH PROTEIN & FIBER

One of the most effective strategies for reducing UPF dependence is stabilizing blood sugar and satiety hormones. Protein and fiber are your weapons here.

- **Protein:** Triggers GLP-1, peptide YY, and reduces ghrelin (the hunger hormone).

- **Fiber:** Slows digestion, balances glucose spikes, feeds beneficial gut microbes.

Together, they **blunt cravings at their root.**

Science check: A 2015 *American Journal of Clinical Nutrition* study found that high-protein breakfasts reduced evening cravings and late-night snacking compared to high-carb breakfasts.

- **Action:**

  o Start your day with 25–30g protein + fiber-rich foods.

  o Build each plate around "protein first."

  o Keep savory, protein-rich snacks (boiled eggs, roasted chickpeas, Greek yogurt) on standby.

Protein and fiber create a biochemical shield against UPFs.

STEP 4 — BREAK THE DOPAMINE LOOP WITH RITUALS

Cravings aren't just chemical. They're a ritual.

- You always reach for chips while watching Netflix.
- You always crave a pastry with coffee.
- You always wander to the fridge at 10 PM.

These are **habit loops**: Cue → Routine → Reward.

Neuroscience shows that breaking the loop doesn't mean eliminating reward. It means substituting it.

Action:

- Replace chips during Netflix with air-popped popcorn + flavored seasoning.
- Swap pastry + coffee for protein bites or a savory option.
- Replace the 10 PM fridge walk with a herbal tea ritual.

The brain craves routine more than it craves food. Change the script.

STEP 5 — PHASE THE EXIT

Trying to quit all UPFs at once can feel overwhelming. Instead, phase them.

Phase 1 (Week 1–2): Remove sugar-sweetened beverages and obvious junk (soda, candy, chips).

Phase 2 (Week 3–4): Replace "health halo" UPFs (granola bars, protein cookies, flavored yogurts) with whole-food alternatives.

Phase 3 (Ongoing): Crowd out with real food—new recipes, batch cooking, community meals.

Phased withdrawal reduces stress and builds momentum.

MARIA'S STORY: THE GRANOLA BAR TEACHER

Maria was a secondary school educator. Her mornings were hurried — shoving granola bars "for energy" in her bag as she rushed to class. By 10 am, she would be shaky with a growling stomach. By 3 pm, she would be crashing and pouring coffee down her throat. Dinner? A lot of times, takeout, because she's too tired to make dinner.

The first time Maria learned about UPFs, she rejected this concept. "But my granola bars are healthy."

After tracking her energy crashes in the form of journaling, Maria had her revelation. It dawned on her that every crash coincided with a UPF. With coaching, she replaced her granola bars with Greek yogurt + berries + nuts. In 2 weeks, her 10 am crash was gone. By week 4, she didn't need the 3 pm coffee.

Maria didn't quit eating. She quit the prescription.

STEP 6 — BUILD A "DEFAULT PLATE"

The most powerful tool in the UPF Exit Plan is the **default plate**— a go-to meal template that makes decision fatigue disappear.

Example:

- Protein (chicken, eggs, lentils, fish)
- Fiber (leafy greens, beans, vegetables)
- Healthy fat (olive oil, avocado, nuts)
- Flavor anchor (herbs, spices, fermented foods)

Once you build 3–5 "default plates," the grip of UPFs weakens because you always know what to fall back on.

Action: Pick one meal you eat often (lunch, dinner). Rebuild it around the default plate. Repeat it until it becomes effortless.

STEP 7 — THE SOCIAL ARMOR

UPFs dominate birthdays, office meetings, and family dinners. Without social armor, even the strongest resolve crumbles.

Action:

- **Preload protein** before events so you're not starving.

- **Contribute a dish** that you can eat confidently.

- **Reframe "no" as "not now."** Research shows polite deferrals reduce peer pressure.

The key is not to isolate—but to enter social spaces armored with clarity and calm.

STEP 8 — REDEFINE REWARD

For decades, food has been tied to comfort and reward. After a long day, the brain expects a dopamine hit. UPFs provide that instantly.

But rewards can be rewired:

- Movement: A brisk walk triggers endorphins.

- Connection: Phone call with a friend lifts dopamine.

- Ritual: Tea, candles, music—signals of reward without sugar.

Action: Pick one reward you currently tie to UPFs. Replace it with a non-food dopamine ritual. Anchor it consistently for 3 weeks.

THE LIBERATION MOMENT

Imagine 30 days from now: You walk into that same supermarket. The candy aisle barely registers. Your eyes move to the fresh produce, and it excites you—because your taste buds have recalibrated. You walk past the bakery, and instead of craving it, you feel compassion for those still trapped in the loop.

This is not deprivation. It's liberation.

STEP 9 — THE LONG GAME

UPF dependence didn't happen overnight. Neither does freedom. But the long game isn't perfection—it's consistency.

Research in *Public Health Nutrition* shows that reducing UPF intake by just **20% lowers the risk of chronic disease significantly.**

That means you don't have to quit 100% to change your health trajectory. You just need to exit the prescription enough to reset your biology.

Action: Track progress in weeks, not days. Celebrate reductions. Focus on the trajectory, not the tally.

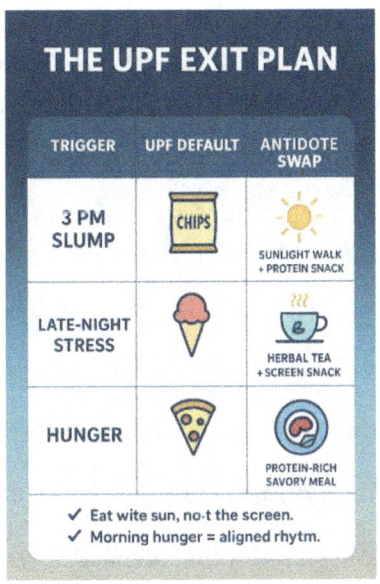

FROM PRESCRIPTION TO FREEDOM

You've experienced a prescription slip written in invisible ink, not by your physician, but by the companies that developed, advertised, and normalized ultra-processed foods. Every bag of chips, every "nutritious" granola bar, every bright neon beverage in the cooler has been specifically crafted – not for your optimal well-being, but for your consumption. The bliss point, the dopamine hit, the quick sugar rise followed by a crash – these were not mistakes. They were the design.

But here's the truth worth emphasizing: you don't have to fill that prescription anymore.

When you substitute the chemical distractions of UPFs with the steady cadence of real food, proteins, healthy fats, high-fiber plant foods, and hearty meals that truly satisfy, the cravings will quiet. Energy will return. Hormones will rebalance. Inflammation will diminish. Sleep will deepen. And most importantly, you will remember what food has always been meant to be: nourishment, connection, and revitalization.

Ultra-processed foods do more than fill grocery store shelves; they also fill hospital beds. They do not just take your money; they also take your vigor. And yet – the antidote is here. Every plate you prepare with intention is a prescription for wellness. Every meal is a vote for vitality.

QUICK-REFERENCE BOX — THE UPF EXIT PLAN

- Reframe the battlefield → control your environment
- Expect the withdrawal curve → it's neuroadaptation, not failure
- Anchor with protein + fiber → biochemical shield
- Break dopamine loops with new rituals
- Phase the exit → junk → "health halo" → reset plates
- Build default plates → eliminate decision fatigue
- Armor for social settings
- Redefine reward
- Play the long game → progress > perfection

If Chapter 4 was a harsh realization of the issue, Chapter 5 will be a gentle transition into the remedy. Because thriving is not just the absence of disease - it is embracing joy.

Let's be straight: food has always been more than just fuel. It is celebration, ritual, culture, family, comfort. The tragedy of the ultra-processed prescription is that it not only damages our biology – it also steals our pleasure and replaces the wholesome satisfaction of real food with empty stimulation.

Thus, the next step of your plan is to rediscover pleasure as you were intended to feel it. To eat in a way that is not about punishment, shame, or fear, but pleasure, freedom, and thriving.

Imagine savoring a meal and really feeling that every bite is delicious and life-giving. Imagine liberating yourself from the guilt of "bad foods" and "cheat days". Imagine eating in sync with your body's natural hunger - not reacting to manufactured cravings.

CHAPTER 5:

THE JOY PRESCRIPTION

HEALING AND THRIVING THROUGH FOOD THAT LOVES YOU BACK

Picture this.

It's midnight. The house is finally quiet. You tiptoe into the kitchen, open the fridge, and there it is — the last square of brownie, nestled in foil. Calling your name. You know you "shouldn't." You told yourself not to eat sugar, that carbs are the enemy, and dessert is a betrayal. But in the silence, you can't resist. You take a bite.

Now pause.

What if, instead of guilt flooding your veins, something else happened? What if you noticed the molten chocolate melting on your tongue, the earthy bitterness of cocoa, the sweetness fading into warmth? What if, instead of being the enemy, this one bite was medicine?

Here's the paradox: the same brownie can be poison or healing. It's not the molecules that change — it's the context. Your body, your brain, and your story about food determine whether that bite fuels inflammation and shame... or satisfaction and release.

We grew up with the idea that pleasure is the enemy. Food should be disciplined, monitored, and punished into submission. But neuroscience is teaching us otherwise. Guilt spikes cortisol, shuts down the digestive tract, and wires the brain to do the very binge we promised we wouldn't repeat. Joy, on the other hand - real joy - is a biological signal of safety, balance, and thriving.

108

So here is the radical prescription: Pleasure is not the enemy of health. Pleasure is the avenue to it.

And you're going to learn how to reclaim joy, not as a guilty indulgence, but as your body's built-in navigation system for healing!

MARIA'S STORY

Maria was still sitting at the same desk long after the last student exited the classroom. The kids had dashed out into the hallway one hour earlier, their joy ricocheting in the distance like an aftershock. The clock read 4:37 p.m. A lunch bag sat folded on her desk, waiting for her.

She was "good" all day. Breakfast: coffee. Lunch: nothing - she had too many papers to grade and, of course, was "saving the calories." By the time the bell rang, her stomach felt like a hollow hole, a banging, dull, dull sound that would not go away.

On the ride home, she tried to be logical. She would wait and make something reasonable: chicken and steamed broccoli. She was disciplined, right?

As soon as the door to her apartment opened, something broke. The tension she had been holding in like a dam burst open. Her eyes landed on a bag of granola bars. Not even her favorites. She opened one. Then another. Fifteen minutes later, she sat contemplating a pile of wrappers, heart racing, shame taking the place of comfort.

I have no willpower, she thought. I really have failed again.

That evening, Maria skipped dinner, in punishment, crawled into bed, and swore tomorrow would be different. Tomorrow came. And the loop continued.

The cultural narrative of guilt

What Maria is stuck in is not unusual. Millions are stuck in it.

We grow up in a food culture that scripts eating as moral: some foods are "good," and the rest are "bad." Eat kale - virtuous. Eat cookies - penance. We speak about ourselves in the language of sin: "I cheated." "I will make it up."

The script is everywhere. Magazine headlines proclaim: "Guilt-Free Desserts." Advertisements sell: "Indulgence - No Remorse." Even our table talk is colonized: "Oh, I shouldn't but just one."

Guilt is the classic invalidating actor when eating has become a moral performance. Guilt is not just an emotion - it is a biochemical cascade. And it backfires.

The neuroscience of guilt eating:

Here is what happens to Maria when guilt eats.

The stress response system is activated. The thought: "I shouldn't be eating this" registers mentally as a threat. Cortisol, the stress hormone, is released.

Digestion is compromised. Cortisol forces blood away from the gut to the muscles involved in "fight or flight." Food consumed at this time is poorly digested - you feel bloated and tired - all because of diverted blood flow and poorly digested food.

Reward circuits are hijacked. Guilt makes the food more rewarding; dopamine, the "wanting" neurotransmitter, spikes, alternating with deprivation and release. For Maria, when she has been restricting herself all day, the first bite is comforting; that comfort is habit-forming.

Neural pathways are reinforced. The brain records the pattern: restrict → binge → guilt → comfort. With each loop, the habit is reinforced, making it increasingly difficult to escape.

To sum up: guilt does not prevent overeating. Guilt programs it.

THE RESEARCH IS CLEAR

Science lines up with what Maria experienced.

- **Shame predicts overeating** — a 2014 study in *Appetite* found women who felt more guilt about eating chocolate were likelier to overeat later.

- **Restriction can fuel bingeing** — classic restraint theory (Herman & Polivy) shows that dieters who set strict rules are more vulnerable when temptation appears.

- **Cortisol and fat storage** — a 2009 paper in *Psychoneuroendocrinology* found people with higher daily cortisol accumulated more abdominal fat, independent of calories.

- **Mindset changes biology** — a 2011 study (Crum et al., *Health Psychology*) gave identical milkshakes labeled "indulgent" or "sensible." Those who had the indulgent shake showed a bigger drop in ghrelin (the hunger hormone). Belief shifted the body's response.

The pattern is consistent: guilt destabilizes the systems that manage hunger and satiety.

A CULTURE OF SILENT SUFFERING

Think about how many Marias exist — teachers, nurses, parents, executives — people who push through long days, discipline themselves, then collapse into shame-driven cycles. These aren't failures of character. They're predictable outcomes of a culture that equates discipline with deprivation and joy with moral failure.

Put another way: piling guilt onto food makes self-control harder, not easier. That's the guilt trap. If we don't change the script, no diet or plan will stick.

ACTION STEP: ESCAPING THE GUILT TRAP (DAY-ONE PRACTICES)

The radical idea: don't get stricter. Rewrite the script.

Practical, immediate steps:

1. **Retire "good vs. bad."** Use neutral language — nourishing, energizing, occasional. Strip the moral score off the plate.

2. **Add, don't subtract.** Instead of "I can't have chocolate," try "I'll have protein and fiber first." Adding nutrients stabilizes blood sugar and reduces binge urges.

3. **Use the guilt-interruption pause.** When guilt rises, pause. Take three deep breaths. Ask: Am I hungry, or am I seeking relief? Pausing slows the dopamine cycle and reintroduces choice.

4. **Celebrate satisfaction.** After eating, note how you feel — energy, mood, digestion — not just taste. That trains the brain to link pleasure with well-being, not punishment.

QUICK-REFERENCE: ESCAPING THE GUILT LOOP

The loop: Restriction → Craving → Binge → Guilt → Restriction.

Break the loop by:

- Dropping moral labels for food.

- Adding protein/fiber before treats.

- Pausing to check hunger vs. relief.

- Noticing satisfaction instead of shame.

Maria's story isn't a moral failure; it's wiring and culture doing what wiring and culture do. Guilt isn't a tool — it's a trap. The brain isn't craving punishment. It's craving safety, stability, and joy. Start there, and the rest follows.

Maria skipped lunch, binged on granola bars, then punished herself, a loop millions know. Guilt doesn't stop overeating; it rewires the brain to keep the cycle going. Try this: drop "good/bad" labels, add protein before treats, pause (3 breaths), and ask if you're hungry or seeking relief. Small changes. Real relief.

THE SCIENCE OF JOYFUL EATING

On a warm afternoon in Florence, the air smells faintly of wood smoke drifting from nearby ovens. Under the wide shade of an olive tree, a group of locals gathers around a spread that looks both simple and abundant: roast chicken finished with a squeeze of lemon, tomatoes glistening under olive oil, still-warm bread, slices of melon so ripe the juice runs as soon as a knife touches it.

Conversation floats easily—glasses of wine clink. Bread is passed around without hesitation, and no one seems to be silently tallying calories or bargaining with themselves over dessert. There's no talk of being "bad" or "earning" indulgence.

And yet, paradoxically, people in cultures that eat way slower meals, food shared with pleasure, have some of the lowest rates of chronic disease. Meanwhile, societies that emphasize restraint, guilt, and constant vigilance around food, like the United States and the United Kingdom, report rising levels of obesity, diabetes, and food anxiety.

The picnic is more than a pleasant image. It's evidence. Joyful eating isn't indulgence; it's a biological advantage.

WHY PLEASURE CHANGES THE BODY

Most of us were taught a different story: pleasure is dangerous, indulgence leads to chaos, and chaos to illness. But neuroscience paints a more nuanced picture.

Dopamine's real role. Often cast as the culprit behind cravings and bingeing, dopamine is actually about learning and motivation.

When we eat slowly, with attention and enjoyment, the brain codes that food as deeply satisfying. Eat the same thing under guilt or distraction, and the signal weakens—leaving us less satisfied and more likely to keep seeking. In other words, joy, not guilt, teaches the brain when "enough" has been reached.

The vagus nerve connection. This bundle of fibers, sometimes called the body's "rest-and-digest highway," is most active when we eat in calm, enjoyable states. When the vagus nerve is switched on, digestion and nutrient absorption improve, and inflammation decreases. Stress, by contrast, shuts the system down.

Hormones of connection. Meals shared with others trigger the release of endorphins and oxytocin, the same chemistry linked to bonding and resilience. Nutrients matter, but the social chemistry matters too.

Hunger and satiety signals. The hormones ghrelin and leptin, which regulate hunger and fullness, respond differently depending on mindset. Joyful, mindful meals tend to stabilize their cycle. Stress-driven meals disrupt it, leaving hunger unpredictable and satiety muted.

WHAT THE RESEARCH SHOWS

Cross-cultural research underscores the point. In the early 2000s, studies compared how French and American participants described food. The French leaned toward words like *pleasure* and *togetherness*, while Americans reached for *health* and *guilt*. Despite higher butter and wine intake, the French reported lower obesity and less overeating.

Other experiments reinforce this:

- When meals were eaten slowly and with presence, participants showed improved blood sugar responses compared to rushed or guilt-driven meals (Sofer et al., 2011).

- A 2011 study led by Alia Crum found that identical milkshakes produced different hormonal responses depending on whether they were labeled "indulgent" or "sensible." Belief alone shifted biology.

- Research at Cornell University in 2015 revealed that people who ate in groups reported greater satisfaction, lower stress, and less snacking afterward than those who ate alone.

The pattern is consistent: joy acts as metabolic leverage.

JOY AT THE TABLE

Contrast Maria's earlier story of eating alone in shame with another evening. Same apartment. Same woman. But this time she sets the table, lights a candle, and puts music on before two friends arrive.

Dinner isn't elaborate: pasta tossed with herbs, a salad, and grilled chicken. They eat slowly, laughing, pouring water, passing bowls back and forth. When dessert arrives—a plate of dark chocolate squares, Maria takes one, enjoys it, and leaves the rest untouched.

The difference isn't willpower. It's context. Joy makes satisfaction possible.

And the biology matches the moment. The same plate of food can land differently depending on how it's eaten. Someone standing at the fridge, alone and guilty, will likely see cortisol spike, digestion falter, and cravings linger. Someone at a lively table, savoring each bite, will see the opposite: cortisol drops, digestion improves, and cravings settle. Same calories. Different outcome.

BUILDING JOY BACK INTO MEALS

If guilt is a trap, joy is the way out, and it can be practiced.

- **Check in with your senses.** Before eating, notice the smell, color, and texture of your food. Anticipation primes the brain for satisfaction.

- **Honor the first bite.** Pay attention to how it tastes. Satiety signals are strongest early on, and noticing them sets the tone.

- **Match pace to the body.** Put utensils down between bites; the body's fullness cues need about 15–20 minutes to surface.

- **Eat with someone.** Whether in person or virtually, meals shared bring hormonal and emotional benefits.

- **Give permission.** Explicitly allow yourself to enjoy food. Paradoxically, permission reduces overindulgence while restriction fuels it.

Quick reminder:

- Joy activates digestion and satiety.

- Stress and guilt disrupt the process.

- Meals with others increase satisfaction and lower overeating.

- Pleasure helps the brain register "enough."

A DOCTOR'S PERSPECTIVE

Dr. Patel, an internist, leaned back in his chair after finishing yet another chart of a patient with prediabetes. "We've told people for decades: eat less, move more. And yet here we are."

He turned to his resident. "What if the missing variable isn't *less*? What if it's joy?"

The resident frowned. "Joy?"

"Yes," Patel said. "Joy is metabolic medicine. And we've starved people of it."

Around the world, long-lived cultures make the same point. Mediterranean families prioritize meals as rituals. Blue Zone communities use food as a source of connection as much as sustenance. In Okinawa, the tradition of *hara hachi bu*—stopping at 80% full—sits inside celebrations, not punishment.

These aren't happy accidents. They're proof that joy is not a luxury in nutrition. It's part of the prescription.

THE BOTTOM LINE

Joy is not the enemy of health; it's the engine of it. The research is clear, but the truth is lived more vividly at tables where laughter and flavor meet presence.

The next time you sit down to eat, remember that your body is wired to respond to joy. And the more you lean into that, the less food feels like punishment—and the more it becomes medicine.

THE JOY PROTOCOL: A PRACTICAL GUIDE TO EATING WITHOUT GUILT

A DINNER TABLE REVOLUTION

On a Tuesday evening in a quiet suburban kitchen, a family sits down to eat dinner. Phones are tucked into a basket by the door, the television is off, and a candle flickers in the center of the table. The food is nothing fancy, just a pot of spaghetti, a bowl of salad, and glasses of water. But the atmosphere has shifted.

The father tells a story about spilling coffee at work, drawing laughter from the kids. Their mother follows with a question, "What was the best part of your day?" that nudges everyone into conversation. The meal moves more slowly than usual. Plates are emptied with less urgency, and when the dishes are cleared, nobody wanders to the pantry for snacks.

The Biology hasn't changed. The food has. Meals framed by presence, humor, and connection trigger the body's "rest-and-digest" response, calm stress hormones, and sharpen satiety signals. This is the foundation of what researchers and clinicians call the **Joy Protocol**, a framework built not on restriction, but on restoring pleasure as a stabilizing force in eating.

At its core is a premise that runs counter to decades of diet culture: **pleasure is not the opposite of discipline. Pleasure is what makes discipline sustainable.**

THE FIVE PRACTICES OF THE JOY PROTOCOL

The framework rests on five practices that blend neuroscience, physiology, and psychology with everyday ritual. Each reshapes not only how food is consumed but how it is experienced.

1. PERMISSION & REFRAMING

For many people, guilt has become the default lens through which food is viewed. A slice of cake becomes a moral failure. A skipped salad earns quiet shame. Yet research shows that restriction often backfires.

In a landmark study (Polivy & Herman, 2002), restrained eaters asked to avoid certain foods later consumed more of them than non-restrained peers. Brain imaging has since confirmed the mechanism: restriction heightens activation in the anterior cingulate cortex, the brain's conflict-monitoring center, which fuels obsession. By contrast, permission engages the prefrontal cortex, the area tied to choice and self-regulation.

On a hormonal level, the difference is just as striking. Restriction amplifies ghrelin, the hunger hormone, while guilt triggers cortisol, which disrupts digestion and encourages fat storage. Permission calms both systems, allowing leptin—the satiety hormone—to signal effectively.

Action step: Write down three foods you've labeled "bad." For one week, introduce them in calm, deliberate settings. Plate the food, eat without distraction, and notice whether cravings lessen when guilt is absent.

2. THE RITUAL OF SLOWING DOWN

Speed is one of the most modern meal's biggest disruptors. Studies from Harvard (2011) found that participants who stretched meals over 30 minutes consumed fewer calories and reported more satisfaction than those who finished in ten.

The biology is simple: hormones like cholecystokinin (CCK) and leptin require 15–20 minutes to register fullness. Eating too quickly floods the stomach before those signals arrive. Slowness, meanwhile, activates the vagus nerve, shifting the body from "fight-or-flight" into "rest-and-digest." Nutrient absorption improves; overeating declines.

This is not merely theoretical. In Okinawa, Japan, centenarians follow *hara hachi bu*, the practice of stopping at 80% fullness. Their meals are unhurried, often social, and strongly correlated with longevity.

Action step: Choose one daily meal to extend to at least 20 minutes. Try the "utensil-down" rule—setting your fork aside between bites—and pay attention to textures as you chew.

3. SAVORING THROUGH THE SENSES

The cephalic phase response—an anticipatory wave of digestive activity—begins before the first bite. When the eyes, nose, and even ears engage with food, enzymes and hormones prime the body for digestion.

Sensory attention also reshapes dopamine release, rather than spiking with volume alone; dopamine peaks when food is anticipated and savored. A 2014 study in *Appetite* found that participants who practiced mindful savoring of snacks ate roughly 25 percent less later in the day.

Action step: Before eating, pause to notice sight, smell, sound, touch, and taste. Name three sensory qualities of the food. Allow flavors to unfold before reaching for the next bite.

4. CONNECTION AT THE TABLE

In Sardinia, Italy, where life expectancy ranks among the highest in the world, meals are rarely solitary. Bread is passed, stories exchanged, wine sipped slowly. Food is as much about people as it is about calories.

Science confirms what tradition has long suggested. Social eating raises oxytocin, the hormone linked to bonding, which in turn lowers cortisol and smooths digestion. Data from the Harvard Family Dinner Project show that children who share regular meals with family have lower rates of obesity and depression. And loneliness, according to psychologist Julianne Holt-Lunstad's 2015 meta-analysis, can raise mortality risk as much as smoking 15 cigarettes a day.

Action step: Commit to one device-free dinner each week. If alone, create a sense of ritual company—through a phone call, music, or journaling.

5. THE JOYFUL AUDIT

Every eater carries a food story. For some, it begins in a grandmother's kitchen, filled with pies and laughter. For others, it begins with being told to "clean your plate" long after hunger had passed.

Psychologists call the process of revisiting and rewriting these narratives "cognitive reframing." The amygdala, which stores emotional memory, plays a powerful role in cravings and avoidance. By identifying shame-based scripts and deliberately cultivating new joyful experiences, people can reset how their brains interpret hunger and satiety cues.

Action step: Write down early food memories, circling moments of joy and underlining moments of shame. Then, each week, create a new positive association: cook with a friend, picnic outdoors, or pair a favorite playlist with dinner.

WHAT CHANGE LOOKS LIKE

For many who adopt these practices, the effects unfold gradually but persistently. Late-night pantry raids become less frequent. Meals leave behind less heaviness and more energy. Digestion steadies; cravings ease.

One composite story, drawn from several participants, captures the shift: a woman who once avoided birthday cake at parties for fear of "being bad" eventually learned to permit herself a slice. "Two bites and I was done," she recalled. "I laughed with my friends, and that was it. I didn't go home and binge. For the first time, food wasn't the enemy."

The Joy Protocol is not another diet. It doesn't ask people to cut carbs, count calories, or grind through hunger. Instead, it reframes eating as a relationship between physiology and psychology, where joy is not indulgence but medicine.

By slowing down, engaging the senses, permitting pleasure, and reclaiming connection, food shifts from a battlefield to an ally. And as the research shows, the benefits reach far beyond the plate— lower stress, steadier metabolism, more resilient health.

In the end, the real prescription is simple: when meals become spaces of joy rather than guilt, the body responds not with chaos, but with balance.

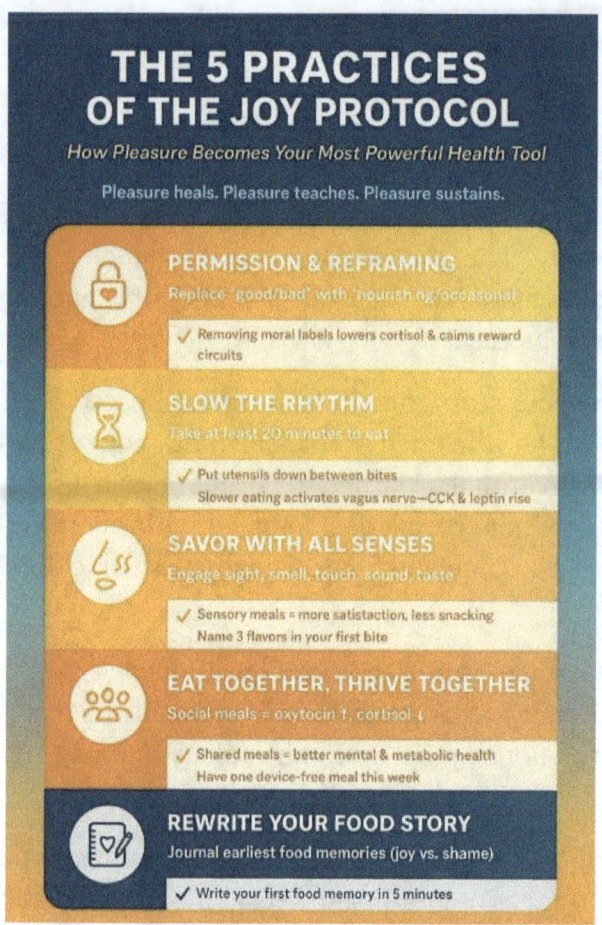

THE 5 PRACTICES OF THE JOY PROTOCOL

How Pleasure Becomes Your Most Powerful Health Tool

Pleasure heals. Pleasure teaches. Pleasure sustains.

PERMISSION & REFRAMING
Replace "good/bad" with "nourishing/occasional"
✓ Removing moral labels lowers cortisol & calms reward circuits

SLOW THE RHYTHM
Take at least 20 minutes to eat
✓ Put utensils down between bites
Slower eating activates vagus nerve—CCK & leptin rise

SAVOR WITH ALL SENSES
Engage sight, smell, touch, sound, taste
✓ Sensory meals = more satisfaction, less snacking
Name 3 flavors in your first bite

EAT TOGETHER, THRIVE TOGETHER
Social meals = oxytocin ↑, cortisol ↓
✓ Shared meals = better mental & metabolic health
Have one device-free meal this week

REWRITE YOUR FOOD STORY
Journal earliest food memories (joy vs. shame)
✓ Write your first food memory in 5 minutes

PART 6 — ACTION STARTER: YOUR JOY PLAN

A DIFFERENT KIND OF RESET

It's Monday morning. The alarm has barely rung, but instead of rolling over in dread, you linger under the blanket for a moment. The thought of food crosses your mind—not with guilt, but with a small curiosity. What would it feel like to begin the day without calculating calories or tallying "slip-ups" from the weekend? What if, instead, the question was: *How can I eat with joy today?*

That pivot, subtle as it sounds, is at the heart of what researchers and clinicians are now calling joy-centered eating. It doesn't postpone contentment until you hit a certain weight or see a particular blood marker improve. Joy can begin in the first bite of breakfast, in the permission you allow yourself to savor, and in the micro-choices that set the rhythm of your day.

Here is a **four-step plan**, grounded in neuroscience and nutrition research, to help rewire the way you approach food—not by restriction, but by steady, deliberate joy.

STEP 1: BUILD YOUR FIRST MEAL AROUND PROTEIN + FIBER

Mornings often unfold on autopilot: coffee clutched in one hand, maybe a piece of toast, or nothing at all until hunger hits like a tidal wave mid-morning. The problem isn't simply "skipping breakfast." It's starting the day without nourishment.

When the first meal of the day emphasizes protein and fiber, the body's systems align differently. Protein blunts ghrelin, the hormone that drives hunger, while also boosting satiety hormones like GLP-1 and PYY. Fiber slows digestion, steadies glucose levels, and feeds the microbiome—an influence that ripples into mood and cravings later in the day.

A randomized trial published in Obesity (Leidy et al., 2013) found that a high-protein breakfast reduced evening snacking by half compared to a lower-protein or no breakfast at all. One participant in a recent lifestyle program described the difference simply: "*By mid-afternoon, I wasn't hunting through the cupboards. I had energy to actually finish my workday.*"

Action Cue: Tomorrow, build your plate with 20–30 grams of protein (eggs, Greek yogurt, salmon, or a protein shake) and at least one fiber-rich plant (berries, avocado, leafy greens). Think of it less as dieting, more as anchoring your day in stability.

STEP 2: SCHEDULE ONE "JOY MEAL" PER WEEK

Most diets falter not because people lack information, but because they slip into a binary rhythm of "good days" and "bad days." That rigid mindset breeds rebellion. Deprivation piles up until it topples.

The alternative is what psychologists call dietary flexibility: deliberately planning a meal each week that is guided by joy, not by rules. There's no calorie counting, no shame, only presence.

Research in the *International Journal of Obesity* (2017) shows that flexible dieting approaches reduce binge episodes and improve long-term adherence compared with rigid dietary rules. As one woman put it after adopting this approach: "*Friday pizza night stopped being my downfall—it became the highlight I looked forward to, without guilt.*"

Action Cue: Pick a weekly ritual—Sunday brunch, Friday dinner, a midweek lunch with friends. Choose food you genuinely love, eat it slowly, and treat it as a celebration rather than a violation. This is not a "cheat meal." It's a joy meal, a pressure valve that sustains consistency.

STEP 3: PRACTICE MINDFUL EATING WITH ONE DAILY SNACK OR MEAL

Much of modern overeating doesn't stem from physical hunger but from distraction—screens glowing, emails pinging, a television murmuring in the background. In those moments, food becomes background noise, and the body never fully registers satiety.

Mindful eating interrupts that pattern. A systematic review in *Appetite* (2014) showed that mindfulness interventions reduced emotional eating, binge frequency, and body weight—all without imposing strict food rules.

Even a small pause can shift physiology. By sitting down, taking a breath, and noticing flavors and textures, you trigger the cephalic phase of digestion—priming enzymes and hormones to sync with the act of eating.

One man who began practicing mindful snacking told researchers, *"I was shocked. I ate half the portion I usually do, but it felt like more because I actually noticed it."*

Action Cue: Select one meal or snack per day to practice mindfully. No screens, no multitasking. Sit down, breathe, and engage your senses—sight, smell, texture, taste. Even three mindful minutes can recalibrate appetite signals.

STEP 4: REPROGRAM GUILT INTO GRATITUDE

Few emotions derail eating behavior like guilt. Research shows that stress-driven guilt spikes cortisol, a hormone that disrupts digestion, encourages fat storage, and intensifies cravings. Gratitude, in contrast, has the opposite effect—shifting the nervous system into parasympathetic "rest and digest" mode.

A study in the *Journal of Positive Psychology* (2019) found that gratitude practices lowered cortisol and improved patterns of eating. Vagus nerve research has also shown that mindful appreciation raises vagal tone, enhancing both digestion and stress regulation.

Several people who adopted this practice describe a similar realization: *"The moment I stopped saying, 'I shouldn't eat this,' and started saying, 'I get to enjoy this,' everything softened. My body responded differently."*

Action Cue: Before your next meal, pause. If an inner voice says, "I shouldn't," reframe it into gratitude: "I get to." Even with a slice of cake, acknowledge the flavor, the moment, the memory. Over time, the emotional landscape shifts—from shame toward genuine satisfaction.

SMALL STEPS, BIG REPROGRAMMING

Joy does not arrive through a sweeping overhaul. It slips in through the small rituals, one protein-rich breakfast, one joy meal savored without guilt, one mindful snack eaten without distraction, one quiet moment of gratitude before a bite.

Repeated daily, these cues reprogram physiology as much as psychology. Ghrelin rhythms normalize. Cortisol softens. Satiety hormones signal more effectively. Cravings lose their urgency.

And slowly, meal by meal, you are not just changing what you eat— you are reshaping your relationship with food itself.

YOUR JOY PLAN
AT A GLANCE

STEP 1

Build Your First Meal (Protein + Fiber)

20-30g protein + one fiber-rich plant
Anchors satiety hormones, steadies energy

STEP 2

Schedule One Joy Meal (Per Week)

Choose one meal you *love* → savor, no gu
Turns flexibility into fuel for long-term succ

STEP 3

Mindful Eating (1 Meal/Snack Daily)

No screens, no multitasking
Chew slowly, notice 3 flavors/textures

STEP 4

Reprogram Guilt → Gratitude

Pause before eating → reframe
From "I shouldn't" → ""I get to nourish mysel

Small daily joy beats big occasional willpower.

PART 7

QUICK-REFERENCE CHECKLIST: THE JOY PRESCRIPTION REMINDERS

A simple compass to keep you anchored in joy, not guilt. Post it on your fridge, desk, or journal.

DAILY COMPASS

- Anchor your first meal with protein + fiber.
- Hydrate before caffeine.
- One mindful moment per meal (pause, breathe, notice).

WEEKLY COMPASS

- Schedule one **"Joy Meal"** → eat what you love, without rules.
- Plan one **nature/connection ritual** → a walk, a shared meal, or dinner outdoors.

MINDSET COMPASS

- **No guilt labels** → there are no "good" or "bad" foods.
- Reframe cravings: **curiosity > criticism**.
- Swap shame for **gratitude** → thank your body before eating.

SCIENCE COMPASS

- Joyful eating → lowers **cortisol**, boosts **digestion**.
- Positive emotions during meals → **activate vagus nerve** for satiety.
- Social meals → mimic **Blue Zones longevity patterns**.

CONSISTENCY COMPASS

- Progress > perfection.

- Even one joyful bite counts.

- Repeat, refine, rejoice.

Post this checklist somewhere visible — your kitchen, journal, or phone lock screen.

Joy isn't a finish line; it's a daily prescription.

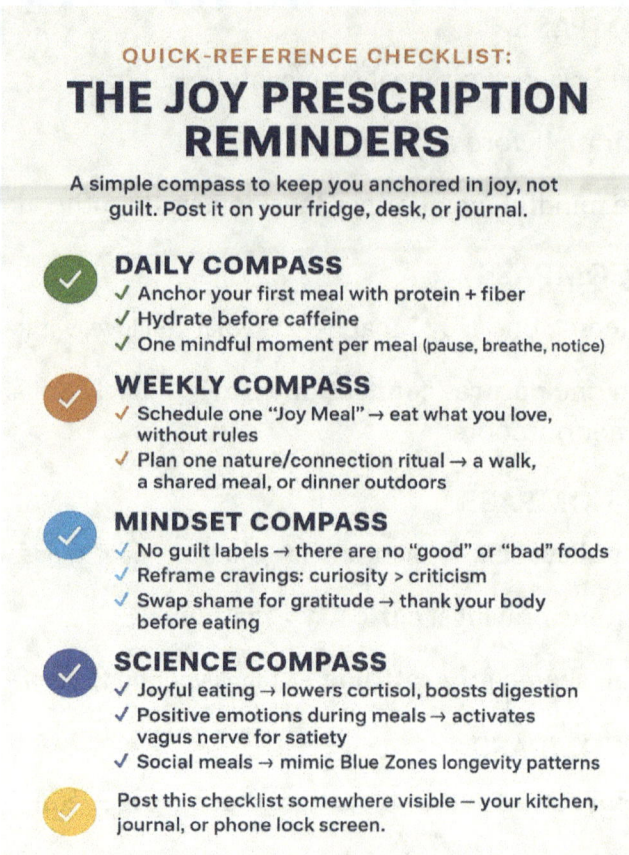

QUICK-REFERENCE CHECKLIST:

THE JOY PRESCRIPTION REMINDERS

A simple compass to keep you anchored in joy, not guilt. Post it on your fridge, desk, or journal.

DAILY COMPASS
✓ Anchor your first meal with protein + fiber
✓ Hydrate before caffeine
✓ One mindful moment per meal (pause, breathe, notice)

WEEKLY COMPASS
✓ Schedule one "Joy Meal" → eat what you love, without rules
✓ Plan one nature/connection ritual → a walk, a shared meal, or dinner outdoors

MINDSET COMPASS
✓ No guilt labels → there are no "good" or "bad" foods
✓ Reframe cravings: curiosity > criticism
✓ Swap shame for gratitude → thank your body before eating

SCIENCE COMPASS
✓ Joyful eating → lowers cortisol, boosts digestion
✓ Positive emotions during meals → activates vagus nerve for satiety
✓ Social meals → mimic Blue Zones longevity patterns

Post this checklist somewhere visible — your kitchen, journal, or phone lock screen.

FROM PRESCRIPTION TO POSSIBILITY

In the past few chapters, we followed the tension of being in survival mode versus thriving, and the tension of cravings cycles versus states of clarity. Along the way, the nuances of food could never be neutral; food can, in some contexts, act as medicine, restoring physiology to equilibrium, and in other contexts, food can act as a disruptor, thus increasing inflammation load and reactive metabolism. Guilt and shame heighten the latter, affirming values of stress and keeping the body in prolonged dysregulation.

What is especially interesting about the research is its counterpoint; when food is consumed more present-ly and less punishment-ly, body physiology begins to change. Now, neuroanatomy is firing more efficiently to support satiation responses, digestion is less disrupted, and hormonal patterns are starting to re-establish equilibrium. Umami eating is an invitation to shift our awareness of food consumption from tension to alignment, leading to tangible biological responses.

This is the intention of the Joy Prescription. It is about not being about restriction or rules, but changing the psychological and physiological context of eating to recalibrate your body's power factor (regulation). When guilt is replaced with present and stress with calm, the output grows beyond our subjective mood. It is seen in the biology of the spores being secreted, in the biology of the reaction of metabolism, and in the biology of the response to the neuronal systems maintaining our regulation of metabolism.

Moreover, over time, the shift in practice adds up, even if it is in little bits. The hunger cues in the morning take a somewhat more reliable rhythm. Post-mealtime energy levels become more consistent; the reduction of cravings moves closer to slowing their intensity. What had been a struggle with food begins to seem more like a collaboration with physiology. These are not abstract changes. They are concrete changes in how our brains and bodies absorb nutrients and regulate appetite.

Moving Toward the Next Layer: Food, Mood, and the Microbiome

The next chapter is determining why the pleasure of eating can be a readily available experience for some people and a more elusive experience for others. A reason resides in a less apparent system — the gut microbiome.

The gut microbiome is more than an ecosystem primarily engaged in digestion; this microbial consortium interacts with the nervous and immune systems of the body in multiple ways. By controlling the production of metabolites, such as short-chain fatty acids, the gut microbes control inflammatory pathways and insulin sensitivity. The microbes make neurotransmitter precursors, which in turn control the quantity of serotonin, dopamine, and gamma-aminobutyric acid (GABA). There are multiple routes these signals take to reach the brain: direct via the vagus nerve, indirect through immune signaling, and other pathways that modulate permeability of the blood–brain barrier.

This bi-directional signaling — often referred to as the gut–brain axis — explains in part why the make-up of the gut microbiome can impact mood states, cognitive states, and cravings. Certain microbiome profiles also provide stability in energy and reduced anxiety. Other microbiome profiles promote systemic inflammation, reduce satiety signals, and consequently compromise the ability to resist cravings for high-sugar, high-fat food.

The remarkable conclusion is simple: food not only feeds human cells. Food feeds microbial populations, and those microbial populations then train human physiology and psychology. Understanding this relationship allows us to shift our understanding of nutrition from one that considers only caloric balance or nutrient intake to understanding that nutrition is now also about ecological balance in our bodies.

As we move into Chapter 6, we will turn the focus from the outer, joy-filled act of eating to the inner, more biological mechanisms that allow joy to be more or less accessible—the key question shifts from what you eat to what your microbiome does with what you eat.

CHAPTER 6:

FOOD + MOOD + MICROBIOME

HOW YOUR INNER GARDEN SHAPES THE WAY YOU FEEL

Imagine this: a woman is sitting in her car outside of a grocery store. The engine is off, and her hands are on the steering wheel. She's not tired from work or rushing between errands. She's frozen. She is frozen because she can't explain why she is feeling like crying for no reason. Yesterday she was just fine: today she is submerged in fog.

Physicians might call this stress. Friends may call it burnout. But, beneath all of it, something far better is in command inside her.

Trillions of tiny organisms - bacteria, fungi, and even viruses - inhabit her gut and are pulling invisible levers that shape her mood, mental cravings, and, more importantly, her clarity. This microscopic metropolis is called the microbiome and is rewriting everything we thought we knew about mental health, energy, and disease.

And here's the kicker: those same microbes do not just digest food. They talk. To your immune system. To your hormones. Even directly to your brain. Their language? Chemical, electrical, hormonal. And depending upon how you've been feeding these organisms, they can make your world feel lighter... or unbearably heavy.

Scientists call this the gut-brain axis. I call it your inner garden. And like any garden, it will either bloom with variety and vitality, or it will wither under neglect and toxic inputs.

And here is the most surprising part: Ultra-processed foods, stress-eating, late nights, and sugar overload aren't just draining your energy. They are literally reprogramming your microbes to demand more of what they've been giving. So this means that late-night cravings, sudden crash moods, even the foggy indecision that often occurs in that 2 PM hour, are not failures of willpower. They are communications from a hijacked ecosystem.

But the good news is this: when you learn to reset your inner garden, mood, and food cease to be adversaries. Anxiety softens. Energy stabilizes. Clarity is restored. And joy - the kind that doesn't require effort—emerges as your natural state.

This chapter details your process for that reset.

PART 1 — THE GUT-BRAIN AXIS:

THE STORY THAT LIVES IN THE GUT

Think about Maria again, the same teacher that we've described in earlier chapters. Maria has a lot of pride when it comes to resilience—she takes no sick days, shows up for her students, and laughs off stress. Lately, however, she has been feeling differently.

Maria is waking up with no appetite and using just enough coffee to fight through the fog, only to find herself crashing hard by the time the afternoon arrives. By dinner time, she is snapping at the kids for nothing and then feeling guilty and apologetic. By the time she puts the kids to bed, she eats cookies in the dark kitchen, not at all because she is hungry, but because, in her words, "It's the only thing that makes me feel better, even if just for a moment."

Maria thinks she has a willpower problem, but her doctor tells her it's stress. But neither explanation fully fits, because the crash-and-crave cycle has been building for months, even as she tries harder to "be good."

What's really happening? Her gut microbiome has shifted. The balance of microbes that once produced calming neurotransmitters like serotonin and GABA has tilted toward species that thrive on sugar and processed starches. These microbes are sending signals through her vagus nerve and bloodstream, demanding the very foods that perpetuate imbalance.

It's not just her mind—it's her microbes calling the shots.

THE SCIENCE OF THE HIDDEN CONVERSATION

Your gut is home to an estimated 100 trillion microbes—more cells than your body has. Collectively, they weigh about 2–3 pounds, the size of your brain. In many ways, they function as a second brain.

Various scientists have coined a term called the gut-brain axis. It consists of a two-way communication network between your digestive system and your nervous system that is always open. Picture a high-speed fibre optic cable kept open to pass a continuous flow of messages back and forth.

Here's how the conversation happens:

- **The Vagus Nerve** → A cranial nerve that runs from your brainstem to your gut, carrying signals in both directions. About **90% of these fibers send information *from the gut to the brain*** (not the other way around).

- **Neurotransmitters** → Gut microbes produce serotonin (about 90% of your body's supply), dopamine, and GABA, all of which directly shape mood and motivation.

- **Short-Chain Fatty Acids (SCFAs)** → Produced when microbes ferment fiber, SCFAs reduce inflammation, stabilize blood sugar, and even cross the blood-brain barrier to influence cognition.

- **Immune Pathways** → About 70% of your immune system lives in the gut lining. Microbial balance dictates whether the immune system calms or inflames. Chronic low-grade inflammation is now recognized as a root cause of depression and anxiety.

This is not "woo-woo." It's biochemistry.

THE MOOD-GUT FEEDBACK LOOP

Now, here's the kicker: it works both ways. Your thoughts, stress, and emotions affect your gut, and your gut affects your thoughts, stress, and emotions.

- Chronic stress increases cortisol, which weakens the gut lining ("leaky gut") and alters microbial diversity.

- An altered microbiome then produces fewer calming neurotransmitters, which worsens anxiety and cravings.

- Anxiety and cravings drive poor food choices (sugar, UPFs).

- Poor food choices further reshape the microbiome.

It's a **feedback loop**—and depending on what you feed it, the loop either spirals down into anxiety and cravings or spirals up into calm clarity.

THE EVIDENCE: GUT MICROBES & MENTAL HEALTH

Science is catching up fast. A few pivotal findings:

- **Serotonin Factory:** About **90–95% of serotonin is produced in the gut**, not the brain (Yano et al., *Cell*, 2015). Without a diverse microbiome, serotonin levels crash.

- **Depression & Microbes:** A landmark study in *Nature Microbiology* (2019) found that people with depression had significantly fewer bacteria that produce butyrate (an SCFA known for anti-inflammatory, mood-stabilizing effects).

- **Anxiety & Gut-Brain Therapy:** Clinical trials show that probiotics containing *Lactobacillus* and *Bifidobacterium* strains reduce anxiety symptoms as effectively as some pharmaceuticals (Wallace & Milev, *Frontiers in Psychiatry*, 2017).

- **Diet & Mood:** The SMILES Trial (Jacka et al., 2017) showed that people with major depression who switched to a Mediterranean-style diet rich in fiber, omega-3s, and unprocessed foods had **significant remission rates** compared to controls.

In short: the microbiome is not a side note to health, it's a **core driver of mood, energy, and resilience**.

THE HIDDEN LABORATORY

Now imagine the "secret lab" inside your belly. Each and every bite you eat is equivalent to a grant application. Fiber-rich vegetables? Beneficial microbes with the intent to protect you from inflammation win their share of funding to continue to flourish. A donut at 11 PM? Sugar-hungry microbes multiply and send signals for more of the same.

Each food choice is like a signal to which microbial "party" rules your inner parliament. Over weeks, the ruling microbes actually change the messages that your body sends to your brain.

- Fiber $\rightarrow$ SCFAs $\rightarrow$ calm, focus, stable mood.
- Sugar/UPFs $\rightarrow$ endotoxins, inflammation $\rightarrow$ anxiety, cravings, brain fog.

The hidden laboratory is always running experiments. The only question is: are you funding the microbes that fuel joy and repair, or the ones that fuel despair and destroy?

ACTION PRIMER: RESETTING THE GUT-BRAIN AXIS

Before we dive deeper into mechanics (circadian alignment, chronic inflammation, etc.), here's your **first small set of moves** to start reclaiming the conversation:

1. Feed the Fiber → Starve the Cravings

a. Every meal: include at least one high-fiber plant (leafy greens, beans, flaxseeds, berries).

b. Why? Fiber is the raw material for SCFAs, which reduce inflammation and balance neurotransmitters.

2. Hydrate Like Your Microbes Matter

a. Dehydration concentrates gut stress and slows digestion. Aim for water first thing in the morning and throughout the day.

b. Herbal teas (ginger, peppermint) also support microbial balance.

3. Mind the Clock

a. Microbes themselves follow a circadian rhythm. Late-night eating disrupts microbial repair cycles.

b. Action: Stop eating 2–3 hours before bed.

4. Ferment for the Win

a. Add one fermented food daily: sauerkraut, kimchi, kefir, yogurt, miso.

b. Live cultures reinforce microbial diversity.

5. Breathe for the Vagus Nerve

a. Two minutes of slow diaphragmatic breathing before meals.

b. Activates the vagus nerve, shifting you into "rest-and-digest" mode, priming the gut-brain axis for balance.

QUICK-REFERENCE BOX

Gut-Brain Reset: First Five Moves

- Fiber fuels calm — every plate, every meal.

- Water is the first "nutrient" your microbes need.

- No late-night snacks: let microbes repair.

- Fermented foods = microbial reinforcements.

- Slow breathing before meals = better digestion + mood.

PART 2 — THE CIRCADIAN HUNGER CLOCK & MICROBIOME

THE NIGHT SNACK THAT BACKFIRES

It's 11:45 PM.

Sam, a 29-year-old nurse who works rotating shifts, collapses on her couch after what feels like a marathon twelve-hour shift. Her body feels empty but wired, like the battery icon on an iPhone blinking red. She knows she shouldn't eat this late—she's read about "late-night eating" — but the call of her cravings is too much to resist. She pulls out a granola bar and a soda, telling herself it's "just a snack."

In no time, the racing thoughts begin to slow down. The sugars and caffeine feel like fuel on her empty tank. But, when the morning comes, the crash comes hard: grogginess, no appetite for breakfast (though she won't miss the morning traffic), and a knot of irritability in her gut. Over a few weeks, this pattern develops into a spiral of disrupted sleep-wake rhythms, strange hunger cycles, and an inescapable sense of anxiety.

Little does Sam know, it really isn't just a "snack". She is feeding her microbes at the wrong time. And when the rhythm of your microbiome's clock is out of sync, so is hers.

THE HIDDEN CLOCK INSIDE YOUR GUT

Your body has not one, but two clocks:

The Master Clock in the brain's suprachiasmatic nucleus (SCN) is set by light and dark.

And Peripheral Clocks, your body's "little timekeepers", are in nearly every cell in your body, including the trillions of microbes in your gut.

These microbial clocks are not "ticking" alone. They are following your meal schedule, as they have been trained to do. When you eat, your gut microbes are metabolizing, fermenting, and essentially splitting into byproducts that enter your blood and eventually, your brain.

The catch? Your microbes expect a "schedule." Think of it as social conditioning: When you eat according to the sun, they thrive. When you eat according to the fridge light at midnight, they riot.

THE MICROBIAL JET LAG

In 2014, a groundbreaking *Cell* study (Thaiss et al.) revealed something extraordinary: gut bacteria themselves have circadian rhythms. Their populations shift in type and activity depending on the time of day.

- During the **day**, microbes specialize in breaking down complex carbs and producing short-chain fatty acids (SCFAs), which fuel colon cells and stabilize mood.

- At **night**, populations shift toward repair and maintenance, reducing digestive activity so the body can rest.

When researchers fed mice at odd hours, their microbial communities became scrambled—like passengers on a flight crossing time zones. This microbial jet lag triggered weight gain, insulin resistance, and inflammation even when calorie counts were the same.

In other words, it wasn't *just what* they ate, but *when*.

CORTISOL, MELATONIN, AND THE GUT

The body's own hormones help keep this internal symphony in time.

- **Cortisol**, the "wake-up hormone," peaks in the morning, helping to stimulate digestion and energy release.

- **Melatonin**, the "sleep hormone," rises at night—not just to cue the brain for sleep but also to tell the gut: *slow down.*

But here's the fun part: when melatonin rises, insulin sensitivity plummets. It means a snack eaten at 11 PM has a vastly different metabolic impact than the very same snack eaten at 11 AM. The blood sugar levels spike higher, fat storage increases, and the microbial diversity decreases.

This is why Sam wakes up sluggish after her midnight granola bar: her microbiome and accompanying hormones are signaling repair, not digestion.

MEAL TIMING AND GLUCOSE CONTROL

The circadian link isn't just a theory. In a study published in *Obesity* (Jakubowicz et al., 2013), participants who ate their largest meal at breakfast lost more weight and improved insulin sensitivity compared to those who ate the same calories at dinner.

Another *Cell Metabolism* study (Zarrinpar et al., 2016) showed that **time-restricted feeding**—confining meals to an 8–10-hour daylight window—restored microbial rhythms and improved metabolic health, even without reducing calories.

The takeaway: your microbiome isn't just passively processing food. It's tracking time.

CRAVINGS AS A CLOCK SIGNAL

Have you ever experienced a 3 PM slump that was more than fatigue? Have you also experienced cravings (often for quick sugar or caffeine)? The cravings are not random or incidental. Your circadian rhythm naturally dips in alertness midafternoon, and whenever meals are out of rhythm, your microbes send you signals of distress that amplify your cravings, which results in weight-gain tendencies.

In Sam's case, night snacking interrupted her microbial clock, which dysregulated her hunger hormones too:

- **Ghrelin** (hunger hormone) spiked at odd times.

- **Leptin** (satiety hormone) dulled, leaving her unsatisfied.

Cravings weren't a failure of willpower. They were her gut's alarm system, telling her rhythm was broken.

THE PARENT, THE ATHLETE, THE WORKER

- **The Parent (Lisa, 42):** Stays up late prepping lunches, often eats dinner at 9:30 PM. She notices bloating and irritability but thinks it's "just stress." In reality, late meals suppress her morning hunger, pushing her circadian rhythm later and compounding fatigue.

- **The Athlete (Jordan, 24):** Trains hard at night, then eats massive post-workout meals at 11 PM. Despite burning thousands of calories, he struggles with brain fog and plateaus. His gut microbes never get a "rest phase," keeping inflammation elevated.

- **The Night-Shift Worker (Ana, 35):** Eats lunch at 2 AM during breaks. Studies show shift workers have significantly lower microbial diversity and a higher risk for metabolic disease. Ana feels she's "always hungry but never satisfied." Her body is living in two time zones at once.

ACTION PRIMER: RESETTING THE HUNGER CLOCK

The good news? Microbial clocks are adaptable. Within a matter of days to weeks, you can begin to resynchronize your gut and hunger cycles.

Here's how:

ANCHOR MEALS TO SUNLIGHT

- Eat your **first meal within 1–2 hours of waking**, ideally with protein and fiber.

- Aim to **finish eating 2–3 hours before bed**.

TIME-RESTRICTED EATING (TRE)

- Start with a **10–12-hour eating window** aligned with daylight.

- Over time, narrow it to 8 hours if sustainable.

FRONT-LOAD CALORIES

- Shift the bulk of calories to earlier meals.

- Research shows bigger breakfasts/lunches improve metabolic health vs. large dinners.

GUT-FRIENDLY SNACKS AT SLUMP TIMES

- Instead of sugar at 3 PM, try fermented foods (yogurt, kimchi) or fiber-protein combos (apple + almond butter). These regulate microbial signaling.

RESPECT REST

- Think of fasting after dinner not as deprivation, but as *microbial sleep hygiene*. Just as you need 7–9 hours of sleep, your microbes need a nightly reset.

Sam, the nurse, didn't realize her late-night snacks were writing her hunger stories. After she started shifting her meals to daylight hours, something extraordinary happened: she woke up hungry again. Her cravings softened, her sleep deepened, and for the first time in years, her energy carried her through her shifts.

The gut had reset its clock.

And here's the deeper magic: the microbiome doesn't just track time. It manufactures the very molecules that sculpt our moods— serotonin, dopamine, GABA. Which means the clock isn't just about hunger; it's about how we feel.

That's where we go next.

PART 3 — MICROBES AND MOOD MOLECULES

THE INVISIBLE PHARMACISTS IN YOUR GUT

If you could visualize a pharmacy hidden inside your body, you might imagine a pharmacy filled with pill bottles, vials, and a location behind the counter for compounding and dispensing measured doses. But in reality, that pharmacy doesn't exist in a white room with a pharmacist in a lab coat — it lives in your gut.

Trillions of microbes respond every hour of every day to the food you provide. They influence your mood, energy levels, and focus — or drag you into anxiety, brain fog, irritability, exhaustion, and all the other facets that make you who you are.

The crazy part is that you don't actually consciously control what they produce. The microbes respond to what you feed them, the rhythms you live in, and the signals your lifestyle sends.

Your gut bacteria are like microscopic pharmacists, compounding neuroactive molecules like serotonin, dopamine, and GABA that determine how your brain feels. The gut-brain axis is a two-way communication pathway, and if your gut makes something, your brain will know about it.

THE CHEMISTRY OF EMOTION

Let's break down the key mood molecules that microbes produce:

1. Serotonin (The Mood Stabilizer)

- Nearly **90–95% of your body's serotonin** is produced in the gut, not the brain (Gershon, 2013, *Nature Reviews Neuroscience*).

- Gut microbes influence serotonin production by fermenting dietary fiber into short-chain fatty acids (SCFAs), which trigger enterochromaffin cells in the intestinal lining to release serotonin.

- **What it does:** stabilizes mood, regulates sleep, improves digestion, and reduces anxiety.

- **What disrupts it:** ultra-processed diets, artificial sweeteners, chronic stress, and disrupted circadian rhythms.

2. Dopamine (The Motivation Molecule)

- Gut microbes synthesize precursors like tyrosine and phenylalanine that fuel dopamine production.

- Dopamine regulates motivation, pleasure, reward-seeking, and motor function.

- **Imbalance:** Too little dopamine = apathy, depression, poor focus. Too much = addiction loops, compulsive eating.

- **Food connection:** Protein-rich foods (eggs, lean meats, legumes) provide amino acids for dopamine. But ultra-processed foods overstimulate dopamine reward pathways, leading to tolerance and a blunted response over time.

3. GABA (The Calm Signal)

- Gamma-aminobutyric acid (GABA) is the brain's main inhibitory neurotransmitter — it calms overactive neurons.

- Certain Lactobacillus and Bifidobacterium strains can produce GABA directly in the gut.

- **What it does:** reduces anxiety, improves sleep quality, and prevents overstimulation.

- **What disrupts it:** antibiotics, low-diversity diets, and chronic alcohol consumption.

4. Short-Chain Fatty Acids (SCFAs)

- Produced when microbes ferment prebiotic fibers.

- Acetate, propionate, and butyrate cross into the bloodstream and even affect brain function.

- SCFAs reduce systemic inflammation (a driver of depression) and regulate the blood-brain barrier.

- **Study highlight:** A 2019 paper in *Nature Microbiology* linked reduced microbial diversity and low SCFA levels with a higher incidence of depression.

5. Inflammatory Molecules (The Dark Side)

- Dysbiosis (imbalanced microbiome) produces lipopolysaccharides (LPS), pro-inflammatory cytokines, and oxidative stress molecules.

- These cross into circulation, reach the brain, and increase the risk of mood disorders.

- **Example:** Elevated LPS has been observed in patients with major depressive disorder (Maes et al., 2012, *Acta Psychiatrica Scandinavica*).

CASE STUDIES: MICROBES AT WORK

CASE STUDY 1: SARAH, THE SHIFT WORKER

Sarah worked rotating night shifts at a hospital, relying on vending machines for meals such as sandwiches, chips, and soda. She had chronic anxiety and did not sleep much during the day. Tests showed disrupted gut microbial diversity and elevated inflammation. After reverting to a more structured meal pattern (high fiber foods during her "daytime," no late-night snacking), her gut-brain signaling normalized, and her anxiety decreased.

CASE STUDY 2: MIGUEL THE ATHLETE

Miguel, a long-distance runner, occasionally forgot to eat and generally relied on energy drinks loaded with simple sugars. Despite being in excellent physical health, he had mood swings and experienced post-race "crashes." A sports nutritionist added fermented foods (kefir, kimchi), resistant starch (green bananas, oats), and more protein to his diet, all of which took little time to incorporate. Within weeks, his recovery improved and his mood stabilized; clearly, athletes need to feed their microbiomes consistently.

CASE STUDY 3: PRIYA THE OVERLOADED PARENT

Priya drank coffee until noon and ate leftovers from her kids at night. She was always bloated, fatigued, and irritable; she felt "broken." Her stool test revealed low levels of Lactobacillus and Bifidobacterium strains. A registered dietitian advised her to eat probiotic yogurt as well as do a daily fiber-based meal, and drink herbal tea in the evening to wind down. Within months, her digestive regime and her sense of calm returned.

SCIENCE SPOTLIGHT: PSYCHOBIOTICS

The term **psychobiotics** refers to probiotics and prebiotics that specifically target mental health.

- **Bifidobacterium longum 1714**: shown to reduce stress and improve memory (Allen et al., 2016, *Translational Psychiatry*).

- **Lactobacillus rhamnosus JB-1**: reduces anxiety-like behavior in animal studies by modulating GABA receptors.

- **Galactooligosaccharides (GOS)**: prebiotic fibers that increase beneficial bacteria and lower cortisol levels in humans.

PRACTICAL ACTION STEPS: FEEDING THE MOOD MOLECULES

1. Start with Fiber First

- Goal: 25–35g fiber/day.

- Sources: lentils, beans, oats, flaxseed, leafy greens.

- Why: fuels microbial fermentation $\rightarrow$ SCFA production $\rightarrow$ serotonin boost.

2. Protein Anchors

- Include complete proteins at every meal (eggs, fish, chicken, tofu).

- Provides amino acids (tryptophan, tyrosine) for serotonin + dopamine synthesis.

3. Fermented Foods Daily

- Yogurt, kefir, kimchi, sauerkraut, miso.

- Introduces live microbes that support GABA and serotonin pathways.

- **Science note:** A 2021 *Cell* study showed fermented foods increase microbial diversity within 10 weeks.

4. Polyphenol Boosters

- Dark berries, cocoa, green tea, and extra virgin olive oil.

- Feed specific bacteria that produce anti-inflammatory metabolites.

- Linked with reduced depression and anxiety symptoms.

5. Circadian Consistency

- Eat meals at consistent times to entrain both microbiome rhythms and hormone rhythms.

- Avoid late-night eating to prevent microbial dysbiosis and cortisol spikes.

6. Stress & Movement Synergy

- Stress hormones reshape microbial balance. Practices like yoga, deep breathing, and walks improve vagal tone, calming both gut and brain.

- Exercise itself reshapes microbiome diversity (Clarke et al., 2014, *Gut*).

Quick-Reference Box: Feeding Your Mood Molecules

Do:

- Prioritize high-fiber, whole-food meals.

- Include protein anchors in every meal.

- Add fermented foods daily.

- Drink polyphenol-rich beverages (green tea, coffee in moderation).

- Stick to regular meal timing.

Avoid:

- Late-night eating.

- Artificial sweeteners (linked to microbiome disruption).

- Over-reliance on ultra-processed snacks.

- Chronic stress without recovery practices.

Your gut is not a silent passenger. It is a living chemical factory influencing your mood. When your microbiome is thriving, it produces the mood molecules that make you feel a sense of resilience, calm, and vitality. When your microbiome you aren't thriving, that neuroscience will be on the side of stress, inflammation, and hopelessness.

The good news? Your microbiome, unlike your genetics, is incredibly malleable. With every meal you eat, your daily rhythms, your daily rituals, you are either providing your microbial pharmacists the toolkit they need to compound healing molecules-or you're leaving them empty-handed.

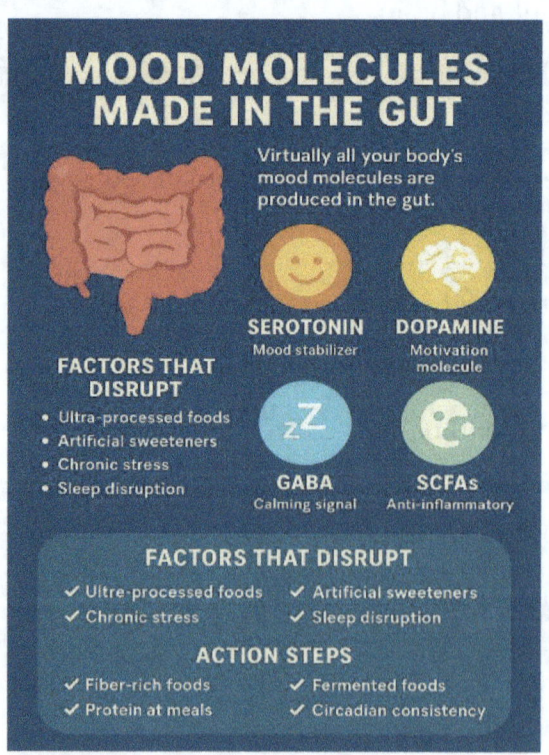

PART 4: THE BROKEN MICROBIOME → MODERN DISRUPTORS

OPENING NARRATIVE: A LIFE OUT OF SYNC

Maria's story continues. After years of teaching late, grading until midnight, living off granola bars and Diet Coke, her gut wasn't just "off" - it was broken. Bloated during afternoon class, sleepless at night, anxiety filled her mornings. When she finally got tested, her microbiome was dominated by Bacteroides and nearly devoid of Bifidobacteria—the kind of imbalance that doctors increasingly recognize as a red flag for anxiety, depression, and metabolic struggles.

Maria's story is not unique. Millions of people walk around with a microbiome that has been silently sabotaged - not only for the use of antibiotics, but also for the daily lifestyle disruptors we have come to accept as normal.

This section is about exposing those lifestyle disruptors - the silent assassins of microbial tranquility.

1. PROCESSED FOODS: FUELING THE WRONG COLONIES

Ultra-processed foods (UPFs) don't just hijack our dopamine circuits (as we explored in Chapter 4)—they also hijack our gut.

- **Low-fiber profiles**: The average Western diet provides <15 g of fiber daily. The microbiome thrives on **prebiotic fibers** (from beans, oats, and vegetables). Without them, beneficial species like *Akkermansia muciniphila* starve.

- **Additives & emulsifiers**: Studies in *Nature* (2015, Chassaing et al.) found that emulsifiers such as polysorbate-80 disrupt gut lining integrity, thinning the mucus layer and promoting leaky gut.

- **Artificial sweeteners**: Research in *Cell* (2014, Suez et al.) revealed that non-nutritive sweeteners (aspartame, sucralose, saccharin) altered glucose tolerance *via microbiome disruption.*

Translation for the reader: Your microbiome is not just what you feed—it's what you starve. Every time you swap fiber-rich foods for ultra-processed snacks, you're selecting for inflammatory bacteria.

2. ANTIBIOTICS & OVER-STERILIZATION

We live in an era of antibacterial soaps, sanitizers, and prescriptions. While lifesaving in acute cases, **antibiotics flatten microbial diversity**.

- A *Nature Reviews Microbiology* (2016) review showed that a single antibiotic course can shift the microbiome for **up to a year**.

- Overuse in childhood is strongly linked to asthma, allergies, and obesity later in life (Bokulich et al., *Cell Host & Microbe*, 2016).

- Sanitizer culture compounds the problem, leaving children's immune systems undertrained and skewed toward hypersensitivity.

Practical Insight: We traded resilience for sterility. Instead of microbial training camps, we built bubble-wrapped ecosystems.

3. CHRONIC STRESS & CORTISOL STORMS

Stress doesn't just live in the mind—it reshapes the microbiome.

- Chronic cortisol surges thin the gut lining, reduce microbial diversity, and allow opportunistic species to thrive.

- Animal studies (Bailey et al., *Brain, Behavior, and Immunity*, 2011) showed that stress reduced levels of *Lactobacillus*, directly altering mood-linked metabolites.

- In humans, work stress correlates with increased IBS symptoms and measurable dysbiosis.

Translation for the reader: The "stress microbiome" looks different under the microscope—it's a less diverse, more inflammatory community that amplifies anxiety.

4. CIRCADIAN MISALIGNMENT (SHIFT WORK, SCREENS, LATE NIGHTS)

The microbiome doesn't run on its own—it follows the **circadian clock**. When we eat, sleep, and are exposed to light at odd times, microbes lose their rhythm.

- *Cell* (2014, Thaiss et al.) showed that jet lag causes microbial shifts that mimic obesity and metabolic syndrome.

- In mice, disrupting light-dark cycles triggered dysbiosis that worsened glucose control.

- Shift workers show a higher risk for obesity, diabetes, and depression—microbiome disruption is now considered one pathway.

Practical Takeaway: When your body clock is broken, your microbiome becomes jet-lagged too.

5. ENVIRONMENTAL TOXINS & CHEMICALS

- **Pesticides**: Glyphosate (Roundup) inhibits the shikimate pathway—deadly to microbes, not just weeds. Some studies link it to reduced beneficial bacterial counts.

- **Heavy metals**: Mercury and lead accumulate and alter gut composition.

- **Plastics (BPA, phthalates)**: These endocrine disruptors also shift microbial metabolism, linking to obesity and hormonal imbalances.

NARRATIVE MINI-STORIES: THE FACES OF A BROKEN MICROBIOME

- **Shift Worker**: Jamal, a nurse, rotates between nights and days. After years, his weight creeps up, mood swings intensify, and his digestion never feels stable. His microbiome sequencing? A mismatch between microbial activity and meal timing.

- **High-Stress Parent**: Sara juggles three kids and a demanding job. She relies on caffeine by day, wine by night. Stress hormones flatten her *Lactobacillus* levels, fueling anxiety and IBS.

- **Athlete**: Marcus trains hard but fuels with processed powders and late-night meals. Despite fitness, he struggles with inflammation and fatigue—his microbiome reveals low diversity.

Each of them feels like their body is betraying them. In reality, it's modern living creating microbial chaos.

ACTION PRIMER: FIRST STEPS TOWARD REPAIR

Before diving into the "Joy Prescription for the Microbiome" in later parts, here's a **starter repair kit**:

1. **Feed the right bacteria daily.**
   Aim for 25–30 g of fiber (beans, oats, chia, vegetables).

2. **Respect microbial rhythms.**
   Anchor meals during daylight hours; finish eating 2–3 hours before bed.

3. **Cut disruptors.**
   Swap sodas/artificial sweeteners with sparkling water or tea.

4. **Stress reset ritual.**
   Even 10 minutes of deep breathing or walking outdoors lowers cortisol and supports microbial stability.

5. **Diversity = resilience.**
   Rotate your plant foods—research suggests 30 different plants per week is a sweet spot (*American Gut Project*).

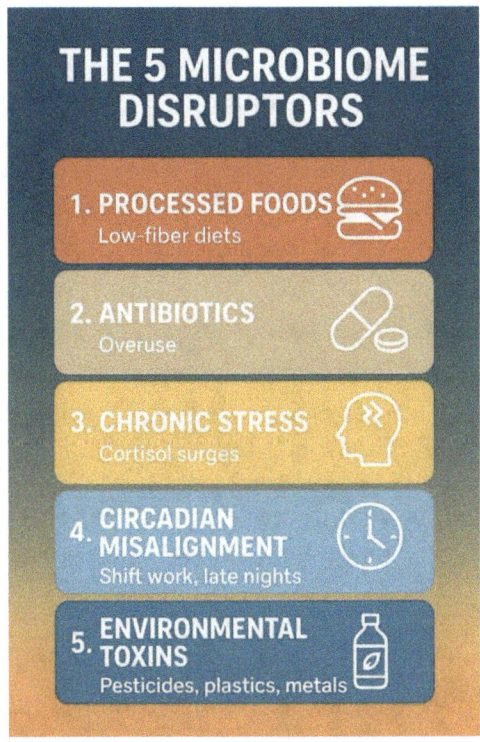

The microbiome is not broken by one deliberate choice—it is broken by a culture. Processed foods, antibiotics, stress, circadian disturbance, and toxins all add up. But because the gut regenerates quickly (microbes can double in 20 minutes), tools for repair are always available. The same system that breaks you down can build you back up, stronger—if you feed it right, time it right, and protect it from disruptors.

PART 5: HEALING THE GUT GARDEN (THE DIET CONNECTION: FEEDING OR STARVING YOUR MICROBIOME)

THE GARDEN THAT WITHERS OR THRIVES

Think of your gut as a beautifully maintained garden. One day, the garden is full of color: bright berries (polyphenols), rich legumes (fiber), flavorful greens (prebiotics). The soil is healthy and full of trillions of tiny gardeners — bacteria, yeasts, and archaea — busy fertilizing, weeding, and maintaining balance. On this day, you are feeling lighter, more focused, and calmer.

Now, think of what happens to that garden if we leave it alone. We do not feed it compost and sunshine, but instead pour synthetic fertilizers, bleach, and asphalt. The soil compacts, the roots suffocate, and the biodiversity decreases. This is what happens when you flood your microbiome with ultra-processed foods (UPFs). We don't just starve our inner garden, we punish it. Instead of resilience, we cultivate fragility.

And the science is becoming clearer: when the gut garden dies, our mood declines, our energy crashes, and our long-term health wanes.

This section will help you identify the foods that starve your microbes, those that nourish them, and how to start healing — one meal at a time.

THE PROBLEM: UPFS AS WEED-KILLERS FOR YOUR MICROBIOME

Modern ultra-processed foods aren't just empty calories. They're **microbial disruptors** — actively eroding diversity in the gut.

- **Low Fiber, High Sugar:** The microbiome feeds primarily on **prebiotic fibers**. UPFs strip these out, leaving microbes starving. What remains? Sugars that feed only a few opportunistic strains (like *Candida* yeasts or certain *Clostridia*). Diversity collapses.

- **Additives and Emulsifiers:** Chemicals designed to make food last longer or creamier (like polysorbate-80 or carboxymethylcellulose) have been shown to thin the gut lining, promoting inflammation and microbial imbalance (Chassaing et al., *Nature*, 2015).

- **Artificial Sweeteners:** Sucralose, aspartame, and saccharin don't just taste sweet. They alter the microbiome in ways that disrupt glucose regulation (*Suez et al., Nature*, 2014).

Study Spotlight: *Sánchez-Villegas et al. Public Health Nutrition*, 2012, showed that people consuming the highest amount of UPFs had a significantly greater risk of depression. The link? Microbial depletion driving systemic inflammation and impaired neurotransmitter production.

THE ANTIDOTE: WHOLE FOODS AS GARDEN FERTILIZERS

The great news is this: the gut responds fast. Within **days of dietary change**, microbial diversity can bloom. Think of it like watering a parched plant — it lifts its head almost immediately.

PREBIOTICS: THE FIBER YOUR GUT CRAVES

- Found in beans, lentils, oats, asparagus, garlic, onions, and bananas.

- Feed beneficial bacteria like *Bifidobacteria* and *Akkermansia*, which produce **short-chain fatty acids (SCFAs)** like butyrate — molecules that reduce inflammation and nourish the gut lining.

Science Check: Butyrate not only repairs the gut but also signals directly to the brain via the vagus nerve, improving mood regulation (*Stilling et al., Front Behav Neurosci*, 2016).

POLYPHENOLS: THE PLANT CHEMICALS THAT SPARK DIVERSITY

- Found in blueberries, dark chocolate, green tea, olive oil, and red grapes.

- Act as **antioxidants** but also feed select microbes that thrive on these compounds, enhancing diversity.

Blue Zone Evidence: In Mediterranean diets, high intake of polyphenol-rich foods correlates with lower rates of depression and higher longevity (*Jacka et al.*, BMC *Medicine*, 2017).

FERMENTED FOODS: REINTRODUCING FRIENDLY GARDENERS

- Yogurt, kefir, sauerkraut, kimchi, miso.

- Deliver **live cultures** (lactobacilli, bifidobacteria) that temporarily reseed the gut.

Study Spotlight: A randomized trial at Stanford (Wastyk et al., *Cell*, 2021) showed that adding fermented foods increased microbiome diversity and decreased markers of inflammation in just 10 weeks.

RESISTANT STARCHES: THE HIDDEN SUPERFUEL

- Cooked and cooled potatoes, green bananas, legumes, oats.

- These starches resist digestion in the small intestine, traveling to the colon where they act like fertilizer for microbes.

- Promote satiety and stabilize blood sugar, cutting off the spikes that trigger mood crashes.

THE HEALING DIET: BUILDING THE MICROBIOME PLATE

Instead of seeing gut health as restrictive, imagine it as **composing a plate that feels like abundance.**

- ½ plate: colorful vegetables + fiber-rich plants (prebiotics).

- ¼ plate: protein (supports satiety and neurotransmitter production).

- ¼ plate: complex carbs (especially resistant starches).

- Side: fermented food (small daily dose).

- Splash: polyphenol booster (olive oil drizzle, handful of berries, or dark chocolate square).

This is **not** about chasing perfection. It's about **daily nourishment and diversity** — because the microbiome thrives on variety.

CASE STORY: MARIA'S GARDEN COMEBACK

Remember Maria, the teacher from Chapter 4? She once lived on protein bars and vending-machine snacks. She came to her doctor not just exhausted, but also describing "brain fog" and "low moods."

Her shift wasn't dramatic. She didn't "go Paleo" overnight or take probiotics in capsules. Instead, she followed one rule: **"Add one fiber food a day."**

Day 1: oats with banana.

Day 2: lentil soup.

Day 3: roasted chickpeas.

Within weeks, Maria reported:

- Clearer mornings.

- Reduced evening cravings.

- More stable moods.

Her microbiome wasn't "healed" instantly — but her inner garden had received water, light, and seeds. And it responded.

ACTION STEP BOX: HEAL YOUR GUT GARDEN

Start Today: Add 1 New Fiber Food Per Day

- Oats for breakfast.

- Beans or lentils at lunch.

- A handful of raspberries or walnuts as a snack.

Within 2 weeks → Notice digestion ease and fewer cravings.

Within 1 month → Energy and mood stability improve.

Long term → Resilient microbiome, lower disease risk, higher joy.

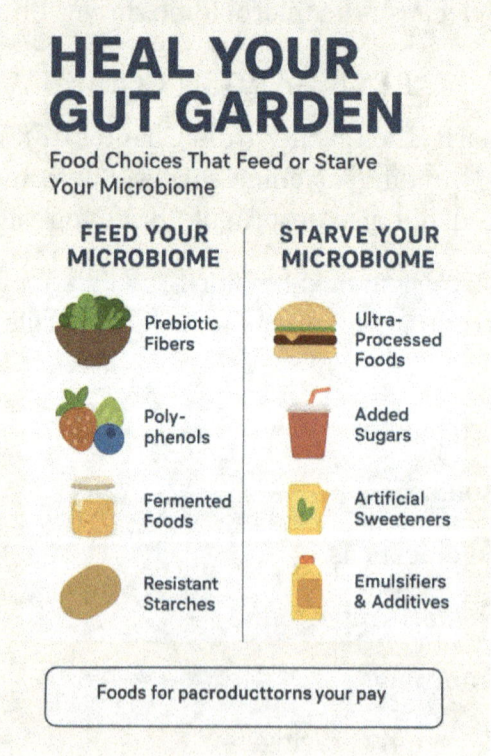

HEAL YOUR GUT GARDEN

Food Choices That Feed or Starve Your Microbiome

FEED YOUR MICROBIOME	STARVE YOUR MICROBIOME
Prebiotic Fibers	Ultra-Processed Foods
Poly-phenols	Added Sugars
Fermented Foods	Artificial Sweeteners
Resistant Starches	Emulsifiers & Additives

Foods for pacroducttorns your pay

Restoring gut health is not a magical supplement regimen. It is about eating the foods that feed your inner ecosystem and not starving it. The microbiome is adaptable, resilient, and fully willing to grow back if you just give it the chance.

The takeaway: Processed foods cause disease. Whole foods prescribe health.

And the easiest prescription of them all? Fiber + diversity + joy.

What you are placing on your plate today is directing your cravings, mood, and resilience for tomorrow. The soil is ready. The garden can grow again.

PART 6 — PROBIOTICS, PREBIOTICS, PSYCHOBIOTICS

THE LIVING PHARMACY INSIDE YOU

Imagine a farmer's market alive and vibrating with activity—rows of stalls filled with vibrant produce—deep-purple eggplants, ruby-red beets, golden squash. The air smells alive: fermented sauerkraut tangling with sourdough bread and earthy herbs. This is not just food—it is a pharmacy for the gut, a living network of compounds and microbes constructed to heal, recalibrate, and signal.

Now imagine the opposite. A sterile aisle in a grocery store with products wrapped up, sealed up, preserved-up—all engineered to last months rather than nourish minutes. A desolate foodscape devoid of microbes, devoid of fibers, devoid of the very signals your gut requires to keep the brain balanced.

Here lies the great divide: the difference between a living gut garden and a desert. And the bridge between the two? Probiotics, prebiotics, and psychobiotics—the new science of food-as-signal for the gut-brain axis.

THE GUT-BRAIN PHARMACY EXPLAINED

For decades, medicine treated mood and digestion as separate issues. Depression—serotonin in the brain. IBS—motility in the gut. Now we know the two are inextricably linked. The gut microbiome acts as a bioactive pharmacy producing neurotransmitters, metabolites, and immune signals that affect the ways you think, feel, and even dream!

PROBIOTICS: THE LIVING ALLIES

- Probiotics are live bacteria that, when ingested in adequate amounts, confer measurable health benefits.

- Not all probiotics are equal. Strain specificity matters.

- For example, *Lactobacillus helveticus* and *Bifidobacterium longum*—tested in a randomized controlled trial—were shown to reduce anxiety and depressive symptoms in healthy adults (Messaoudi et al., *Br J Nutr*, 2011). Participants reported calmer moods, and cortisol levels dropped measurably.

- These microbes don't just colonize; they communicate, sending metabolites and short-chain fatty acids (SCFAs) like butyrate into circulation, directly influencing brain chemistry.

PREBIOTICS: THE FERTILIZER

- Prebiotics are fibers and compounds that feed your gut bacteria—essentially **soil nutrients for the microbial garden**.

- Common examples: inulin (from chicory root), galacto-oligosaccharides (GOS, found in beans and lentils), resistant starches (in cooled potatoes, oats, and green bananas).

- They increase the production of SCFAs, which reduce systemic inflammation and modulate stress responses.

- A 2015 trial (Schmidt et al., *Psychopharmacology*) found that GOS prebiotics reduced the cortisol awakening response—a key marker of stress physiology. Translation: feeding your microbes helps calm your nervous system.

PSYCHOBIOTICS: THE NEXT FRONTIER

- Coined less than a decade ago, **psychobiotics** are specific probiotics or prebiotics that directly impact mood and cognitive function.

- This includes strains like *Lactobacillus rhamnosus* (shown to modulate GABA receptors in the brain and reduce anxiety in rodent studies).

- Human studies are growing: targeted combinations of psychobiotics are now being tested for depression, PTSD, and even Alzheimer's prevention.

- What makes them different? They don't just improve digestion—they **change the chemical signals your gut sends to your brain**.

FERMENTED FOODS: THE ANCESTRAL PSYCHOBIOTICS

Long before the term "psychobiotic" was coined, cultures worldwide leaned on fermentation. From Korean kimchi to Ethiopian injera, from kefir in the Caucasus to Japanese miso, fermented foods were humanity's way of both preserving nutrition and cultivating microbial diversity.

Today, science is validating what tradition always knew.

- A 2021 Stanford study (*Cell*) led by Wastyk et al. showed that eating **fermented foods daily increased microbial diversity and reduced markers of inflammation** in healthy adults.

- Sauerkraut, yogurt, kombucha, kefir—they're not just culinary add-ons, but microbial delivery systems that reseed the gut with beneficial organisms.

- Compare this with ultra-processed foods (UPFs), which are sterile and laden with preservatives designed to **kill microbes, not feed them.**

CASE STUDIES: THE HUMAN SIDE

CASE 1: SARAH, THE OVERWHELMED PARENT

Sarah lived on protein bars, coffee, and takeout dinners. Always tired, mood swinging, digestion sluggish. When she added one daily fermented food (kefir smoothie in the morning) and rotated fiber foods weekly (beans one week, oats the next), within a month she noticed fewer sugar crashes, more stable moods, and even lighter mornings—less brain fog.

CASE 2: MARCO, THE STRESSED ATHLETE

Training twice a day, Marco relied heavily on protein powders and energy gels. His gut was wrecked—bloating, stress diarrhea, constant anxiety. A sports dietitian introduced resistant starches (cooked-cooled rice and potatoes) and a probiotic strain with documented stress benefits (B. *longum* 1714). Not only did digestion improve, but Marco reported calmer pre-competition nerves.

THE SCIENCE DEEP DIVE

- **SCFAs (Short-Chain Fatty Acids):** Produced when microbes ferment fiber. Butyrate, propionate, acetate → anti-inflammatory, protect the blood-brain barrier, enhance neuroplasticity.

- **Neurotransmitters:** 90% of serotonin is made in the gut. Dopamine precursors are heavily influenced by microbial metabolism of amino acids.

- **The Vagus Nerve:** Microbes stimulate the vagus nerve, sending "safety" signals to the brain. Yogurt containing L. *rhamnosus* has been shown in rodents to reduce stress responses via vagal pathways.

- **HPA Axis Modulation:** Probiotics can blunt stress hormone spikes, balancing cortisol rhythms.

- **Diversity = Resilience:** Studies on Blue Zones show diverse, fiber-rich, fermented diets support microbial richness, which correlates with longevity and lower rates of depression and cognitive decline.

THE ACTION PLAN: REBUILDING YOUR MICROBIAL SYMPHONY

STEP 1: DAILY PROBIOTIC FOOD

- Choose one fermented food per day: kefir, sauerkraut, miso, kimchi, kombucha.

- Rotate to expand microbial exposure.

STEP 2: FIBER ROTATION

- Add **one new fiber food daily**: beans, lentils, oats, resistant starches.

- Aim for 30+ plant-based fibers per week (the "diversity count").

STEP 3: TARGETED PSYCHOBIOTICS (OPTIONAL)

- If struggling with anxiety, sleep, or mood, consider a tested strain supplement (consult medical provider).

- Look for strains with published research (L. *helveticus* R0052, B. *longum* R0175).

STEP 4: GUT-FRIENDLY RITUALS

- Eat slowly to activate vagus nerve signaling.

- Avoid artificial sweeteners (aspartame, sucralose), which disrupt microbiota (Suez et al., *Nature*, 2014).

- Pair protein + fiber at each meal to stabilize blood sugar and feed microbes.

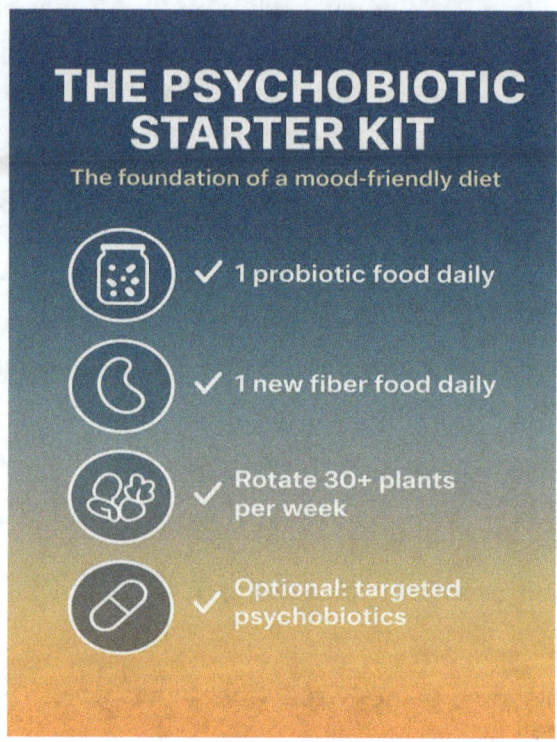

THE PSYCHOBIOTIC STARTER KIT

The foundation of a mood-friendly diet

- ✓ 1 probiotic food daily
- ✓ 1 new fiber food daily
- ✓ Rotate 30+ plants per week
- ✓ Optional: targeted psychobiotics

Quick-Reference Box — The Psychobiotic Starter Kit

- 1 probiotic food daily (kefir, miso, kimchi, sauerkraut).

- 1 new fiber food daily (beans, oats, resistant starch).

- Rotate 30+ plants per week.

- Optional: targeted psychobiotic strains.

- Protect vagus nerve: slow eating, mindful meals.

This is where food becomes medicine, not by depriving, but by activating an army of living allies.

When you're feeding microbes, you're feeding mood molecules. When you seed a gut garden, you're restoring brain chemistry.

This is not just a dietary adjustment—it's a reprogramming of the gut-brain symphony.

PART 7 — THE MOOD-FOOD FEEDBACK LOOP

THE LOOP YOU DON'T SEE

Maria sat in her car staring at the steering wheel.

She had just dropped her students off for recess; meanwhile, she should have walked back inside to prepare lesson plans, but instead she ripped into the "emergency" chocolate stash she kept in her glove compartment.

The first bite of chocolate delivered waves of calmness; relief even.

By the second, her shoulders relaxed.

By the third, her heart sank — she was feeling relief now, but she knew what came next: the foggy crash, the guilt, and the hunger would return, but most likely even stronger.

Maria wasn't broken.

She was simply stuck in a cycle. A cycle that millions of people are stuck in each day.

Low mood leads to cravings for quick-fix junk food → the junk food disrupts the gut microbiome, which creates inflammation in the body → now with altered biology, you slip deeper into low mood → the low mood leads you to crave more junk food.

This is not a weakness.

This is just biology going round and round in circles.

And the reality is, the cycle can be broken.

THE SCIENCE OF THE MOOD–FOOD LOOP

1. Depression Feeds Cravings

When mood dips, brain chemistry shifts:

- **Dopamine deficiency** → the brain seeks quick spikes (sugar, refined carbs, fried foods).

- **Serotonin drops** → cravings for comfort foods rise, because carbohydrate-rich foods briefly increase serotonin activity.

- **Cortisol surges** under stress → appetite is dysregulated, pushing us toward calorie-dense foods.

Study Spotlight:

A 2017 study in *Scientific Reports* (Knüppel et al.) found that people consuming the highest levels of added sugars had a **23% higher risk of developing depression** over five years. The more sugar, the stronger the cravings, the deeper the mood spirals.

2. Cravings Worsen the Microbiome

Ultra-processed foods (UPFs) don't just fill the stomach; they **starve the gut garden**:

- Sugar feeds pathogenic bacteria and fungi (like *Candida*), outcompeting beneficial microbes.

- Emulsifiers and additives thin the gut lining → inflammation signals reach the brain.

- Lack of fiber means no fuel for microbes that produce **butyrate**, the short-chain fatty acid linked to reduced inflammation and improved mental resilience.

Study Spotlight:

A 2015 *Nature* paper (Suez et al.) showed artificial sweeteners altered gut microbiota and impaired glucose tolerance, illustrating how "fake sugar" rewires not just metabolism but mood-regulating microbes.

3. Microbiome Disruption Deepens Low Mood

When the gut suffers, so does the brain:

- **Less serotonin:** 90% of serotonin is produced in the gut—a starved microbiome = reduced serotonin signaling.

- **Leaky gut → systemic inflammation:** inflammatory cytokines cross into the brain, suppressing mood circuits.

- **Reduced GABA:** certain probiotic strains (e.g., *Lactobacillus rhamnosus*) stimulate calming GABA. Without them, anxiety spikes.

Study Spotlight:

Jacka et al. (2017, *BMC Medicine*) found that switching to a Mediterranean diet high in fiber, legumes, and fish reduced depressive symptoms significantly in just 12 weeks compared to a control group.

The Loop Visualized

1. **Low Mood** → Stress hormones spike.

2. **Cravings** → Reach for sugar, fried foods, UPFs.

3. **Gut Damage** → Microbial imbalance + inflammation.

4. **Brain Impact** → Lower serotonin, dopamine disruption.

5. **Worse Mood** → Loop resets, cravings intensify.

This isn't psychology alone. It's **biopsychology**: the gut-brain-microbiome loop in real time.

NARRATIVE DEEP DIVE: MARIA'S LOOP

Maria's day followed a pattern she couldn't explain until she saw it mapped:

- **Morning:** Skipped breakfast → caffeine + leftover pastry on the way to school.

- **Afternoon:** Energy dip → granola bar, quick sugar lift, then a slump.

- **Evening:** "I deserve it" dinner → fast food, fries, soda.

- **Night:** Anxiety, cravings → chocolate binge, restless sleep.

Each day, the loop reinforced itself. She wasn't just eating poorly — she was **being programmed by her biology**.

When Maria shifted to a **savory protein breakfast** (eggs + spinach + beans), she noticed the first crack in the loop. Cravings hit later. Afternoon fog lightened. By week three, her evening "emergency stash" had dust on it.

BREAKING THE MOOD–FOOD FEEDBACK LOOP

Step 1: Anchor the Morning

- Eat within 1–2 hours of waking.

- Prioritize **protein (20–30g) + fiber**.

- Why? Stabilizes dopamine and serotonin precursors early, preventing 10 AM sugar dives.

Research: A 2013 study in *Obesity* showed that high-protein breakfasts reduced evening cravings in overweight women.

Step 2: Reframe Cravings as Signals

- Instead of judging cravings as weakness → interpret them as **feedback from your microbiome and hormones**.

- Ask: "Am I truly hungry, or am I seeking a dopamine hit?"

Step 3: Insert a Gut-Healing Snack

- Replace candy/granola bars with fermented or fiber-rich foods:
  - Kefir, kimchi, miso.
  - An apple + handful of almonds.
  - Roasted chickpeas.

- These stabilize microbes and smooth mood fluctuations.

Step 4: The Evening Savory Shield

- End the day with a **balanced dinner**: lean protein + healthy fats + fiber (not refined carbs).

- Why? Keeps ghrelin low, prevents the 10 PM craving wall.

Step 5: Sleep + Sunlight

- Morning light exposure → anchors circadian rhythm.

- 7–9 hrs quality sleep → lowers cortisol and resets appetite hormones.

Research: Short sleep raises ghrelin and lowers leptin, driving cravings (Taheri et al., PLoS Med, 2004).

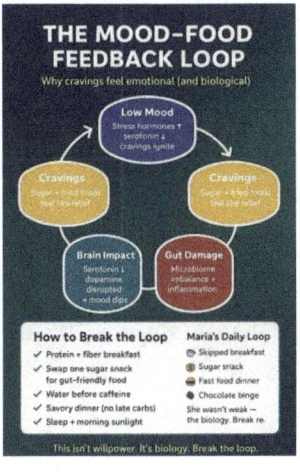

ACTION STEP BOX

The Mood–Food Reset (Day One Starter):

- Start the day with a savory protein + fiber breakfast.

- Replace one "quick sugar snack" with a gut-friendly option.

- Drink water before caffeine to blunt cortisol spike.

- Eat dinner 2–3 hours before bed, balanced and savory.

- Prioritize one "joy practice" (gratitude, walk, journaling) instead of an evening snack.

Breaking the cycle isn't about discipline. It's about re-engineering the signal flow from your gut to your brain, to your plate.

Imagine:

Waking up balanced instead of jangled.

Having lunch without the redux of craving dessert in an hour.

Wrapping up the day fulfilled instead of ashamed.

This isn't fantasy. It's what can happen when you take control of your feedback loop and reprogram it.

In the next sections of Chapter 6, we bring all of this together: how to build a daily microbiome rhythm so that joy, clarity, and resilience become your new defaults.

THE JOYFUL GUT: BLUE ZONE LESSONS

A TABLE IN OKINAWA

The sun rises over Okinawa, and a few of the older women with wide-brimmed hats, kneeling, pulling purple sweet potatoes from the soil. At mid-morning, the village is full of clinking bowls and the light chatter of neighbors.

The table fills with simple, colorful foods: a soup of miso, fermented tofu, stir-fried greens, and a few dishes of pickled vegetables. There is no need to rush. They sit together, laugh together, eat slowly, and when they are satisfied, they all stop.

No calorie counting. No meal tracking apps. No guilt.

And yet - Okinawa has one of the highest concentrations of centenarians in the world. Lives to age 100 and not just alive, but thriving.

This is not by chance.

This is a design.

WHAT BLUE ZONES TEACH US

Dan Buettner and his team identified **five regions of extraordinary longevity**, known as the *Blue Zones*:

- Okinawa, Japan
- Sardinia, Italy
- Nicoya, Costa Rica
- Ikaria, Greece
- Loma Linda, California (Seventh-day Adventist community)

On the surface, these places couldn't be more different: island villages, mountain towns, small farming regions, and one modern American city.

But look deeper, and patterns emerge — not just in *what* they eat, but *how*.

THE MICROBIOME SIGNATURE OF LONGEVITY

Science is catching up with cultural wisdom.

1. Microbial Diversity

- Populations in Blue Zones show **higher microbial diversity** than typical Western populations.

- More species = more resilience. Diversity protects against inflammation, infection, and mood disorders.

Study Spotlight:

Research in *Nature* (2016) revealed that centenarians had **richer gut microbiota and more unique strains** capable of producing anti-inflammatory compounds.

2. Short-Chain Fatty Acids (SCFAs)

- Blue Zone diets are naturally high in **fiber**: beans, lentils, whole grains, and vegetables.

- Fiber → fermented by microbes → SCFAs like butyrate, acetate, propionate.

- SCFAs reduce systemic inflammation, strengthen the gut barrier, and influence brain health.

Study Spotlight:

A 2020 paper in *Cell* showed SCFAs directly stimulate the vagus nerve, improving mood and stress resilience.

3. Fermented Foods = Microbial Allies

Every Blue Zone has its version of fermented foods:

- Okinawa: miso, tofu, pickled daikon.

- Sardinia: sourdough bread, sheep's milk cheese.

- Ikaria: homemade wine, goat yogurt.

- Nicoya: corn tortillas (nixtamalization), beans.

- Loma Linda: less fermentation, but nuts and plant-based staples sustain gut richness.

Study Spotlight:

Wastyk et al. (*Cell*, 2021) showed that increasing fermented food intake for just 10 weeks boosted microbial diversity and lowered inflammation markers.

CULTURAL WISDOM BEYOND FOOD

The microbiome doesn't only respond to what's on the plate, but also to *how life is lived around it.*

1. Shared Meals = Parasympathetic Activation

In every Blue Zone, eating is communal.

- Talking, laughing, and slowing down → activates the **vagus nerve**.
- This shifts the body into **rest-and-digest mode**, improving nutrient absorption and lowering stress hormones.

2. Eating Slowly = Better Digestion

Meals are unhurried, often stretching over an hour. Chewing well allows more satiety hormones (like **CCK and GLP-1**) to be released, preventing overeating.

3. Purpose and Rhythm

- In Okinawa, the concept of **"ikigai"** (reason for living) is as important as miso soup.
- In Sardinia, wine is sipped with friends at dusk — not chugged from stress.
- In Ikaria, meals are tied to festivals, traditions, and joy.

NARRATIVE: MARIA'S BLUE ZONE EXPERIMENT

At home, in her suburban kitchen, Maria gazed down at the jar of miso paste she purchased after reading about Okinawa. It seemed strange. It felt daunting. But she scooped a spoonful into some hot water, added some tofu and scallions, and sat down at the table instead of standing at the counter.

For the first time in years, she was not scrolling on her phone while she ate. She let the warmth linger, savoring each bite. The meal lasted ten minutes longer than usual. She did not feel heavy. She did not feel guilty.

She felt steady.

That night, she slept more deeply. The next morning, she noticed her cravings were not as sharp. A small shift, but a big one: she took that step on the path of the Joyful Gut.

BLUE ZONE PILLARS FOR THE JOYFUL GUT

Pillar 1: Plant-Forward Eating

- Beans and legumes are at the center of meals.
- Vegetables daily, seasonal, and local.
- Whole grains over refined.

Pillar 2: Fermented Staples

- Add miso soup, kefir, kimchi, sauerkraut, sourdough, or yogurt.
- Aim for one fermented food daily.

Pillar 3: Minimal Processing

- Rarely any packaged snacks, refined oils, or additives.
- Foods look like they did in nature.

Pillar 4: Slow, Shared Meals

- No screens.

- Sit with others when possible.

- Use conversation as a digestive medicine.

Pillar 5: Rhythm Over Restriction

- Eating windows aligned with daylight.

- No rigid counting. Instead: natural pauses, smaller portions, mindfulness.

Science + Longevity Connection

- **Inflammation:** Blue Zone diets reduce inflammatory biomarkers (CRP, IL-6).

- **Mood:** Fiber + fermented foods improve serotonin and dopamine pathways.

- **Longevity:** Microbial richness is linked with slower biological aging.

Meta-Analysis: 2021 review (*Nutrients*) found adherence to Mediterranean-like, plant-forward diets correlated with reduced depression risk and improved life satisfaction.

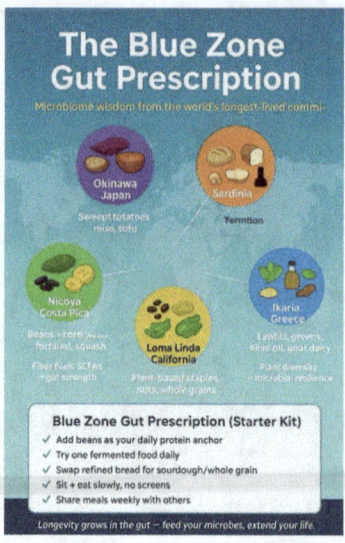

The Blue Zone Gut Prescription

Microbiome wisdom from the world's longest-lived communities

Okinawa Japan
Sweet potatoes, miso, tofu

Sardinia
Fermentation

Nicoya Costa Rica
Beans + corn (nixtamalized), squash
Fiber feeds SCFAs, gut strength

Loma Linda California
Plant-based staples, nuts, whole grains

Ikaria Greece
Lentils, greens, olive oil, goat dairy
Plant diversity = microbial resilience

Blue Zone Gut Prescription (Starter Kit)
✓ Add beans as your daily protein anchor
✓ Try one fermented food daily
✓ Swap refined bread for sourdough/whole grain
✓ Sit + eat slowly, no screens
✓ Share meals weekly with others

Longevity grows in the gut — feed your microbes, extend your life.

ACTION STEP BOX: THE JOYFUL GUT STARTER

Adopt 1 Blue Zone Practice Weekly:

- Add beans (black beans, lentils, chickpeas) as your protein anchor.

- Try fermented food daily (miso soup, sauerkraut, kefir, kimchi).

- Replace refined bread with sourdough or whole grain.

- Sit at the table, no screens, chew slowly.

- Share one meal per week with friends or family.

The Blue Zones are not strange lands — they are laboratories of happiness, rhythm, and microbial harmony.

You do not have to relocate to Okinawa or Ikaria to take advantage of their lessons. You only need to take their wisdom into your kitchen, your food system, your rhythm.

One meal at a time, one shared giggle at a time, one new high-fiber food at a time, your microbiome shifts. Your mood shifts. Your future shifts. And your body thrives.

The Joyful Gut is not about restriction; it is about remembering the most ancient of truths: health was always in the context of food; it was never just about the food; it's about how we ate, when we ate, and who we ate with.

PART 9 — THE ACTION STARTER: GUT RESET DAY

RESET IN REAL TIME

It's 6:30 AM. Maria wakes up not to the buzzing anxiety of her alarm but to shining coals of warm light emanating from her kitchen window. Today is different. She is not reaching for a bowl of cereal or scrolling through her phone while moving through coffee and a pastry.

She is doing something radical, something deceptively simple: she is giving her gut a reset.

One day. One rhythm. One whole-body experiment in the experience of feeling when food works with her instead of against her.

This is The Gut Reset Day: a one-day prescription for your microbiome, your mood, and your cravings.

Why a Reset Day?

Think of it like rebooting your system.

We live most of our days in noise: processed snacks, late-night eating, constant scrolling, irregular rhythms. A reset day not only cancels out the noise; it lets your body and microbiome "hear" its natural signals again.

For your gut: a reset day allows you to slowly reintroduce fiber, fermented foods, and slow eating.

For your brain, it allows you to feel what stable energy and calm digestion actually feel like.

For your circadian rhythm, a reset day allows you to realign eating windows to daylight.

And the coolest part? You don't need weeks of commitment to notice a change. One day will always be enough to remind you what is possible.

THE SCIENCE OF ONE-DAY SHIFTS

This isn't just a motivational trick. Even a single day of dietary rhythm can create measurable effects:

- **Gut Microbes Respond Quickly:** Studies in *Nature* (David et al., 2014) showed that microbiota composition shifts within 24 hours of a diet change. A plant-rich day boosts microbial diversity.

- **Blood Sugar Stability:** A high-protein, fiber-rich breakfast reduces glucose spikes for the rest of the day (*Diabetes Care*, 2015).

- **Cortisol & Hunger Hormones:** Eating meals at regular times with no late-night snacks supports the natural cortisol awakening response and reduces ghrelin dysregulation.

- **Mood Shifts:** Even one meal rich in tryptophan (eggs, oats, beans) increases serotonin synthesis pathways (*Am J Clin Nutr*, 2006).

THE BLUEPRINT OF THE GUT RESET DAY

We're going to walk through this day **hour by hour**, so you not only know *what* to do, but also *why it works*.

Morning: 6 AM – 10 AM

Theme: Align with cortisol + ghrelin.

What to Do:

- Hydrate with water or herbal tea.

- Breakfast: savory, protein + fiber-based. Examples:
    - Scrambled eggs with spinach + side of steel-cut oats.
    - Greek yogurt with flaxseed + blueberries.
    - Tofu scramble with veggies + avocado.

Why It Works:

- Protein stabilizes blood sugar and increases satiety hormones (GLP-1, PYY).
- Fiber feeds gut microbes, producing SCFAs that set the tone for mood regulation.
- Savory > sweet = fewer midmorning cravings.

Science Spotlight: A 2013 study in *Obesity* found that high-protein breakfasts reduced evening cravings by 60%.

Micro-Practice: Before the first bite, place your fork down. Breathe deeply three times. This activates your vagus nerve and primes digestion.

Midday: 10 AM – 2 PM

Theme: Leverage insulin sensitivity.

What to Do:

- Make this your largest meal of the day.
- Fill half your plate with vegetables, a quarter with lean protein, and a quarter with beans, lentils, or whole grains.
- Example meals:
    - Lentil stew with salmon + roasted vegetables.
    - Chicken, black beans, avocado, and quinoa bowl.
    - Tofu stir-fry with brown rice + broccoli.

Why It Works:

- Midday is when your body is most efficient at handling glucose and metabolizing nutrients.

- Bigger meals here → smaller, lighter meals at night → better circadian alignment.

Science Spotlight: A study in *Diabetes Care* (2013) showed that eating the majority of calories earlier improved weight loss and metabolic health versus eating them later.

Micro-Practice: Eat slowly enough that your meal takes 20 minutes. Satiety hormones (CCK, GLP-1) need at least that long to activate.

Afternoon: 2 PM – 6 PM

Theme: Beat the cortisol dip.

What to Do:

- Instead of a sugary snack, get **movement + light exposure**.
  - 10–15 minutes outside.
  - Stretch or walk.
- If you need food:
  - Fermented snack (kefir, sauerkraut, kimchi, miso broth).
  - Pair with a small protein source (nuts, boiled egg, hummus).

Why It Works:

- Sunlight resets the circadian rhythm, lowering cravings.

- Fermented foods provide live microbes that strengthen the gut.

- Protein steadies blood sugar and prevents "energy crash."

Science Spotlight: Wastyk et al. (*Cell*, 2021) found fermented foods significantly increased microbial diversity in just weeks.

Micro-Practice: Pause before reaching for food. Ask: *Am I hungry, or just tired?* If it's tiredness, movement is the medicine.

Evening: 6 PM – 10 PM

Theme: Wind down digestion.

What to Do:

- Eat a **lighter meal**, 2–3 hours before bed.
- Example meals:
  - Grilled fish with leafy greens.
  - Lentil soup with vegetables.
  - Tofu and steamed broccoli with tahini sauce.

Why It Works:

- Late eating disrupts melatonin, sleep quality, and microbiome repair cycles.
- A light dinner allows ghrelin to fade naturally, preventing nighttime cravings.

Science Spotlight: Research in *Cell Metabolism* (2017) showed time-restricted eating improves circadian alignment, reduces inflammation, and enhances sleep.

Micro-Practice: Close the kitchen after dinner. Signal to your body that the eating window is over.

Night: 10 PM – 6 AM

Theme: Repair and restore.

What to Do:

- Only water or herbal tea (chamomile, rooibos).

- Begin a wind-down ritual:

  o Gratitude journaling.

  o Low light, no screens.

  o Breathing exercise or stretching.

Why It Works:

- No food = gut microbes switch to **repair and recycling mode**.

- Sleep is deeper and more restorative without digestion competing.

Science Spotlight: Cortisol levels are lower and sleep efficiency is higher when no food is consumed within 3 hours of bedtime (*Nutrients*, 2019).

Micro-Practice: Write down three things you're grateful for before sleep. Gratitude activates the parasympathetic system, improving rest and digestion.

MARIA'S FIRST GUT RESET

By the time Maria's day ended, she realized she hadn't experienced the usual rollercoaster. No frantic afternoon crash. No desperate evening craving. She slept through the night without waking, and in the morning, she noticed something surprising:

She woke up hungry — but not for sugar or coffee. She wanted real food.

That's the **signal of alignment**: when your hunger feels like an invitation to nourish, not a trap to escape.

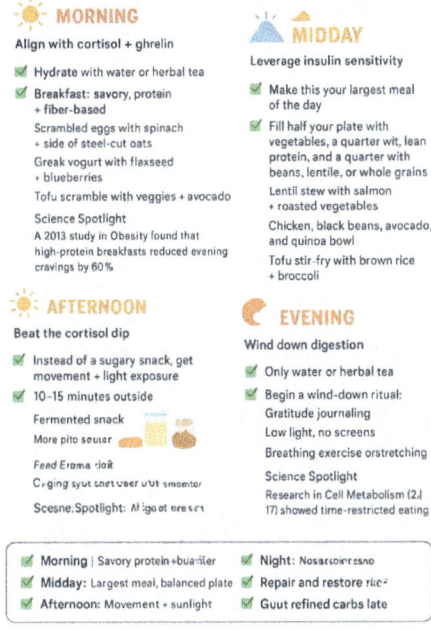

GUT RESET DAY CHECKLIST

☀ MORNING

Align with cortisol + ghrelin

☑ Hydrate with water or herbal tea

☑ Breakfast: savory, protein
+ fiber-based

Scrambled eggs with spinach
+ side of steel-cut oats

Greak yogurt with flaxseed
+ blueberries

Tofu scramble with veggies + avocado

Science Spotlight
A 2013 study in Obesity found that
high-protein breakfasts reduced evening
cravings by 60%

☀ AFTERNOON

Beat the cortisol dip

☑ Instead of a sugary snack, get
movement + light exposure

☑ 10-15 minutes outside

Fermented snack
More pito seuser

Feed Eroma dolk
C.ging syot cnet user u'bt smomter

Scesne:Spotlight: Al igu ot ore s rt

⛰ MIDDAY

Leverage insulin sensitivity

☑ Make this your largest meal
of the day

☑ Fill half your plate with
vegetables, a quarter wit, lean
protein, and a quarter with
beans, lentile, or whole grains

Lentil stew with salmon
+ roasted vegetables

Chicken, black beans, avocado,
and quinoa bowl

Tofu stir-fry with brown rice
+ broccoli

🌙 EVENING

Wind down digestion

☑ Only water or herbal tea

☑ Begin a wind-down ritual:
Gratitude journaling
Low light, no screens
Breathing exercise orstretching

Science Spotlight
Research in Cell Metabolism (2.I
17) showed time-restricted eating

☑ **Morning** | Savory protein+buantier
☑ **Midday:** Largest meal, balanced plate
☑ **Afternoon:** Movement + sunlight

☑ **Night:** Nosarsoixresno
☑ Repair and restore ruc²
☑ Guut refined carbs late

QUICK-REFERENCE BOX: GUT RESET DAY CHECKLIST

Morning 📷

- Savory protein + fiber breakfast
- Hydrate before coffee
- Breathe before eating

Midday ☼

- Largest meal, balanced plate
- 20-minute meal pace

Afternoon ☁

- Movement + sunlight > snacks
- Fermented snack if needed

Evening 🔅

- Light dinner, 2–3 hrs before bed
- Avoid refined carbs late

Night 🌙

- Herbal tea + gratitude ritual
- No late eating

The Gut Reset Day isn't a diet. It isn't punishment. It's a taste of what your body feels like when you live in rhythm with your biology.

It's proof that change is possible. It's evidence that cravings don't control you — they dissolve when your gut and brain are nourished. It's the doorway into the bigger journey: a microbiome that thrives, a mood that stabilizes, a body that feels light and clear.

And all it takes is one day to begin.

The Gut Reset Day is not a diet. It is not a punishment. It is an experience of what your body feels like with rhythmic biology.

It's a confirmation that change is possible.

It's proof that cravings don't run you. They dissolve when your gut and brain are fueled.

It is a gateway to the larger adventure: a thriving microbiome, a stabilizing mood, a light and clear feeling in your body.

And it starts with just one day.

You've come a long way through the hidden pathways of the gut— the interior garden that is ever present below every choice, every craving, and every emotional current.

We started with the gut–brain axis as more than a metaphor—not a notion, but an actual two-way superhighway shared by electrical impulses, chemical messengers, and microbial whispers. We traced

184

its rhythms—how the circadian hunger clock tells our microbes when to feast or fast, and how the hormonal output from microbes lets us know if we enter the day in homeostasis or in craving.

We learned about mood molecules, serotonin and dopamine, produced not only in the brain but also in the trillions of organisms that inhabit the folds of our intestines. We witnessed what happens when the system breaks down—when processed foods, artificial sweeteners, antibiotics, and long-term stress disrupt diversity and mute the voices of good microbes. Depression deepens. Anxiety sharpens. Fatigue sets in.

And then, we built a pathway forward. The healing garden: whole foods, fermented foods, fibers, and polyphenols that nourish microbial life, much like rain to dry land. Probiotics, prebiotics, and psychobiotics are more than buzzwords—they are tools to nurture this hidden organ within an organ. We ventured into Blue Zones—a region where the diversity of microbes flourishes, and joy is woven into the fabric of food culture. Finally, we presented a "Gut Reset Day", pragmatic, easy, and immediate, so that healing could begin not in some distant future, but within 24 hours.

THE GUT AS YOUR EMOTIONAL REGULATOR

The gut isn't just in the background of your journey; it is, in fact, your emotional regulator, resilience creator, and mood stabilizer. Each meal either calms or ignites a storm in your nervous system. Each bite is a vote for diversity, or depletion. Each day, the gut votes with its remarkable wisdom on how clearly your mind can think, how high your mood can lift, and how deeply your body can rest.

When you nourish it well, you are building your physical body and your emotional resilience. When you ignore it, you are sabotaging the foundational relationship between the source of wisdom in a mind-body dialogue.

A BRIDGE TO WHAT'S NEXT

But here's the kicker: just nurturing the gut isn't enough.

Because even when you are eating the intervention foods, even when you are providing your microbes with a feast of fiber and fermented gifts, there is one stealthy culprit, powerful enough to unravel the entire gut system—stress.

Stress floods the gut with cortisol, halts digestion, triggers cravings, and inflames the very lining we've been trying to heal. It's like static on the signal between brain and belly—a distortion that leaves the messages scrambled, the rhythms broken, and the moods unstable.

If the gut is your second brain, the invisible hand of stress can silence it.

So as we close this chapter, it's time to recognize what you have unlocked already: a new relationship with food—a relationship based on joy, rhythm, and bacterial harmony rather than deprivation or control. You now understand the gut is not a liability—it is an ally. Allies need protection.

In order to protect your gut's delicate balance, in order for your second brain to speak with its true voice, you need to conquer stress.

This is where we go next.

PART III

ENERGY, MOVEMENT, AND RECOVERY

CHAPTER 7:

THE STRESS PRESCRIPTION

PART 1: — WHEN STRESS BECOMES THE OPERATING SYSTEM

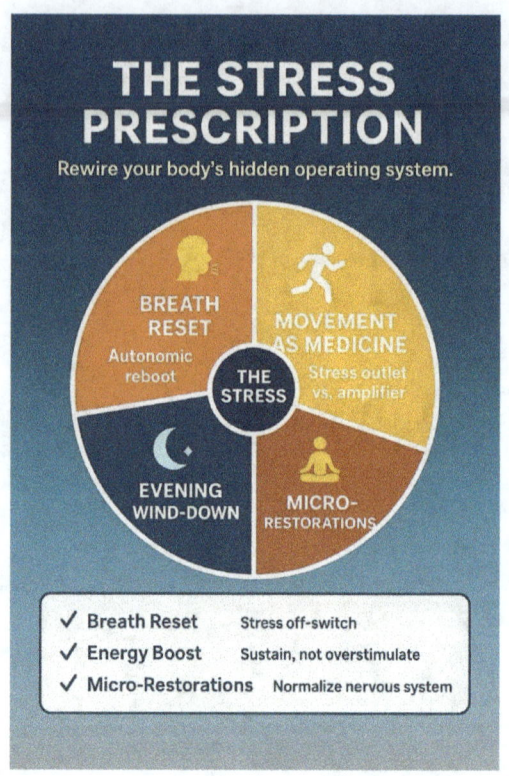

It's dark in the room, but not in your head. You've been laying down there for hours, heart racing as though you just finished a marathon. Your body feels heavy, but your brain is on fire, reviewing the email you forgot to send, the bill you haven't paid, or the fight you had with your partner. You turn over in bed, grab your phone for distractions, and there it is, the screen gently glowing and reminding you it's already 3 a.m. again. Tomorrow will hurt.

But here's the twist: your body doesn't know the difference between running to save your life from a tiger and worrying about your inbox. To your nervous system, stress is stress. And when stress becomes your default operating system, everything else in your biology—from your gut to your sleep to your cravings—starts unraveling.

THE HIDDEN OPERATING SYSTEM

We like to think we are in control, that our decisions are rational and thought-through, but underneath our thinking mind is a faster, older command center. It is our "hidden operating system," the stress response, which is the constant back-and-forth between the sympathetic ("fight-or-flight") and the parasympathetic ("rest-and-digest") branches of your autonomic nervous system.

When your life is balanced, these two branches alternate paths like skilled dancers: you ramp up when it is time to, then go to calm. In modern life, that dance is messed up. You stay stuck in sympathetic overdrive and keep your foot on the gas. Your cortisol never resets. Your adrenaline stays in the blood. Your parasympathetic brake—the one that helps you digest, repair, sleep, and lessen the danger signals—is getting weaker every day.

And this isn't just "feeling stressed." Chronic stress has measurable, body-wide effects:

- **Metabolic Chaos** → Elevated cortisol spikes blood sugar and insulin, driving belly fat and energy crashes.

- **Gut Disruption** → Stress hormones alter gut motility, permeability, and microbial diversity. IBS flares. Bloating worsens.

- **Immune Breakdown** → Chronic cortisol suppresses immunity, leaving you inflamed but defenseless.

189

- **Neurochemical Drain** → Stress depletes dopamine and serotonin, tilting the brain toward anxiety, depression, and cravings.

Stress isn't just in your head. It's in your cells, in your gut, in your mitochondria. It *is* your operating system.

MARIA IN SURVIVAL MODE

You are acquainted with Maria, the teacher who works very hard, with students and her children keeping her busy. Let's get back to her.

It is Thursday afternoon. She has not consumed anything since a hurried bagel at 7:00 a.m. Staff meeting drags on, and her phone dings with three emails from parents! Her jaw tightens. Her chest constricts. By the time she returns home, she is fatigued, but strangely wired. At dinner, she picks at her kids' pasta; however, later that night, while standing at the pantry, she consumes half a sleeve of cookies without even recognizing it.

She didn't crave; her brain was under stress. The cortisol was running the process. And the stress operating system hijacked her cravings, her digestion, and her sleep in one sweep.

Maria is not weak. She is not broken. Her body is running a program that millions of us are stuck in.

SCIENCE SPOTLIGHT: THE CORTISOL AWAKENING RESPONSE

Here's something most people don't know: your stress operating system literally writes your day before you've even had coffee.

In a healthy rhythm, cortisol rises steeply in the first 30–45 minutes after waking. This surge wakes you up, primes your metabolism, and sets your energy baseline. But in people stuck in chronic stress, this curve flattens—or worse, inverts. That means instead of a strong morning rise and calm evening dip, you get sluggish mornings and wired nights.

Research from the *Journal of Endocrinology and Metabolism* (2010) shows that a dysregulated cortisol curve predicts fatigue, depression, obesity, and even cardiovascular disease. In other words, when stress is the operating system, your entire biology shifts into survival mode.

THE PRESCRIPTION BEGINS

But here's the good news: just like your computer's operating system can be updated, so can your stress biology. The body has built-in switches—vagus nerve activation, breath regulation, light exposure, movement—that can reboot the system and restore balance.

This chapter is not about eliminating stress (that's impossible). It's about learning to rewire your hidden operating system so that stress no longer hijacks your biology. Instead, you'll have tools to:

- Flip your nervous system from "fight-or-flight" into "rest-and-digest" on command.

- Restore your cortisol rhythm to match daylight, not deadlines.

- Protect your gut and brain from stress-driven sabotage.

- Build resilience so you can *feel stress without being ruled by it*.

The Stress Prescription is about reclaiming sovereignty over the one operating system you can't afford to ignore.

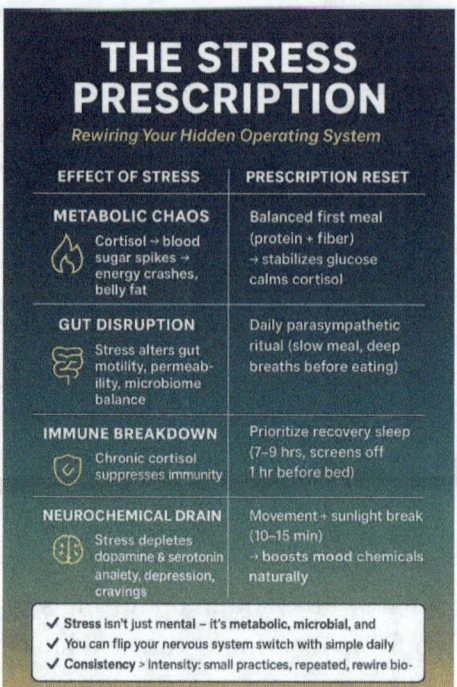

PART 2 — THE PHYSIOLOGY OF STRESS: DECODING THE HIDDEN OPERATING SYSTEM

THE INVISIBLE SWITCHBOARD

Imagining this, you are sitting in traffic. Just ahead of you, a red sea of brake lights stretches ahead. You're late for work, your phone starts buzzing with a reminder of looming deadlines, and all of a sudden, a jolt of adrenaline kicks in. Palms sweat, breath is suddenly shallow, teeth locked together.

What just happened?

You did not choose to make your heart race. You did not consciously tell your sweat glands to start working. A hidden operating system — the stress circuitry of your body — made the call for you.

This circuitry, shaped over millions of years of evolution, is designed for our survival. The issue? It hasn't updated for modern life. Instead of fleeing from predators, we now face inboxes, traffic, bills, and social media scroll fatigue — Yet our body responds as if we are in the wilderness, fleeing for our lives.

Welcome to the HPA axis, the autonomic nervous system, and the delicate balance between stress and calm.

THE HPA AXIS: YOUR STRESS COMMAND CENTER

The **HPA axis** (hypothalamic–pituitary–adrenal axis) is the body's central stress-response network. Think of it as your **internal alarm system**, spanning brain to adrenal glands:

1. **Hypothalamus** → Detects threat and signals "go."

2. **Pituitary gland** → Releases ACTH (adrenocorticotropic hormone).

3. **Adrenal glands** → Release **cortisol**, the primary stress hormone.

Cortisol, often vilified, is not inherently bad. In fact, you *need it*:

- It mobilizes glucose for quick energy.

- It sharpens focus.

- It suppresses non-urgent functions (digestion, reproduction, long-term immunity) to conserve resources for "fight or flight."

But here's the catch: cortisol was designed for *short bursts*. Modern life has turned it into a **chronic drip feed**, leaving our operating system jammed in survival mode.

CORTISOL RHYTHMS: THE DAILY TIDE

Healthy stress physiology isn't about *avoiding stress*, but *riding its natural rhythms*. Cortisol is meant to follow a **circadian curve**:

- **Morning Surge (6–8 AM):** Cortisol peaks, helping you wake up, feel alert, and fuel your brain.

- **Gradual Decline:** Levels should steadily fall throughout the day.

- **Evening Low:** Cortisol dips, making way for melatonin (sleep hormone) to rise.

Now, what happens under **chronic stress**?

- Cortisol stays **elevated at night**, disrupting sleep.

- Morning peaks are **blunted**, leaving you groggy and "wired but tired."

- The system may even **burn out** — leading to flat cortisol curves, fatigue, weight gain, and a higher risk for depression.

Research Snapshot:

A 2003 study in *Psychoneuroendocrinology* showed that individuals with flat cortisol rhythms had **double the risk of early mortality**, compared to those with healthy peaks and valleys.

THE AUTONOMIC NERVOUS SYSTEM: GAS VS. BRAKE

Parallel to the HPA axis is the **autonomic nervous system (ANS)** — the rapid-response switchboard that manages stress in milliseconds.

It has two main branches:

1. Sympathetic Nervous System (SNS) → the "gas pedal."

    a. Increases heart rate and blood pressure.

    b. Diverts blood to muscles.

    c. Shuts down digestion and long-term repair.

2. Parasympathetic Nervous System (PNS) → the "brake."

    a. Slows heart rate.

    b. Enhances digestion and nutrient absorption.

c. Promotes healing and recovery.

Healthy stress response = **dynamic balance** between gas and brake. Chronic stress = **pedal jammed on the gas**.

THE VAGUS NERVE: YOUR BUILT-IN RESET BUTTON

Enter the **vagus nerve** — the body's longest cranial nerve, running from the brainstem through the lungs, heart, and gut.

It's the **command line of the parasympathetic nervous system**. Stimulating it is like hitting "reset" on your internal alarm.

- **Deep diaphragmatic breathing** → stimulates vagal tone, lowering heart rate and blood pressure.

- **Cold exposure (face dunk or shower)** → triggers the dive reflex, activating vagal pathways.

- **Humming, chanting, or singing** → vibrates the vagus, boosting calm.

Science Snapshot:

- A 2010 study in *Biological Psychiatry* showed that people with higher vagal tone had **greater emotional resilience** and lower inflammation.

- Clinical vagus nerve stimulation (VNS) is now FDA-approved for treatment-resistant depression.

Translation? You don't need a prescription or an implant. You have a built-in anti-stress lever — and every breath is a chance to pull it.

WHY STRESS FEELS DIFFERENT TODAY

Your ancestors faced **acute stress**: chase, escape, survive. Stress hormones rose, did their job, then reset.

We face **chronic micro-stresses**:

- Inbox overload.

- Social media comparison.

- Lack of sleep.

- Processed foods.

- Financial strain.

Instead of a jagged peak-and-reset curve, we live in a **low-grade storm**. Cortisol never fully shuts off. The vagus is underused. The body forgets how to come back to baseline.

The result? Anxiety, depression, digestive issues, weight gain, insulin resistance — all flowing from one overloaded operating system.

ACTION PRIMER: FIRST RESET STEPS

Before we dive deeper into the four pillars (breath, movement, wind-down, micro-restorations), here are **Day One resets** you can start today:

- **Morning light + movement:** Step outside within 30 minutes of waking. Anchors cortisol rhythm.

- **1:2 breathing:** Inhale for 4 seconds, exhale for 8. Repeat x5. Instant vagus activation.

- **Caffeine curfew:** Last cup before noon. Prevents cortisol disruption at night.

- **Evening dimming:** Lower lights 2 hours before bed. Tells cortisol to step down, melatonin to rise.

Your stress physiology isn't broken — it's overloaded. The HPA axis, cortisol rhythms, the vagus nerve — these aren't abstract science terms. They are the switches and levers that determine whether your body is locked in survival... or free to heal, focus, and thrive.

The next sections will show you how to use this knowledge — turning biology into practice, and stress from enemies into an ally.

PART 3 — SUNLIGHT + NATURE

A DIFFERENT KIND OF MEDICINE

Picture this: it's 7 a.m., and instead of scrolling your phone while rushing coffee into your system, you step outside. The world is calm, the sky is blossoming gold. You feel the fresh air against your skin, and you feel the warmth of the sun hitting your face. You are not just observing light - you are taking a prescription that is older than any pill bottle.

For millions of years, humans have been syncing their biology with the rhythm of the sun's circadian/evolutionary light. Morning light told our brain, "Wake up, align, reset." Evening darkness gently told our brain, "Slow down, repair." In a world filled with the ugliness of fluorescent bulbs, phone screens, and concrete walls, we have lost that dialogue with the light. And the end result? Cortisol rhythms flatten, melatonin release gets delayed, inflammation increases - and stress multiplies.

Let's walk back outside. Let's reclaim humanity's most primal prescription - sunlight and nature!

THE SCIENCE OF LIGHT AND STRESS

Your body has a master clock — the **suprachiasmatic nucleus (SCN)** in your brain. Think of it as the conductor of your circadian orchestra. It takes its cues from light entering the retina, particularly the **blue wavelengths of morning sunlight**. When that light hits your eye:

- **Cortisol Awakening Response (CAR):** Within 30–45 minutes, cortisol rises naturally. This isn't "bad stress" — it's your system's fuel injection, setting you up for focus, energy, and resilience.

- **Melatonin Shutoff:** Morning light tells your pineal gland to stop melatonin production, signaling your body that night is over.

- **Neurotransmitter Boost:** Sunlight exposure also boosts **serotonin**, which acts as a precursor for melatonin later at night — syncing both ends of your day.

Study Spotlight: A 2017 study in *Sleep Health* found that office workers who received more morning sunlight had **lower cortisol variability, better sleep quality, and fewer symptoms of depression**.

THE STRESS RESET IN NATURE

It's not just sunlight — it's the *setting*. Forests, parks, rivers — these environments engage your nervous system in ways no treadmill or LED-lit gym can.

- **Forest Bathing (Shinrin-Yoku):** Japanese researchers have shown that spending just 2 hours in a forest lowers **cortisol by 16–20%**, reduces **blood pressure**, and decreases **inflammatory cytokines**.

- **The Vagus Nerve Connection:** Natural settings stimulate the vagus nerve — your parasympathetic "rest-and-digest" superhighway — slowing heart rate and improving variability (HRV), a marker of resilience.

- **Immune Boost:** A landmark study (Li et al., *Public Health*, 2010) found that phytoncides — aromatic compounds from trees — increase **natural killer cell activity** in humans, strengthening immune defense.

Nature isn't just "pretty." It's biochemical medicine.

MINI-STORY: DAVID'S COMMUTE SWAP

David, our stressed-out office worker from Chapter 1, used to start his day hunched over his laptop with a double espresso. His stress baseline was already high before he left the house. When his coach challenged him to spend just **10 minutes outside each morning** before checking email, the shift was profound. Within 2 weeks:

- His mid-afternoon crash eased.

- His sleep tracker showed longer deep sleep.

- He reported feeling "less clenched" — a direct sign of nervous system recalibration.

The light didn't just wake him. It reprogrammed his stress rhythm.

PRACTICAL ACTION STEPS: THE SUNLIGHT + NATURE PRESCRIPTION

STEP 1: MORNING LIGHT DOSE

- Aim for **10-15 minutes outside within 1 hour of waking**. No sunglasses if possible (unless medically necessary).

- Cloudy? Doesn't matter. Even diffuse daylight is **10-50x stronger** than indoor light.

STEP 2: MIDDAY MOVEMENT BREAK

- Step outside for **5-10 minutes at lunch**. Sunlight at this time stabilizes serotonin and keeps cortisol in check.

STEP 3: GREEN SPACE THERAPY

- Once a week, schedule at least **30-60 minutes in a natural setting** (park, beach, forest).

- No agenda. Walk slowly. Breathe deeply. Let your senses take over.

STEP 4: SUNSET RITUAL

- Watch the sky darken. The shift in light temperature (from blue to amber) signals melatonin production.

- This is a natural "dimmer switch" for your stress system.

QUICK-REFERENCE BOX: THE SUNLIGHT + NATURE RESET

- **Morning Light:** 10–15 minutes outside → Cortisol & serotonin aligned.

- **Midday Break:** 5–10 minutes outdoors → Keeps energy stable.

- **Nature Immersion:** 30–60 min weekly → Cortisol ↓, immune system ↑.

- **Sunset Cue:** Watch the evening sky → Melatonin on time.

Bottom Line: Stress is not just about what you subtract. It's also about what you *add back*. Sunlight and nature aren't luxuries — they're the original prescriptions for balance.

PART 4 — THE BODY UNDER SIEGE: STRESS + MICROBIOME

THE WAR YOU CAN'T SEE

Imagine a teacher, drained after a grueling day of grading, staff meetings, and tending to two kids at home, collapses onto the couch with a plate of dinner still in hand, half-eaten. Her stomach hurts—not food poisoning, not malaise, but something much more insidious. It's the stress. And while she feels tension in her shoulders and her mind racing, something else is happening invisibly, deep inside: her gut microbes are fighting for survival.

Stress doesn't just make your heart race or your jaw tighten. It rewrites your inner ecosystem.

THE GUT-BRAIN STRESS LOOP

The gut and brain are hardwired together through the **gut-brain axis**, a superhighway of nerves, hormones, and immune messengers. When stress surges, the **hypothalamic-pituitary-adrenal (HPA) axis** releases cortisol — a survival hormone designed to sharpen your senses and mobilize energy. But when cortisol is elevated too often, it triggers collateral damage in the gut.

- **Thinning the Gut Lining:** Chronic cortisol exposure reduces proteins that hold gut lining cells together. The result? A more permeable gut — often called "leaky gut."

- **Microbial Shifts:** Stress hormones change the composition of the microbiota, reducing beneficial bacteria like **Lactobacillus** and increasing pro-inflammatory species.

- **Reduced SCFA (short-chain fatty acid) production:** Normally, gut microbes produce SCFAs like **butyrate**, which fuel colon cells and regulate inflammation. Under stress, SCFA output drops, weakening gut resilience.

Study Spotlight: A 2011 paper in PNAS showed that stressed mice had reduced microbial diversity and increased gut permeability, leading to systemic inflammation. Human studies mirror this — medical students under exam stress show shifts in microbiome composition after just a few weeks (*Stress*, 2013).

HOW STRESS FEEDS DYSBIOSIS

Stress changes gut behavior in at least three layers:

1. **Nervous System Signals:** Stress increases sympathetic "fight-or-flight" tone, which slows digestion and alters gut motility. Food lingers too long or passes too fast, creating imbalances.

2. **Hormonal Messages:** Cortisol and adrenaline change bile acid release, altering which microbes thrive.

3. **Immune Shifts:** Stress elevates inflammatory cytokines that directly suppress microbial diversity.

This trifecta creates **dysbiosis** — a microbial imbalance linked to anxiety, depression, metabolic disease, and even autoimmune conditions.

MARIA'S EXAM GUT

Maria, a graduate student, would eat a nutritious diet, engage in regular exercise, and sleep reasonably well—until finals season. In just two weeks of late nights studying and constant stress, she noticed bloating and irregular digestion, along with sudden intolerances to certain foods. After undergoing lab work, she had markers that indicated elevated levels of gut permeability and decreased markers of protective bacteria. Her gut was not 'broken'— it was overwhelmed with stress signals.

STRESS, SCFAS, AND MOOD

Why does this matter for mood? Because SCFAs like **butyrate** are not just gut fuel—they're neuroactive. They cross the blood-brain barrier, dampen inflammation, and even support **BDNF (brain-derived neurotrophic factor)**, a molecule critical for resilience against depression.

When stress lowers SCFA production, it sets off a chain reaction:

- Gut lining weakens → inflammation rises.

- Microbial diversity drops → mood-regulating pathways weaken.

- The brain receives more "distress" signals via cytokines and the vagus nerve.

Study Spotlight: A 2020 review in *Frontiers in Immunology* highlighted that stress-induced dysbiosis increases risk for depression via reduced SCFA signaling and neuroinflammation.

ACTION STEPS: DEFENDING YOUR GUT UNDER STRESS

☑ 1. MICROBIOME-FRIENDLY STRESS BUFFERS

- Add fermented foods (yogurt, kefir, kimchi) 3–5x per week → shown to increase microbial resilience.

- Boost SCFA production with resistant starches (green bananas, oats, beans).

☑ 2. CORTISOL COOL-DOWN RITUALS

- Practice paced breathing (inhale 4, exhale 6) for 5 minutes → activates vagus nerve and lowers cortisol.

- Evening wind-down: dim lights, herbal tea → signals HPA axis to shut down.

☑ 3. PROTECT THE LINING

- Omega-3s and polyphenols (flax, walnuts, blueberries, olive oil) support tight junction proteins.

- Avoid "stress-snacking" on UPFs → they amplify permeability and inflammation.

QUICK-REFERENCE BOX: THE GUT UNDER STRESS

⚠ Stress → Cortisol ↑ → Gut lining thins, microbes shift.

⚠ Dysbiosis → Less SCFA → Mood regulation ↓.

- Buffer with fermented foods + resistant starch.

- Reset daily with vagus nerve rituals.

- Feed lining with omega-3s + polyphenols.

Bottom Line: Stress is not just a mental weight. It's a microbial earthquake. Protecting your gut during stress isn't optional—it's the frontline defense for mood, energy, and resilience.

PART 5 — THE STRESS PRESCRIPTION (THE REWIRE PROTOCOL)

Stress is not merely something to be eliminated — it is a code to be reprogrammed. The body is not broken. It is adaptive. But when stress signals remain stuck in "high alert," it scrambles your body's hidden operating system — the HPA axis, your vagus nerve, and your circadian cortisol rhythms. The result? You live in survival mode.

This is your prescription to rewire stress, not in a way that numbs you, but one that retrains your biology to respond resiliently. Think of it as a five-step protocol: breath, movement, light, micro-restoration, sleep.

1. BREATH RESET (AUTONOMIC REBOOT)

Picture yourself sitting in traffic after a brutal day. Horns blaring, emails still pinging in your head, shoulders tight, breath shallow. Your nervous system reads this as danger. Heart rate up. Cortisol dripping. Fight-or-flight engaged.

Now picture something different: you place your hand on your belly, inhale slowly for four counts, exhale for 6. Within 90 seconds, your vagus nerve signals your brain: *The danger is gone.* Heart rate slows. Cortisol curve flattens.

SCIENCE:

- Slow, diaphragmatic breathing lengthens the exhale → stimulates the vagus nerve → increases parasympathetic tone.

- **HRV (heart rate variability)** rises, a direct biomarker of resilience.

- A 2017 meta-analysis (Frontiers in Psychology) confirmed that paced breathing enhances vagal activity and reduces cortisol.

ACTION STEPS:

- Practice the **4-6 Breath Reset**: Inhale 4 counts, exhale 6 counts. Repeat for 2–5 minutes.

- Layer with posture: Sit upright, shoulders soft, belly expanding.

- Cue it with triggers: stoplights, email checks, and before meals.

Why it works: Your autonomic nervous system can't tell the difference between a lion in the savannah and a deadline email — unless you give it a signal to reset. Breath is that signal.

2. MOVEMENT AS MEDICINE

Two stressed professionals, two very different outcomes.

- John, after his 12-hour day, thrashes through an intense HIIT session. Heart pounding, adrenaline raging — he feels a short high, but sleep is wrecked.

- Maria, equally stressed, takes a 30-minute brisk walk outdoors. Her cortisol dips, her mood lightens, and her sleep later is deep.

SCIENCE:

- Exercise modulates the HPA axis. **Moderate-intensity movement** reduces cortisol and inflammation.

- But **overtraining** or late-night HIIT elevates cortisol, prolonging stress.

- A 2015 review in *Neurobiology of Stress* showed that consistent aerobic exercise improved stress resilience, while excessive anaerobic loads amplified stress response.

ACTION STEPS:

- **Identify your outlet, not amplifier,** if you feel wired after training, swap intensity for rhythm (walking, yoga, cycling).

- **Daytime movement > evening movement.** Cortisol naturally declines at night — honor that curve.

- Use the **10-Minute Rule:** Even 10 minutes of walking outdoors lowers cortisol (Harvard T.H. Chan study, 2018).

Why it works: Movement isn't about burning calories here — it's a neural reset. Done right, it teaches your stress circuits: *There is safety in motion.*

3. SUNLIGHT + NATURE

A corporate manager wakes in darkness, rushes to work under fluorescent lights, eats lunch at her desk, scrolls indoors until bed. Her body doesn't know the time of day. Cortisol misfires, melatonin is suppressed, and cravings spike.

Contrast that with a gardener who steps into the morning sun, feels light on her skin, breathes in green air. Her body's stress rhythm resets naturally: cortisol rises with the dawn, fades with dusk.

SCIENCE:

- **Morning light exposure** anchors the cortisol awakening response → aligns circadian rhythm.

- **Forest bathing (shinrin-yoku)** reduces cortisol, lowers blood pressure, and decreases inflammatory cytokines (Park et al., Environmental Health & Preventive Medicine, 2010).

- Green spaces buffer psychological stress and improve microbiome diversity via environmental exposure.

ACTION STEPS:

- **Sunrise Rule:** Step outside within 30 minutes of waking. No sunglasses. 5–10 minutes is enough.

- **Nature Micro-Dose:** Add 10–20 minutes of outdoor walking, especially in green or blue spaces.

- **Digital Swap:** Replace one scroll break/day with a nature break.

Why it works: Light and nature are original medicines. They don't just "calm you" — they tune your cortisol dial, reprogram your circadian code, and remind your body what safe rhythms feel like.

4. MICRO-RESTORATIONS

Stress isn't only about the big crises. It's the thousand micro-cuts: endless notifications, small conflicts, rushing, multitasking. Each drip adds to the cortisol pool. Without recovery, you drown in it.

SCIENCE:

- Even 1–5 minutes of intentional "pattern interrupt" lowers cortisol and resets brain waves.

- **Polyvagal theory:** Micro-restorations activate safety cues (warmth, slow breath, visual rest).

- A 2016 study in *Psychoneuroendocrinology* found that brief mindfulness breaks on workdays lowered cortisol trajectories.

ACTION STEPS:

- **90-Minute Rule:** Every 90 minutes, insert a reset: look at the horizon, stretch, deep breath, step outside.

- **Sensory Rest:** Try earplugs for 3 minutes, or soft eye closure — it signals the nervous system to shift gears.

- **Micro-joys:** A song, a laugh, a gratitude note. Tiny but potent stress interrupts.

Why it works: Stress is cumulative. So is recovery. By stacking tiny restorations, you prevent the dam from breaking.

5. EVENING WIND-DOWN RITUALS

Picture two evenings.

- In one, you scroll in bed under blue light, answer "just one more" email, and snack late. Cortisol remains high, and melatonin is delayed. You wake groggy, cravings sharp.

- In the other, you dim the lights after dinner, sip herbal tea, stretch, breathe. Cortisol recedes. Melatonin rises. Sleep becomes deep medicine.

SCIENCE:

- **Sleep is the ultimate cortisol reset.** Sleep deprivation magnifies cortisol surges, impairs glucose control, and heightens anxiety circuits.

- Evening rituals cue the nervous system into parasympathetic dominance.

- A 2019 study in *Sleep Medicine Reviews* found that consistent pre-sleep routines improved cortisol rhythms and reduced insomnia.

ACTION STEPS:

- **Screens-off Rule:** No bright screens 60 minutes before bed. Use the amber light if needed.

- **Dinner Timing:** Finish eating 2–3 hours before bed → avoids cortisol spikes from late digestion.

- **Anchor Ritual:** Choose two calming cues: herbal tea, stretch, journaling, or prayer.

- **Consistency > Perfection:** Same sleep/wake times anchor the cortisol-melatonin cycle.

Why it works: Evening rituals tell your body the war is over. You've survived the day. Now it's time to repair.

SYNTHESIS OF THE REWIRE PROTOCOL

Breath, movement, light, micro-restoration, sleep. Five simple practices.

But together, they are not just habits — they are **code rewrites**. They send your nervous system one message: *You are safe. You can thrive.*

When practiced daily, this prescription doesn't erase stress. It trains your body to meet stress, process it, and recover stronger. This is resilience — not from willpower, but from biology.

Imagine yourself weeks from now: you face the same traffic, deadlines, noise — but your body feels different. Less braced, more grounded. Your breath is slower. Your cravings are softer. You sleep more deeply. This isn't fantasy. It's what happens when you practice the Stress Prescription.

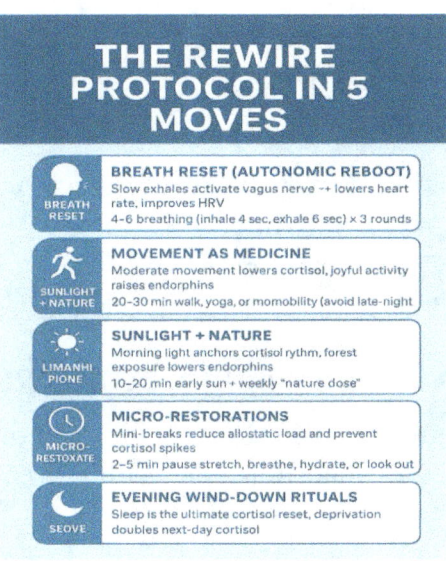

THE REWIRE PROTOCOL IN 5 MOVES

BREATH RESET (AUTONOMIC REBOOT)
BREATH RESET
Slow exhales activate vagus nerve → lowers heart rate, improves HRV
4-6 breathing (inhale 4 sec, exhale 6 sec) × 3 rounds

MOVEMENT AS MEDICINE
SUNLIGHT + NATURE
Moderate movement lowers cortisol, joyful activity raises endorphins
20-30 min walk, yoga, or momobility (avoid late-night)

SUNLIGHT + NATURE
LIMANHI PIONE
Morning light anchors cortisol rythm, forest exposure lowers endorphins
10-20 min early sun + weekly "nature dose"

MICRO-RESTORATIONS
MICRO-RESTOXATE
Mini-breaks reduce allostatic load and prevent cortisol spikes
2-5 min pause stretch, breathe, hydrate, or look out

EVENING WIND-DOWN RITUALS
SEOVE
Sleep is the ultimate cortisol reset, deprivation doubles next-day cortisol

PART 6 — THE STRESS-FOOD FEEDBACK LOOP

Maria sits in her car in the school parking lot; the day is finally over. She has papers to grade in the passenger seat, her phone buzzing with emails she can't face, and a body humming with the invisible current of adrenaline. She hasn't eaten since lunch, but now, it isn't a balanced dinner that she craves; it is the bright orange bag of chips she left in her desk for "emergencies."

She rips it open before she even leaves the lot. The salt and crunch and quick hit of starch dull the edges of her exhaustion for a moment. But that night, sleep was fitful and scattered. By morning, her heart is pounding before her alarm clock even sounds. The next day will begin, and she is already behind.

This isn't a matter of willpower. This is the feedback loop of the stress-food cycle, or, as I like to call it, the stress-food cycle, one of the most common and most damaging cycles of modern life.

THE SCIENCE OF THE LOOP

1. STRESS SPARKS THE CRAVING

When the body senses threat, the **HPA axis** (hypothalamus-pituitary-adrenal) surges, flooding the body with cortisol and adrenaline. Cortisol isn't just a "stress hormone"—it also primes the brain to seek **quick energy**. The reasoning is ancient: in times of danger, we needed calories fast.

Modern translation? Stress makes you crave **processed, calorie-dense foods**—chips, sweets, drive-thru meals. The brain's reward system, especially the **dopamine circuits**, lights up even brighter under stress, making these foods feel irresistible.

2. PROCESSED FOODS DEEPEN THE STRESS LOAD

Ultra-processed foods (UPFs) are engineered to give a dopamine spike but leave blood sugar crashing. Within hours, insulin surges, glucose dips, and cortisol rise again. Instead of calming the system, stress-eating winds it tighter.

At the same time, emulsifiers, additives, and refined sugars disrupt the **gut microbiome**—eroding microbial diversity and suppressing **short-chain fatty acids (SCFAs)**, which normally help regulate inflammation and mood. Stress eating literally reprograms the gut–brain loop against resilience.

3. POOR SLEEP AMPLIFIES IT ALL

Maria's chips don't just add calories—they sabotage sleep. High-sugar, high-fat snacks eaten late blunt melatonin release and increase overnight cortisol. Studies show sleep deprivation magnifies cravings for processed foods the next day (Greer et al., *Neuron*, 2013).

It's a vicious circle:

Stress → Processed foods → Gut disruption + poor sleep → Higher stress tomorrow.

THE HUMAN COST

This loop doesn't just sap energy—it builds into chronic illness:

- **Metabolic strain:** Blood sugar spikes drive insulin resistance.

- **Mood volatility:** Microbiome imbalance worsens anxiety and depression risk.

- **Cardiovascular load:** Stress hormones and inflammatory foods accelerate vascular aging.

Maria's story is one, but millions live this loop daily—grabbing food to soothe stress, only to feel heavier, more restless, and more stressed tomorrow.

BREAKING THE LOOP: BEFORE THE FORK

The good news? The loop isn't unbreakable. But here's the critical insight: **you can't break it at the point of food choice alone.** Telling Maria to "just resist the chips" ignores the biology driving the craving.

Instead, the loop has to be rewired **before the fork touches the plate**:

- **Breathing resets** lower cortisol before it hijacks hunger.

- **Movement micro-doses** replace the dopamine hit of processed foods.

- **Sunlight anchors** the body clock, making real hunger easier to distinguish from stress hunger.

- **Micro-restorations** keep stress from building until it overflows.

By calming the stress system upstream, cravings lose their grip. The chips stop calling like sirens. The body remembers how to ask for real food.

PART 7 — ACTION STARTER: YOUR STRESS RESET DAY

Imagine giving your body and brain a 24-hour "operating system reboot." Not through willpower. Not through restriction. But by nudging your biology back into its natural rhythm—one small step at a time.

This is **Your Stress Reset Day**: a practical, day-long experiment to feel what it's like when your stress response starts working *for* you instead of against you. Think of it as a rehearsal for resilience.

MORNING: BREATH + SUNLIGHT

PROTOCOL:

- Begin the day not with your phone, but with your lungs.

- 2 minutes of slow, deliberate breathing (inhale 4 sec, exhale 6 sec, repeat).

- Step outside for at least 5 minutes of natural light, even if it's cloudy.

Science: Morning light anchors the circadian clock, setting cortisol to rise naturally early in the day (instead of spiking unpredictably). Slow exhale breathing activates the vagus nerve, lowering resting heart rate and stabilizing heart rate variability (HRV)—a marker of stress resilience.

MIDDAY: WALK IT OFF

PROTOCOL:

- After lunch, take a 10-minute walk—outside if possible.

- Keep it easy-paced, not exercise intensity.

Science: Light post-meal movement blunts glucose spikes (Colberg et al., *Diabetes Care*, 2016), which means fewer mid-afternoon crashes that feed stress cravings. Walking also lowers circulating cortisol and raises endorphins, converting stress energy into recovery fuel.

AFTERNOON: THE STRESS SNACK SWAP

PROTOCOL:

- Instead of reaching for chips, soda, or candy, swap in protein + fiber.

- Examples: Greek yogurt + berries, hummus + veggies, a handful of nuts, or an apple with almond butter.

Science: Processed snacks spike insulin and worsen stress reactivity. Protein and fiber stabilize glucose, sustain energy, and signal satiety hormones like GLP-1 and PYY—calming the body instead of pushing it further into the stress loop.

EVENING: WIND-DOWN RITUAL

PROTOCOL:

- One hour before bed, go **tech-free.**

- Dim lights, brew herbal tea, stretch, or read.

Science: Blue light and late-night stimulation delay melatonin, keeping cortisol elevated past its natural curve. A tech-free buffer restores the circadian wind-down, ensuring that sleep becomes the ultimate "cortisol reset button."

NIGHT: GRATITUDE JOURNAL

PROTOCOL:

- Write down three things that went well today.

- Keep it simple and specific ("I finished my report," "My daughter laughed at dinner").

Science: Gratitude practices reduce cortisol by as much as 23% (Redwine et al., *Spirituality in Clinical Practice*, 2016) and increase parasympathetic activity. In short, they hardwire the nervous system for calm and connection, priming tomorrow to start lighter.

QUICK-REFERENCE BOX

ONE DAY TO RESET YOUR OPERATING SYSTEM.

- Breath reset + sunlight → cortisol synchronizer

- Midday walk → metabolic stress buffer

- Snack swap → break cravings loop

- Wind-down ritual → restore melatonin, reset cortisol

- Gratitude → calm the nervous system before sleep

This single day isn't perfection—it's **proof of concept**. You'll feel what it's like when stress eases its grip, when food stops being a crutch, when sleep feels restorative again. And once you've felt it, you'll know how to return to it, day by day.

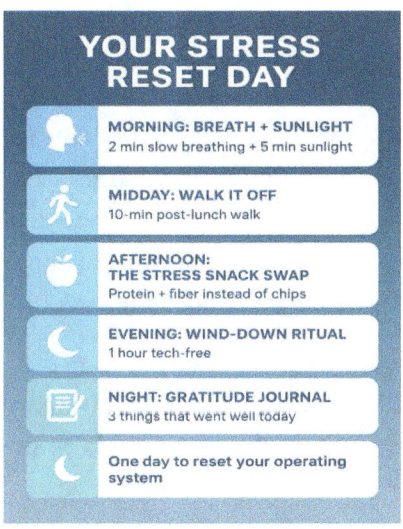

QUICK-REFERENCE CHECKLIST

THE STRESS PRESCRIPTION REMINDERS

☑ **Cortisol is not the enemy — imbalance is.**

Your stress hormone keeps you alive. It only harms you when it runs unchecked without recovery.

☑ **Stress is full-body, not just mental.**

Every surge touches your gut, heart, immune system, and brain. It's physiology, not just psychology.

☑ **Daily micro-restorations > occasional vacations.**

Five minutes of calm daily beats a single "escape" once a year. Stress resets are cumulative.

☑ Sleep is your best stress prescription.

One night of restorative sleep does more for cortisol balance than any supplement.

☑ Consistency rewires your operating system.

Tiny daily practices are what retrain the nervous system — not heroic, one-off efforts.

Stress is not your enemy. It is your operating system. Just as the software on your phone or computer quietly runs processes in the background — giving breath, heart rate, digestion, and blood pressure — But just like software, it can get buggy. Under too much load, with no updates, the system crashes.

The reality is, you cannot simply uninstall stress. You were never meant to. Stress is wired in your being to help you adapt, focus, and survive. What you can do is patch it. Upgrade it. Change the wiring. Each breath reset, every walk in sunlight, every micro-restoration is like giving your system a new update — replacing glitchy coding with resiliency programming.

Imagine your day as a loop of feedback: if you never break the cycle, it continues to rerun the same script — stress → cravings → sleep → stress. But as soon as you put just one reset ritual into place, the feedback loop changes. The system begins to stabilize. Energy stabilizes. Cravings decrease. Recovery expands.

This is the Stress Prescription: not to eliminate stress, but to teach your body to run it wisely, so it no longer runs you.

If stress is your operating system, then movement is your power source. Not punishment. Not burning calories. True life-giving fuel.

Because the way you move — or don't move — tells your nervous system whether you are thriving or under threat. In the next chapter, we will learn how to turn movement into medicine, into joy, and into momentum.

Chapter 8: Move to Thrive, Not to Burn Calories is when you will learn how to stop exercising out of guilt — and start moving as if your life depends on it. Because it does.

CHAPTER 8:

MOVE TO THRIVE, NOT TO BURN CALORIES

PART 1 — WHY WE GOT MOVEMENT WRONG

IT STARTS WITH A TREADMILL.

You've witnessed this scenario a hundred times before:

A late-thirty-something years old man, sweat dripping down his temples, gasping for air, his eyes fixed not on the world outside or the rhythm of his breath but on a glowing red digital number: Calories Burned.

He clenches his jaw as the screen ticks from 298 to 299, waiting for the triumphant flip into the 300s. His body feels like lead, his knees ache, his mind whispers, Almost there. Burn more. Earn it.

And he stops. He gulps down water, limps to the locker room, and an hour later, he is shoving a muffin and a latte into his mouth, which more than negates any "progress" achieved while working out. That treadmill session wasn't joyful, renewing, or even energizing. It was a transaction—a desperate bargain with the calorie counter.

Now, imagine this:

A sixty-something years old woman, walking down the street in her neighborhood at dawn. She is not wearing the latest hybrid shoe technology, nor is she gripping a smartwatch. She walks with freedom and takes in the cool morning air. She encounters her neighbor, who waves to her, and she waves back. When walking by, she stops to pull a weed from her own garden. Grass rustles and birds chirp above her. She does not burn calories; she gathers life.

They both move their bodies.

One is just surviving.

The other is thriving.

MOVEMENT AS PUNISHMENT VS. MOVEMENT AS NOURISHMENT

Somewhere along the way, many of us were taught that movement is a debt payment.

- Did you eat the pizza? Do the spin class.

- You want dessert? Add 30 minutes on the treadmill.

- You're not thin enough? Sweat harder.

We've been conditioned to think of exercise as a math problem, not a love letter to the body. The result? Gyms filled with exhausted, burnt-out people chasing numbers while dreading every step.

But here's the truth that science and anthropology keep shouting back at us: **movement was never meant to be punishment.**

Movement is the most primal signal to your body that you are alive, safe, and thriving.

Your ancestors didn't "work out." They moved because life demanded it — walking miles for water, gathering food, carrying children, dancing around the fire. Movement was not separated from life. It *was* life.

Today, we've broken that bond. We outsource movement to machines, count calories instead of moments, and then wonder why it feels like suffering.

THE CULTURAL PROGRAMMING THAT BROKE US

Think about your first memory of exercise. Was it joy? Play? Or was it gym class drills, weigh-ins, or being told you were too slow, too heavy, too weak?

For many, movement is tied to shame.

- The gym became the place to fix what was "wrong" with your body.

- Fitness magazines told you to "torch fat" or "earn your cheat meal."

- Ads promised a six-pack if you just suffered long enough.

This mindset created an entire generation of movers who equate sweat with suffering, calories with morality, and workouts with penance.

But what if you stripped all that away? What if you stopped counting? What if you didn't move to lose — but to live?

THE SCIENCE THAT CHANGES THE STORY

Here's where the narrative shifts.

Science now tells us that **movement is medicine** far beyond calorie math:

- **Myokines**: Every time your muscles contract, they release signaling proteins called *myokines*. Scientists call them "hope molecules" because they literally bathe your organs and brain in resilience chemistry. They fight inflammation, protect against cancer, boost immunity, and even stimulate new brain cell growth.

- **BDNF (Brain-Derived Neurotrophic Factor)**: Movement releases this powerful molecule that acts like fertilizer for your brain. It improves memory, focus, and mood — literally rewiring your brain for clarity and resilience.

- **Endocannabinoids & Dopamine**: The so-called "runner's high" is real — not just for runners. Even walking or dancing floods your system with feel-good chemicals designed to reduce stress and heighten joy.

- **Mitochondrial Biogenesis**: Movement signals your cells to build new mitochondria — the "power plants" of energy. Translation? You don't just burn fuel; you create energy capacity. You age more slowly. You feel younger.

None of this has to do with a treadmill calorie counter. It's not about burning. It's about **building.**

A STORY THAT MIRRORS US ALL

MEET DAVID.

At 42 years old, a mid-level manager with two children, David is experiencing stress. Every January, he decides to "get fit." He buys a gym membership, downloads a calorie counter app, and forces himself to do tough workouts at five o'clock in the morning. He is burned out by March, his knees hurt, and he's eating junk food to cope with his tiredness. By April, he quits.

David doesn't lack the willpower to be 'conditioned.'

He's trapped in a broken frame.

He was told movement = punishment.

Here is Aisha, a 39-year-old school teacher. Aisha doesn't chase after the ideal at the gym; she walks with her colleague every morning before class, she practices fifteen minutes of bodyweight strength three times a week at home, she dances with her children in the living room on Friday, and she stretches before bed. Every month, she lives feeling stronger, she sleeps better, and her stress goes down.

Aisha isn't "exercising."

She's thriving.

THE EMOTIONAL COST OF THE WRONG FRAME

When movement is punishment, here's what happens:

- You dread it.

- You quit it.

- You build resentment toward your own body.

When movement is nourishment, here's what happens:

- You crave it.

- You keep it.

- You build trust with your body.

One is survival mode.

The other is Thrive Mode.

WHAT IF MOVEMENT WAS JOY?

Pause here.

Take a moment to ask yourself: When was the last time that I moved and I felt joy?

Was it chasing down your child in the yard? Dancing at the wedding? Laughing through a hike with friends? Or perhaps stretching in the morning sun?

Your body remembers those moments. The laughter, the rhythm, the aliveness. That is the blueprint. That is what your biology craves.

This chapter will not teach you how to burn calories. It will not demand that you suffer through endless reps. It will not guilt you into exercise.

This chapter will show you how to move to thrive. To move in a way that signals safety to your nervous system, power to your muscles, clarity to your mind, and joy to your spirit.

The truth is this: Your muscles are not calorie-burning machines; they are longevity organs. They are our shield from illness, our pharmacy of hope molecules, and our passport to a vibrant old age.

And you don't need hours in a gym to unlock them. You need the right frame for it to make sense. You need the Thrive frame.

In the following sections, we will debunk the myth of calorie-counting and explore the science of movement as medicine. We will examine how the body responds differently to punishment vs nourishment. We will deconstruct why the old paradigm fails, and how the new model can literally rewire your brain, your stress response, your energy, and your aging.

And we will begin to create the Thrive Movement Prescription - a model of not restriction, but restoration.

Imagine this: getting up, not dreading your workout, but welcoming the message your body needs to receive. Imagine exercise as play, as power, as joy. Imagine movement as the medicine that adds not just years to your life, but life to your years.

That's where we are headed.

And it begins by rewriting the story.

PART 2 — THE BIOLOGY OF MOVEMENT AS MEDICINE

MOVEMENT AS A SIGNAL, NOT JUST A BURN

Here's the great myth of modern exercise: that its purpose is to erase.

Erase last night's dessert. Erase the softness around your waist. Erase guilt.

But biology tells a different story. Your body doesn't register movement as subtraction. It registers it as **communication.** Every step, every contraction, every stretch whispers signals into your cells, your brain, your immune system.

To your muscles, movement says: "*Build.*"

To your heart, it says: "*Strengthen.*"

To your brain, it says: "*Grow.*"

To your immune system, it says: "*Protect.*"

The burn doesn't erase; it programs. And when you understand that, the treadmill number becomes meaningless. The question isn't "How many calories did I burn?" but **"What message did I send to my body today?"**

THE MUSCLE AS A SECRET PHARMACY

Scientists now call muscle an **endocrine organ** — not just tissue that moves bones. When you contract a muscle, you don't just lift a weight; you release chemical messengers into your bloodstream called **myokines.**

Think of myokines as text messages from your muscles to the rest of your body. Over 600 have been identified so far. Here's what they do:

- **Irisin**: Released during exercise, it stimulates the browning of fat cells, turning them into energy-burning factories (Boström et al., *Nature*, 2012).

- **IL-6 (in its exercise form)**: Lowers inflammation instead of raising it. Unlike the IL-6 released in chronic stress, the exercise-induced form is protective (*Petersen & Pedersen, J Appl Physiol*, 2005).

- **BDNF (Brain-Derived Neurotrophic Factor)**: Encourages neurogenesis — literally the growth of new brain cells. Movement fertilizes your brain.

Each contraction acts like a prescription pad signed by your own body: "Here's a dose of anti-inflammatory, here's a neuroprotective boost, here's a little anti-depressant."

No pharmaceutical company could design such a cocktail. Yet your body does it for free — if you move.

ENERGY FACTORIES AND THE MITOCHONDRIA REBOOT

Your cells carry little power plants called mitochondria. They determine how much energy you feel, how well you burn fuel, and how young your body behaves.

Sedentary living sends these mitochondria a message: "*We don't need much power. Shut it down.*" Movement sends the opposite: "*We need more. Build capacity.*"

This is called **mitochondrial biogenesis** — the creation of new mitochondria. Research shows that endurance activity and strength training both trigger this process (Holloszy, J *Biol Chem*, 1967; later confirmed by Hood et al., J *Physiol*, 2009).

The result?

- More energy.
- Slower cellular aging.
- Greater resilience against fatigue and disease.

Movement doesn't drain your energy. It manufactures it.

THE PARENT WHO FOUND POWER AGAIN

Rina, a 44-year-old woman with three kids, had spent almost all of her life avoiding exercise. "I don't have time," she said, "and I honestly hate it." In the past, exercise was always about punishment. Punishing to lose weight and punishing to burn off the day's stress.

Then one day, at her son's soccer practice, she noticed she could hardly climb the bleachers without wheezing. Later that evening, she decided to try something different. No counting calories. No HIIT workouts that feel like punishments. She simply walked laps around the practice field while her kids practiced, 20 minutes, three times a week.

After two months, she made a surprising discovery: she had more energy at night. She no longer crashed after work. She played with her kids instead of simply watching from the couch. Her blood pressure was lower. Depressive symptoms lifted.

Rina's body didn't respond positively to "calories burned." It responded to a signal. A signal saying: "Build mitochondria. Release myokines. Reset the stress loop."

She was not punishing her body. She was programming her body to live. Of course, when your body is fully thriving and you find out that you enjoy HIIT, without the feeling of punishing yourself, go ahead and maximize it as long as you are enjoying yourself.

MOVEMENT AND THE BRAIN: YOUR ANTIDEPRESSANT IN DISGUISE

Why does a simple walk make you feel better? Because movement rewires your brain chemistry in real time.

- **Endorphins**: The body's opioids, dulling pain and elevating mood.

- **Endocannabinoids**: Molecules similar to cannabis, giving you calm and pleasure without substances.

- **Dopamine**: The motivation molecule. Movement recalibrates dopamine pathways, increasing drive and satisfaction.

- **Serotonin**: Modulated by rhythmic, repetitive exercise — stabilizing mood.

One landmark study (Blumenthal et al., JAMA, 1999) compared exercise to antidepressant medication in patients with major depression. The results? Exercise was **just as effective** at reducing symptoms. Even more powerful, relapse rates were lower in the exercise group months later.

Your body isn't just moving. It's producing a pharmacy of mood stabilizers and resilience boosters.

THE STRESS RESET BUTTON

Modern life keeps us in **sympathetic overdrive** — the fight-or-flight state. Movement, done right, taps the **parasympathetic nervous system** through the vagus nerve.

Slow walks, yoga, swimming, and breathing-based movement activate vagal tone — measured by **HRV (heart rate variability).** Higher HRV = greater resilience to stress.

Animal studies confirm this: voluntary wheel running in rodents reduces HPA-axis hyperactivity (Greenwood et al., *Neuroscience*, 2003). In humans, even light activity buffers cortisol spikes.

When you move, you don't just sweat. You send a message to your nervous system: *"We are safe. We can shift out of crisis mode."*

MOVEMENT AS AN ANTI-INFLAMMATORY PRESCRIPTION

Chronic inflammation underlies nearly every modern disease: diabetes, heart disease, cancer, Alzheimer's.

Sedentary lifestyles fuel it. But exercise acts as a regulator.

Research: Petersen & Pedersen (*Nat Rev Immunol*, 2005) showed that muscle contractions release anti-inflammatory myokines and suppress inflammatory cytokines like TNF-alpha.

Translation?

- Fewer inflammatory sparks.

- Lower risk of chronic disease.

- A body that heals instead of degrades.

Movement isn't just "fitness." It's immune training.

THE LONGEVITY EFFECT

Every long-lived culture on Earth — from Okinawa to Sardinia — has one thing in common: **movement woven into daily life.** Not gyms, not marathons, but continuous, low-intensity, functional activity.

The **Blue Zones** research (Buettner, 2008; Poulain et al., *Exp Gerontol*, 2004) shows that elders who garden, walk, and move naturally into their 90s maintain stronger bodies, sharper minds, and greater social connection.

It isn't about sets, reps, or calories. It's about a lifetime of motion as ritual.

THE SHIFT WORKER

Take Miguel, a 52-year-old nurse. Night shifts left him drained, eating junk food at odd hours, and battling creeping blood pressure. He thought he needed a hardcore workout plan, but he didn't have the time or energy.

Instead, his doctor recommended "movement snacks": 10 squats before every break, two minutes of stair climbing between rounds, and a five-minute stretch before bed.

Six months later, his labs improved. His sleep deepened. His mood stabilized.

Miguel didn't "burn" much. But he **signaled** enough — to his mitochondria, to his immune system, to his brain. His operating system was rewired.

FROM BURN TO THRIVE: THE REFRAME

When you zoom out, the truth crystallizes:

- Movement is not about erasing what you ate.

- It's about instructing your biology to adapt, heal, and thrive.

Every step, squat, or stretch is a data packet your body processes: build more mitochondria, release protective myokines, grow new neurons, balance stress.

The Thrive Frame doesn't ask: *"How many calories did you burn?"* It asks: *"What medicine did you dose your body with today?"*

Now that you've seen how movement works at the molecular and systemic level, the next question is: **Where should you start?**

The answer doesn't begin with a gym membership or an hour of HIIT. It begins with understanding *which kinds* of movement deliver which signals — and how to blend them into a prescription that feels like joy, not punishment.

That's where we go next: **Sunlight + Nature** — the overlooked movement medicine hiding in plain sight.

PART 3 — SUNLIGHT + NATURE: THE FORGOTTEN PRESCRIPTION

THE MOMENT YOU STEP OUTSIDE

Close your eyes for a second and imagine this:

It's 7:00 a.m. You step outside barefoot onto the cool grass. The air carries that faint bite of morning chill, and the horizon glows with first light. Your eyes meet the rising sun. Within minutes, your biology begins to shift.

- Cortisol rises naturally, syncing your wake-up signal.

- Melatonin, the sleep hormone, is shut off.

- Dopamine and serotonin pathways are activated.

- Your body clock — the circadian rhythm — locks into gear.

This is not just "fresh air." This is medicine—a prescription written not by a pharmaceutical company but by four billion years of evolution.

WHY LIGHT IS THE MASTER SWITCH

Your body runs on a 24-hour cycle. At its center is the **suprachiasmatic nucleus (SCN)** in your brain — your biological "master clock."

The SCN takes its orders from **light.**

When light hits the retina, it travels through a dedicated pathway to the SCN, telling your brain: *"It's morning. Time to wake up. Reset everything."*

Here's what happens next:

- **Cortisol rises** in the morning — not the "toxic stress" cortisol, but the healthy surge that gives you energy and focus.

- **Melatonin drops** so your body knows it's daytime.

- **Peripheral clocks** in your liver, pancreas, gut, and muscles synchronize with the master clock.

Research confirms: even **10 minutes of outdoor morning light** stabilizes circadian rhythms (Khalsa et al., *J Clin Invest*, 2003).

The modern problem? Most people wake up and look at their phone before they look at the sky. Screens don't carry the same full-spectrum cues as sunlight. The result: circadian drift. Foggy mornings. Cravings at night. A weakened stress response.

THE OFFICE WORKER

Let's talk about a woman named Elena, a 36-year-old graphic designer. She habitually woke up feeling tired. She would gulp down coffee at her desk, and then as dusk approached, she'd become wired and spend hours doomscrolling in bed.

230

Then, to her surprise, her doctor proposed an odd solution: "Before you open your laptop, try opening your front door."

So every morning, regardless of the weather, she went outside for 10 minutes. And after a few weeks, she started noticing a kind of weird phenomenon.

She woke up feeling more natural.

The dreaded energy drop in the afternoons disappeared.

The late-night snack cravings dwindled.

Her sleep deepened.

Her body wasn't just "getting air," but was instead syncing her body clock to the oldest form of life: the sun.

THE STRESS BUFFER OF NATURE

Beyond light, **nature itself** rewires the stress response. The Japanese call it **Shinrin-yoku** — forest bathing. Simply being among trees lowers cortisol, heart rate, and blood pressure.

A landmark study (Park et al., *Environ Health Prev Med*, 2010) measured cortisol in participants who walked in forests vs. city streets. Results? Cortisol dropped 15% more in forest walkers.

Other findings:

- Natural settings lower sympathetic nervous system activity (fight-or-flight).

- They increase parasympathetic tone (rest-and-digest).

- Immune function rises, with higher natural killer cell activity (Li et al., *Int J Immunopathol Pharmacol*, 2009).

The prescription is simple: green time, not just screen time.

SUNLIGHT AND MOOD MOLECULES

Light doesn't just regulate sleep. It programs your **mood**.

- **Serotonin**: Morning light boosts serotonin, stabilizing mood and appetite (Lambert et al., *Lancet*, 2002).

- **Dopamine**: Light exposure to the retina modulates dopamine in brain circuits — crucial for motivation.

- **Seasonal Affective Disorder (SAD)**: Caused by lack of winter sunlight; treated successfully with light therapy boxes mimicking morning sun.

Translation? Your body literally "drinks" light the way it drinks water. Without it, mood wilts.

THE INFLAMMATORY LINK

Stress and inflammation walk hand in hand. Sunlight helps break the cycle.

- **Vitamin D**: Produced by UVB rays, regulates over 200 genes, many linked to immune and mood function (Holick, NEJM, 2007).

- **Nitric Oxide Release**: Sunlight triggers nitric oxide from skin, lowering blood pressure (Liu et al., *J Invest Dermatol*, 2014).

- **Cytokine balance**: Outdoor exposure reduces inflammatory cytokines that rise during chronic stress.

It's not just the forest. Even the **sun on your skin** is part of the anti-stress pharmacy.

ACTION STEP 1: THE 10-MINUTE RULE

Tomorrow morning, before screens, go outside for **10 minutes**. No sunglasses, no glass between you and the sky. Look toward the horizon, not at the sun directly.

Science suggests this is enough to:

- Boost cortisol at the right time.
- Lock the circadian rhythm.
- Improve mood within a week.

ACTION STEP 2: THE GREEN BREAK

Set a 5-minute alarm at lunch. Go outside, even if it's just standing by a tree in a parking lot. Drop your phone in your pocket. Breathe.

Your nervous system doesn't need wilderness. It needs *anything living: a* tree, a patch of grass, a garden bed.

ACTION STEP 3: THE WEEKEND FOREST DOSE

Once a week, replace one indoor activity with an outdoor one: hiking, gardening, beach walking, or cycling. Studies show that as little as **120 minutes in nature per week** significantly improves well-being (White et al., *Sci Rep*, 2019).

Movement is medicine. But when you take it **outside, in light and nature**, the dose multiplies. You're not just burning calories or building strength; you're syncing with the rhythm of the planet, dialing down inflammation, and reminding your nervous system what safety feels like.

And here's the kicker: the benefits compound. The more consistently you anchor your body in sunlight and nature, the more resistant you become to the storms of stress.

But what happens when stress is unrelenting — when it doesn't just stay in your mind but seeps into your biology, your gut, your immune system?

That's the next frontier: **The Body Under Siege.** Stress doesn't just make you tense — it rewrites your inner ecosystem.

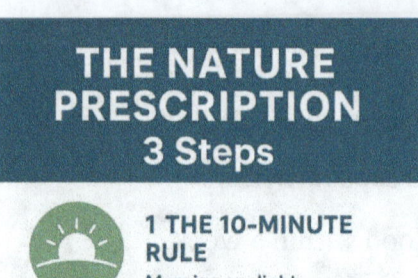

THE NATURE PRESCRIPTION
3 Steps

1 THE 10-MINUTE RULE
Morning sunlight, before screens

2 THE GREEN BREAK
5 minutes outside at lunch

3 THE WEEKEND FOREST DOSE
120 minutes outside a week

PART 4 — THE BODY UNDER SIEGE

THE SILENT WAR WITHIN

Picture this: Maria, our beloved middle-school teacher we've introduced in these chapters, arrives home after a long day. She leaves her bag by the door and sits back on the couch. Her smartwatch buzzes, displaying 3,142 steps for the day. She sighs, fully aware of how far away she is from her long-ago goal of 10,000 steps. She scrolls through her phone, eats dinner while watching TV, and remains seated until sleep calls.

Under the surface, Maria's night looks entirely harmless. But within her own body, a much different reality is unfolding:

Muscles that have been unused for hours are now messaging her brain that the priority is about energy storage, not energy burning.

Blood sugar from the pasta she had for dinner will rise higher and stay elevated longer because her leg and core muscles, which are the body's largest glucose "sinks," are inactive. Her gut microbes sense the sedentary lull, producing fewer mood-supportive short-chain fatty acids.

Cortisol, which was already high after a stressful day of teaching, can't be cleared as efficiently because the body isn't getting the movement it normally uses as a buffer.

It's almost as if Maria's body is under siege, but not by an invader, but rather the very absence of movement.

THE PHYSIOLOGY OF INACTIVITY: A BREAKDOWN

1. Metabolic Gridlock

a. When muscles are idle, glucose transporters (GLUT-4) in muscle cells remain locked inside, instead of coming to the surface to draw sugar out of the bloodstream.

b. This means blood sugar lingers, insulin spikes harder, and over time, cells grow resistant to insulin's call.

c. A landmark NASA study in the 1970s showed that even young, healthy men confined to bed rest developed insulin resistance and lost muscle mass within days.

2. Inflammatory Cascade

a. Sedentary living triggers the release of pro-inflammatory cytokines — tiny "fire signals" in the bloodstream.

b. Without muscle contraction, the body misses out on *myokines* — anti-inflammatory molecules secreted during movement. Myokines like IL-6 (in its exercise form) calm inflammation and support brain health.

c. Without them, the balance tilts toward chronic, smoldering inflammation — the kind that underlies heart disease, diabetes, and depression.

3. Circulatory Stagnation

a. Movement acts as a second heart: contracting muscles squeeze veins, helping pump blood back to the chest. When you sit too long, circulation slows, blood pools, and clotting risks rise.

b. After just 90 minutes of uninterrupted sitting, markers of vascular function decline measurably (Thosar et al., *Medicine & Science in Sports & Exercise*, 2015).

4. Neurochemical Fallout

a. Movement boosts dopamine and serotonin, neurotransmitters that stabilize mood and motivation. Without it, the brain's chemical balance tilts toward fatigue, irritability, and cravings.

b. Chronic inactivity is linked with hippocampal shrinkage (the brain's memory center), while regular activity enhances neurogenesis (new brain cell growth).

THE WRONG KIND OF MOVEMENT: OVERDRIVE AS A STRESS AMPLIFIER

The siege doesn't only come from stillness. Sometimes, it comes from too much of the wrong type of movement.

- **HIIT at the wrong time:** Late-night high-intensity workouts spike cortisol, delay melatonin release, and impair sleep.

- **Overtraining syndrome:** Chronic high-volume training without recovery drives up inflammatory cytokines and suppresses immune function.

- **The paradox of punishment workouts:** Many people, especially when stressed, turn to punishing exercise as a "detox" for food guilt. Instead of relieving stress, this amplifies it, embedding movement in the same shame cycle as food.

Science echoes this balance: movement is medicine, but dose and timing matter. Like any prescription, too little fails to heal, too much harms.

SCIENCE SPOTLIGHT: THE SIEGE TIMELINE

- **Day 1 of Sedentary Life:** Blood sugar spikes higher, insulin works harder.

- **Day 2–3:** Muscles lose measurable insulin sensitivity; calorie burn drops.

- **Week 1:** VO_2 max (a measure of fitness) declines; triglycerides rise.

- **Week 2–3:** Inflammatory markers increase, and HDL cholesterol declines.

- **Month 1+:** Mood worsens, sleep deteriorates, and microbiome diversity shrinks.

BREAKING THE SIEGE: MOVEMENT AS ARMOR

If inactivity wages war, then movement is armor. But the key insight is this: armor doesn't need to be forged in heroic, hour-long gym sessions. It can be woven from minutes of light walking, stretching, or stair climbing throughout the day.

- A 2-minute walking break every 30 minutes restores blood sugar control to near-normal levels (Dunstan et al., *Diabetes Care*, 2012).

- Light activity after meals lowers post-meal blood sugar as effectively as some medications.

- Even "non-exercise activity thermogenesis" (NEAT) — fidgeting, standing, carrying groceries — contributes to resilience against the siege.

MARIA'S PIVOT

Let's return to Maria. One week, she decides to experiment: instead of collapsing on the couch after dinner, she takes a ten-minute walk in the neighborhood. Initially, it feels insignificant. But by the end of the week, she notices a change: less bloating by the evening, deeper sleep, and a reduction in morning sensitivity.

Beneath the surface, the siege is easing:

Glucose is being cleared more efficiently.

Cortisol is decreasing with the sunset.

Her gut microbes are producing more butyrate, a mood-stabilizing short-chain fatty acid.

Maria is no longer just surviving the siege. She is building her armor.

We've seen how the absence (or misapplication) of movement places the body under siege, transforming stress into chronic disease and eroding resilience. But if movement is medicine, and the wrong movement is poison, then how do we prescribe it correctly?

That leads us directly into **Part 5: The Movement Prescription — Practical Frameworks for Thriving.**

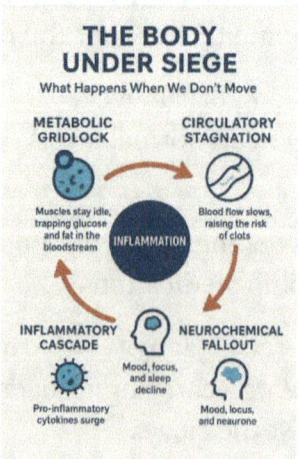

PART 5: THE MOVEMENT PRESCRIPTION —
PRACTICAL FRAMEWORKS FOR THRIVING

For many, the word "exercise" conjures images of treadmills whirring away in fluorescent-lit gyms, sweat pooling on a yoga mat, or the relentless voice of a fitness influencer repeating, "No more excuses!"

But what if exercise were not something we have to do?

What if it was something your biology craved, a prescription written not by a trainer, but by your cells, your heart, and your brain?

That is the reframing of The Movement Prescription; it is not punishment, and not calorie calculations or guilt. It is medicine, coded into your DNA, waiting to be unlocked. And we will unpack the dose, frequency, and type.

This section is your blueprint. It scaffolds ancient wisdom with modern science, stitching together the stories of everyday individuals who have rebuilt their health, revitalized their energy, and transferred their well-being with sustainable and enjoyable patterns of movement that transform into thriving regimens.

FRAMEWORK 1: THE DAILY RHYTHM RESET (CIRCADIAN ANCHORING WITH MOVEMENT)

One of the most powerful levers you have isn't just *what* kind of movement you do—it's *when* you do it. Your muscles, mitochondria, and metabolism run on circadian clocks. Just like your brain syncs to light, your muscles sync to motion.

THE SCIENCE

- A 2019 study in *Cell Metabolism* found that exercising in the morning improved insulin sensitivity and fat oxidation more effectively than the same workout at night.

- Conversely, strength gains may peak in the late afternoon, when body temperature and reaction times are highest (*Frontiers in Physiology*, 2018).

THE PRESCRIPTION

- **Morning Movement:** 5–15 minutes of low-intensity movement (walk, mobility, yoga). Anchors your cortisol awakening response, stabilizes appetite hormones.

- **Afternoon Strength:** If you lift or train, late afternoon may give you peak performance.

- **Evening Calm:** Gentle stretching or walking after dinner helps digestion and prevents blood sugar spikes (*Diabetes Care*, 2016).

NARRATIVE

Maria, the teacher from earlier chapters, had tried "bootcamp" workouts at 9 p.m.—they left her wired and sleepless. Once she shifted to morning walks and afternoon bodyweight sessions, her cravings decreased, and her sleep deepened.

FRAMEWORK 2: MOVEMENT SNACKS (MICRO-DOSES THAT ADD UP)

Forget the "hour at the gym" rule. Your mitochondria don't keep score in 60-minute blocks.

THE SCIENCE

- Sitting for more than 30–60 minutes stiffens blood vessels and reduces glucose uptake in muscles (*Diabetologia*, 2014).

- A 2–3 minute walking break every half hour lowers blood sugar and blood pressure (*British Journal of Sports Medicine*, 2020).

THE PRESCRIPTION

- **Every 30–60 min:** Stand, stretch, walk to refill water.

- **2–5 min snacks:** Bodyweight squats, calf raises, desk push-ups, or stair climbs.

- **Daily baseline:** Aim for at least 6,000–8,000 steps, even if broken up.

NARRATIVE

Think of your day like a symphony. Instead of waiting for one grand crescendo at the gym, movement snacks are the beats and rhythms that keep the music alive.

FRAMEWORK 3: THE STRESS RESET (MOVEMENT AS EMOTIONAL MEDICINE)

Exercise isn't just for muscles—it's for your mind. Movement metabolizes stress.

THE SCIENCE

- Moderate aerobic activity reduces cortisol and increases brain-derived neurotrophic factor (BDNF), which improves resilience against depression (PNAS, 2011).

- Exercise stimulates endocannabinoids ("the runner's high"), which regulate mood and pain perception (*NeuroReport*, 2003).

THE PRESCRIPTION

- **When anxious:** Try rhythmic movement (walking, cycling) for 10–20 minutes.

- **When angry:** Channel with intensity—boxing bag, sprint intervals.

- **When low:** Gentle stretching, restorative yoga, or even dancing in your living room.

NARRATIVE

James, a firefighter, used to drink whiskey after stressful shifts. Now, he takes a 15-minute walk around the block instead. He calls it "bleeding the stress valve."

FRAMEWORK 4: FUNCTIONAL LONGEVITY TRAINING

Forget six-pack abs. What keeps you independent at 80? Strength, balance, and mobility.

THE SCIENCE

- Resistance training improves insulin sensitivity, lowers the risk of type 2 diabetes, and preserves bone density (*Journal of Bone and Mineral Research*, 2017).

- Grip strength is one of the strongest predictors of longevity (*The Lancet*, 2015).

THE PRESCRIPTION

- **2–3x per week:** Strength training (bodyweight, resistance bands, weights).

- **Daily:** Balance and mobility work (single-leg stance, hip openers).

- **Rule of thumb:** Train movements, not just muscles: push, pull, squat, hinge, carry.

NARRATIVE

In Okinawa, one of the Blue Zones, elders squat to the ground multiple times per day into their 80s and 90s. Their "functional training" is embedded in life.

FRAMEWORK 5: JOYFUL MOVEMENT (THE PLAY PROTOCOL)

Exercise you hate is medicine you'll never take. The most powerful prescription is the one you *look forward to.*

THE SCIENCE

- Enjoyment predicts long-term exercise adherence better than weight-loss goals (*Health Psychology*, 2014).

- Dancing has been shown to improve memory, coordination, and reduce dementia risk (*Frontiers in Human Neuroscience*, 2017).

THE PRESCRIPTION

- **Choose joy > calories.** Pick what excites you—tennis, swimming, gardening, or salsa.

- **Anchor in community.** Group activity doubles adherence.

- **Play weekly.** At least one session purely for fun, not fitness metrics.

NARRATIVE

Remember being a kid, playing tag until the streetlights came on? That's the spirit to reclaim. Maria started Zumba once a week—not to burn fat, but to laugh and move with friends.

ACTION STEP BOX: THE 5 MOVES OF THE MOVEMENT PRESCRIPTION

☑ Anchor movement to your circadian rhythm (morning, afternoon, evening).

☑ Snack on movement every 30–60 minutes.

☑ Use exercise as a stress reset tool.

☑ Train for longevity: strength, balance, mobility.

☑ Prioritize joy: if you hate it, you'll quit it.

The Movement Prescription is not about punishment. It's about freedom—freedom from the chair, freedom from chronic disease, freedom from the shame-driven fitness narrative.

Your body doesn't want perfection. It wants rhythm, variety, and joy. The same way a garden thrives with sun, water, and care, your body thrives when you feed it movement—daily, consistently, with gratitude.

This is how you move not to burn calories, but to **thrive**.

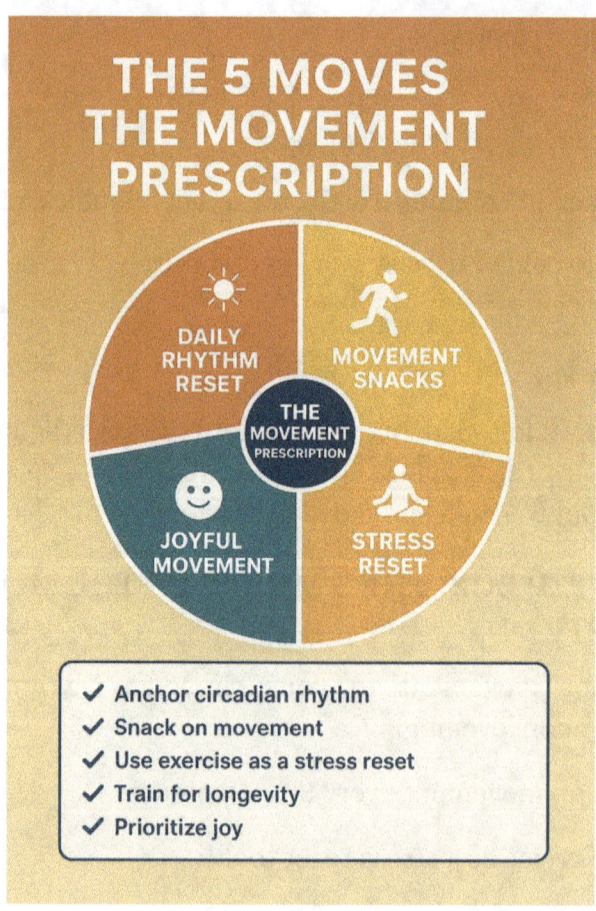

PART 6 — ACTION STARTER: YOUR MOVE TO THRIVE DAY

You don't need a gym membership to start thriving body movements. You don't need a spreadsheet of calories. What you need is one single day to prove to your body what's possible. One day to feel the electricity of movement the way it was meant to be: not punishment, not debt repayment, but communication. A conversation between you and your biology.

Think of this as a *reset script* for your nervous system, your hormones, your microbiome, and your brain. It's a way of sending signals that whisper: *You're alive. You're safe. You're meant to thrive.*

MORNING: SUNLIGHT + MOBILITY WAKE-UP

- **Action:** Step outside within 30 minutes of waking. Walk for 5–10 minutes in the morning light. Then, roll your shoulders, open your chest, and do a simple mobility stretch (hip circles, spinal twists, or a yoga sun salutation).

- **Why it works:**

    o Morning light anchors your *circadian clock*, balancing cortisol rhythms and setting up better sleep at night (Huberman, 2021).

    o Gentle stretching and walking awaken lymphatic circulation, decrease stiffness, and prime dopamine pathways for motivation.

- **Narrative:** Picture Maria (our teacher). Instead of scrolling her phone in bed, she slips outside, coffee in hand. The cool air on her face, the first rays of light hitting her eyes — her brain registers "*daytime.*" Her cortisol spike is synced instead of chaotic. Already, her body feels steadier.

MIDDAY: THE STRENGTH SNACK

- **Action:** Between classes, meetings, or emails, drop into a "strength snack": 1–2 minutes of bodyweight movement (push-ups against a desk, squats, resistance band pulls).

- **Why it works:**

  o Strength work activates *myokines* — signaling molecules from muscle that lower inflammation and boost brain-derived neurotrophic factor (BDNF), supporting mood and memory (Pedersen, Nat Rev Endocrinol, 2019).

  o "Snacks" of exercise are shown to improve metabolic flexibility as effectively as longer sessions spread across a week.

- **Narrative:** At 1:15 p.m., Maria shuts her laptop, pushes her chair back, and does a slow set of squats. Her heart rate rises, her posture opens, her brain fog lifts. That one minute wasn't "burning calories." It was telling her metabolism to stay flexible.

AFTERNOON: NEAT BREAK (NON-EXERCISE ACTIVITY THERMOGENESIS)

- **Action:** Take the stairs, stand during a call, walk while dictating a note. Aim for at least one 5–10 minute "moving break" in the afternoon slump.

- **Why it works:**

  o NEAT (incidental movement) accounts for hundreds of daily calories burned without ever "exercising." But more importantly, it stabilizes glucose levels and reduces post-lunch crashes (Levine, Science, 2005).

  o Short bouts of walking after meals reduce blood sugar spikes as effectively as certain diabetes medications.

- **Narrative:** Maria feels the mid-afternoon fog rolling in. Instead of grabbing chips, she takes a phone call outside, pacing up and down the sidewalk. By the time she returns, the craving storm has passed, her blood sugar is steadier, and her mood feels reset.

EVENING: PLAYFUL MOVEMENT

- **Action:** Replace "end-of-day collapse" with 15–30 minutes of playful movement—dance in the living room. Kick a soccer ball with your kids. Stretch out in yoga.

- **Why it works:**

  o Evening movement lowers sympathetic nervous system activity, easing stress while raising serotonin and endorphins.

  o Playful exercise activates *mirror neurons* and reward circuits — making the brain associate movement with joy, not punishment.

- **Narrative:** Instead of collapsing on the couch with Netflix, Maria puts on music while she cooks dinner. She and her daughter laugh as they dance barefoot across the kitchen tiles. Her body gets its workout, but more importantly, her nervous system gets its joy prescription.

QUICK-REFERENCE CHECKLIST

☑ **Morning:** 10-min sunlight walk + stretch

☑ **Midday:** 1-2 min "strength snack" (push-ups, squats, bands)

☑ **Afternoon:** NEAT break — stairs, walking call, movement micro-dose

☑ **Evening:** Playful movement (dance, yoga, sports, family activity)

💡 *Remember: Move to send life signals, not calorie math.*

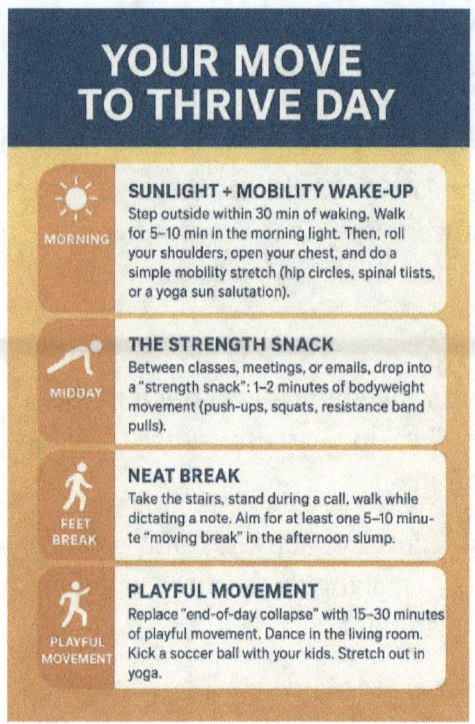

Movement isn't just about strength, endurance, or burning calories—it's communication. Every step, every stretch, every deep breath after a hill climb tells your biology a story: *"I am alive. I am capable. I am safe."*

When you move, you're not punishing your body—you're affirming its resilience. Your muscles become chemical messengers, releasing myokines that calm inflammation, sharpen focus, and elevate mood. Your heart rate variability rises, signaling adaptability. Your bones, joints, and connective tissue quietly remodel, whispering, *"We are preparing for tomorrow."*

Think about that: your body listens to every signal. It interprets stillness as fragility and decline, but it interprets movement as vitality and hope. The difference between decay and thriving is often the difference between stagnation and motion.

And here lies the real prescription: **movement is medicine, and your muscles are your fountain of youth.** Every time you choose to walk after dinner instead of scrolling, to stretch before bed instead of collapsing into exhaustion, or to play with your kids instead of watching from the sidelines, you are rewriting the script of your future.

This is not about being an athlete. It's about being *human*, in alignment with the blueprint we evolved for. It's about reclaiming the birthright of strength, mobility, and energy that our modern sedentary culture quietly robs from us.

So as we close this chapter, remember: **your movements are your medicine, and the more you prescribe them daily, the more your body thrives.**

But movement is only half the story. Imagine having a powerful switch inside your body—one that could reset inflammation, restore insulin sensitivity, repair cellular damage, and sharpen your mind. A switch our ancestors used daily, but we have almost forgotten in our modern, always-fed world.

That switch is **fasting**—an ancient biological superpower now being rediscovered by science.

In the next chapter, we'll explore **The Intermittent Fasting Blueprint: Healing Effects of Fasting and Rediscovering an Ancient Superpower**—how aligning with nature's rhythm of eating and pausing can heal, energize, and unlock resilience you didn't know was inside you.

MOVEMENT AS MEDICINE RECAP

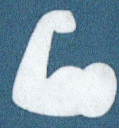
MUSCLES
Myokines strengthen and heal

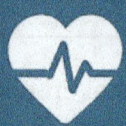
HEART
HRV rises, signaling adaptability

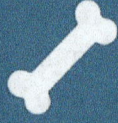
BONES
Resilience, strength, and repair

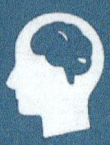
BRAIN
Mood boost, sharper cognition

CHAPTER 9:

THE INTERMITTENT FASTING BLUEPRINT

PART 1: THE FORGOTTEN SUPERPOWER

The fire has nearly quenched. The shadows dance on the stone walls while distant creatures stir in the night. A small group of early humans huddles together in the warmth. Their bellies are empty, but their senses are alert. They have not eaten since yesterday. This time tomorrow, they will wander in a wide arc across the savanna, spears and woven nets in hand, to hunt for game or gather roots. They will continue for hours with little to show for it. But they will not swoon in frailty. They do not panic. Their bodies are not designed to collapse from hunger. They are built to sharpen.

In this nightly cadence of sleep-rise-search-eat-rest-repeat, fasting was not a choice. It was life. And it was not only survivable. In those long hours without food, the body orchestrated a hidden symphony: sharpening attention, mobilizing fat stores, preserving muscle, and activating cellular repair. Hunger was not an enemy but a signal — one that tuned their body for survival.

Fast forward 50 thousand years, and we can imagine one of those humans from the distant past wandering into an ultra-modern kitchen in the midnight hour. Fluorescent lights shine bright. The refrigerator hums, overflowing with leftovers, sodas, condiments, and cheese sticks. A few feet away, the pantry moans under the weight of chips, crackers, and granola bars. In the corner, a glowing rectangle stands by offering delivery of pizza, ice cream, or curry in a blink, all without stepping outside. In this world we are living today, fasting is no longer the baseline of life. It is nearly extinct.

THE GREAT REVERSAL

What was a normal cycle of fasting and eating has now flipped. We eat from the moment that we rise until minutes before we sleep. Some have snacks at their bedside. Data from food logging apps show the average person grazes for 15-16 hours per day, and only has a sliver of "fasting" at night, often only 7-8 hours. Our ancestors' bodies, forged in scarcity and rhythm, are now flooded with round-the-clock abundance.

AND HERE LIES THE TENSION:

The body you live in was designed for fasting. The only thing unnatural is the endless feeding we now call "normal."

This is the forgotten superpower — fasting not as deprivation or a diet trend, but as a biological rhythm baked into human evolution. A switch that activates repair. A pause that restores balance. A cycle that keeps us resilient.

FASTING AS A RHYTHM, NOT A FAD

In the modern world, "fasting" has been hijacked by hashtags and headlines. You've seen it: 16:8 *Intermittent Fasting Will Melt Fat*, *The One Meal A Day Hack*, *Fast Like Celebrities*. This packaging makes fasting sound like a Silicon Valley invention or a biohacker's experiment. But strip away the marketing gloss, and fasting is as ancient as fire. Every creature on Earth — from fruit flies to elephants — lives in cycles of eating and not eating. Cells depend on these cycles. Genes activate in these cycles. Hormones rise and fall in these cycles.

When you fast, you're not doing something extreme. You're returning to baseline. You're aligning with the same rhythm that allowed your ancestors to thrive, the same rhythm that let your body evolve into what it is today.

WHY FASTING DISAPPEARED

If fasting is so natural, why do we seem to struggle with it today? The answer is brutal, but straightforward: our environment has been rewired against us. The modern food environment is so hyper-optimized and engineered to obliterate pauses. Processed snacks are sold as "mini-meals." Coffee shops open at 5 a.m. and offer muffins the size of a child's head. Gas stations promise "fuel" at every corner, though most of it is sugar and seed oil. Work culture rewards hustling at your desk with energy bars instead of meals. The kitchen light never turns off.

For most people, the longest fasted window isn't even intentional; it's just the stretch of sleep between late-night snacks and breakfast. That is not rhythm. That is decay. And the cost of these decays manifests in ways such as insulin resistance, obesity, extreme fatigue, unstable moods, and chronic systemic inflammation. Our biology is screaming for a pause button, and instead we just keep hitting "play."

A BODY BUILT FOR PAUSE

Consider what occurs when you don't eat breakfast. The body doesn't shut down. It doesn't self-destruct immediately. The body merely does what it was designed to do. Switches fuel sources, uses up glycogen and fat, sharpens attention, boosts norepinephrine and growth hormone, and turns on repair pathways like autophagy. That quiet biological movement, the metabolic switch, is not starvation. It's survival architecture. It's resilience.

In fact, many of today's health issues, from type 2 diabetes to fatty liver, from brain fog to premature aging, are not from hunger but from its absence. From never letting the body access that second gear. From forgetting the rhythm of feast and fast.

THE REDISCOVERY

Around the world, fasting traditions never fully disappeared. Muslims observe Ramadan. Christians have Lent. Jews fast for Yom Kippur. Buddhists often avoid evening meals. These rituals are not accidents; they echo ancient wisdom that fasting is not only survivable but purifying. Modern science is now catching up, showing that time-restricted eating, intermittent fasting, and longer fasting protocols can:

- Improve insulin sensitivity

- Reduce inflammation

- Enhance cellular repair (autophagy, mitophagy)

- Boost mental clarity through ketone production

- Even triggering the immune system "reboots" in certain conditions

In other words, the "fad" is actually the foundation.

THE BLUEPRINT AHEAD

This chapter is about remembering. About taking fasting out of the domain of gimmick diets and placing it where it belongs: as one of your body's deepest biological blueprints for resilience.

We'll walk through the science of what happens hour by hour in a fast. We'll explore how fasting affects men and women differently, and how to choose rhythms that honor those differences. We'll decode how fasting taps into the molecular machinery of repair and longevity. And most importantly, we'll give you a practical roadmap to begin reclaiming this rhythm — without turning it into punishment, obsession, or self-denial.

This is not about white-knuckling hunger. It's about rediscovering an ancient superpower.

Your body already remembers how to fast. It's waiting for you to remember, too.

PART 2 — THE BIOLOGY OF FASTING

(WHAT HAPPENS WHEN YOU STOP EATING)

Imagine this: Dinner is done at 7:00 PM—a hearty meal of salmon, roasted vegetables, and quinoa. You tidy up your dishes, brush your teeth, and settle into the evening. This is when the clock starts. Not the wall clock — your internal metabolic clock. From this moment on, a quiet cascade of biological shifts begins to unfold.

The story of fasting is not about absence. It's about a choreography. Hormones, enzymes, and genes turn on and off in sequence, like instruments coming in and out in a symphony.

Now let's walk through the timeline.

HOUR 0–4: THE FED STATE — THE "ENERGY STORAGE" WINDOW

After eating, your body prioritizes digestion and storage. Blood glucose rises, insulin is released, and cells are encouraged to pull nutrients in.

- **Insulin surge:** Insulin acts like a traffic cop, directing glucose into muscle and liver, and steering excess into fat cells.

- **Nutrients flood:** Amino acids from protein are shuttled into the muscle. Fatty acids are packaged into triglycerides. Glycogen stores in the liver and muscles top off.

- **Metabolic note:** Your body is "in storage mode." This is why constant grazing prevents fasting's benefits — insulin never gets a break.

Science snapshot: A 2017 review in *Cell Metabolism* showed that insulin spikes not only regulate blood sugar but also actively suppress fat breakdown (lipolysis). Only when insulin falls does fat burning accelerate.

HOUR 4–12: THE POST-ABSORPTIVE PHASE — SWITCHING FUELS

By 4–6 hours after your last bite, digestion winds down. Insulin begins to drop. The body transitions from burning mostly glucose to tapping stored fuels.

- **Glycogen drawdown:** The liver releases glucose to maintain blood sugar.

- **Fatty acids released:** With low insulin, fat cells are unlocked, releasing fatty acids into circulation.

- **Brain on alert:** Rising norepinephrine (noradrenaline) sharpens attention — an ancient survival mechanism during hunger.

Case vignette: Tom, a night-shift worker, once feared skipping meals would wreck his focus. Yet when he allowed a 12-hour overnight fast, he noticed his mornings were sharper, not foggier. His brain wasn't "shutting down" — it was flipping to a built-in alert system fueled by stored fat.

HOUR 12–16: THE METABOLIC SWITCH — FAT BURNING IGNITES

Around the 12-hour mark, the body switches into 'fasting mode.' Glycogen stores begin to deplete, and fat metabolism starts to ramp up.

- **Ketone trickle:** The liver begins producing ketone bodies (beta-hydroxybutyrate, acetoacetate) from fatty acids.

- **Hormone shift:** Growth hormone rises, preserving muscle and mobilizing fat.

- **Repair genes awaken:** SIRT1, often called the "longevity gene," is upregulated, enhancing DNA repair and anti-inflammatory pathways.

Science spotlight: A 2019 *New England Journal of Medicine* review (de Cabo & Mattson) detailed how fasting activates adaptive cellular stress responses — improving mitochondrial function, antioxidant defenses, and DNA repair.

HOUR 16–24: KETONES CLIMB, AUTOPHAGY SPARKS

This is where the real magic begins. By 16–20 hours, ketone levels rise more significantly. Your body begins deep maintenance work.

- **Autophagy activation:** Cells begin recycling damaged proteins and organelles, clearing debris that, if unchecked, leads to disease.

- **Immune modulation:** Inflammatory cytokines decline, while immune surveillance improves.

- **Mental clarity:** Many fasters report a mental "lift" — ketones provide stable energy to the brain, often described as clean, focused fuel.

Narrative vignette: *Maria, the teacher we've followed, first feared fasting would trigger her late-night binges. But when she extended her eating pause to 16 hours, she noticed a paradox — cravings shrank. Instead of collapsing into chips, her evenings became calmer, her mind clearer. The pause was not punishment. It was permission to reset.*

HOUR 24–48: DEEP REPAIR MODE

At the 24-hour mark and beyond, the fasting state enters deeper layers of repair.

- **Autophagy intensifies:** Misfolded proteins are dismantled. Damaged mitochondria are recycled. This "cellular housekeeping" is central to fasting's anti-aging reputation.

- **Stem cell activation:** In longer fasts, stem cells in the gut and immune system show signs of renewal (Longo et al., *Cell Stem Cell*, 2014).

- **Growth hormone peak:** Up to 5x baseline, preserving lean tissue.

- **Insulin sensitivity reset:** With glycogen depleted, muscles become more responsive to insulin once refeeding occurs.

Science spotlight: Yoshinori Ohsumi won the 2016 Nobel Prize in Medicine for his work on autophagy, showing how this cellular "self-eating" process is essential for survival and longevity.

HORMONES IN THE FASTING SYMPHONY

INSULIN

- Falls steadily, allowing fat burning and autophagy.
- Chronic high insulin (from grazing) blocks this switch.

GLUCAGON

- Rises as insulin falls, telling the liver to release glucose and produce ketones.

CORTISOL

- Gently rises in the morning, in a fasted state — not a stress problem, but part of the circadian rhythm that sharpens wakefulness.

GHRELIN

- The "hunger hormone." Interestingly, ghrelin rises in waves, then falls — meaning hunger comes in pulses, not a straight climb. Studies show ghrelin adapts within days of fasting, making hunger easier to manage.

GROWTH HORMONE

- Surges during fasting, countering muscle breakdown and supporting fat mobilization.

THE GUT'S ROLE IN FASTING

The microbiome doesn't sit idle. During fasting windows:

- Certain microbial populations flourish, especially those linked to fat metabolism.

- Fasting strengthens the gut lining, reducing "leaky gut" permeability.

- Animal studies show fasting cycles increase microbial diversity, a hallmark of resilience.

MISCONCEPTIONS ABOUT FASTING

1. **"Fasting means muscle loss."**
   Wrong — short-term fasting increases growth hormone and preserves lean mass—only prolonged, extreme fasting risks muscle breakdown.

2. **"Skipping meals crashes metabolism."**
   Evidence shows the opposite: metabolic rate slightly increases during the first 2–3 days of fasting due to norepinephrine rise (Mansell et al., *Metabolism*, 1990).

3. **"Hunger will just build and build."**
   Studies show hunger plateaus and even declines after 24–36 hours due to ketones and ghrelin adaptation.

CASE STUDIES

- **Shift worker:** Tom improved focus and energy after aligning fasting with circadian cues, reducing late-night snacking.

- **High-stress parent:** Maria found fasting gave structure and peace, reducing guilt-driven binges.

- **Athlete:** David, a runner, used fasted training to enhance fat adaptation — improving endurance and recovery. Research backs this: fasted exercise boosts mitochondrial biogenesis.

THE CORE TRUTH

When you stop eating, you are not starving your body. You are awakening ancient programs written into your DNA. Programs that sharpen, repair, clean, and reset. Programs are designed for cycles, not nonstop intake.

Fasting isn't about absence. It's about unlocking the hidden operating system of your biology.

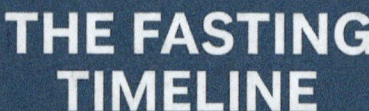

THE FASTING TIMELINE
What Happens Hour by Hour

0-4 HOURS
Post-meal digestion and energy storage

4-12 HOURS
Switch to fat burning
Drop in insulin and rising brain energy

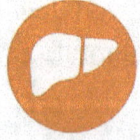

12-16 HOURS
Deep fasted state
Rise in ketones and growth hormone

16-24 HOURS
Cellular repair
Autophagy and immune function

THE HOURGLASS OF HEALING

Think of fasting not as starvation, but as turning over an **hourglass of biology**. Every hour that ticks by without food is not empty — it's **full of signals, switches, and healing cascades**.

Your body is not shutting down. It's waking up.

HOUR-BY-HOUR TIMELINE OF FASTING

0–4 HOURS: THE FED STATE

- **Fuel Source:** Glucose from your last meal.

- **Insulin:** Elevated, shuttling sugar into cells.

- **Glucagon:** Suppressed (no need to mobilize stored energy yet).

- **Gut:** Busy digesting, blood flow directed to intestines.

- **Brain:** Reward circuits are satisfied by dopamine from eating.

NARRATIVE:

Maria, the middle-school teacher, eats her 8 a.m. bagel. For the next few hours, she feels steady — her body is busy with digestion, her insulin acting like traffic police, directing glucose into muscle and fat.

4–8 HOURS: TRANSITION ZONE

- **Fuel Source:** Glycogen (stored glucose in the liver and muscles).

- **Insulin:** Dropping.

- **Glucagon:** Rising, telling the liver to release glucose.

- **Cortisol:** Helps maintain blood sugar balance.

- **Ghrelin ("hunger hormone"):** Peaks in waves, then falls if you don't eat.

NARRATIVE:

At 11 a.m., Maria's stomach growls — ghrelin spikes. But by noon, after drinking water and refocusing on her students, the wave passes. Her body switches from "where's my snack?" to "let's use reserves."

8–12 HOURS: METABOLIC SHIFT

- **Fuel Source:** Glycogen stores are nearing depletion.

- **Insulin:** Now low — "unlocking" fat burning.

- **Glucagon & Catecholamines:** Increasing, mobilizing fatty acids.

- **Growth Hormone:** Starts rising, protecting lean muscle.

- **Brain:** Ketone levels trace upward, though still low.

HEALING EFFECT:

Fatty acids begin to be released → early lipolysis (fat burning).

12–16 HOURS: FAT BURNING & KETONE RISE

- **Fuel Source:** Fatty acids + early ketones.

- **Autophagy (cellular cleanup):** Switches on in some tissues.

- **Inflammation markers (IL-6, TNF-α):** Begin to decline.

- **Mitochondria:** Start upregulating efficiency.

NARRATIVE:

At 2 p.m., Maria feels surprisingly clear-headed. The fog of constant snacking is gone. Her body has crossed the threshold into fat-burning, and ketones are beginning to fuel her brain with steady energy.

16–24 HOURS: AUTOPHAGY MODE

- **Fuel Source:** Fat + ketones dominate.

- **Autophagy:** Old proteins are tagged and recycled into building blocks.

- **Immune Reset:** Damaged white blood cells cleared.
- **BDNF (Brain-Derived Neurotrophic Factor):** Rising → improves synaptic plasticity, resilience.
- **Insulin Sensitivity:** Improving.

HEALING EFFECT:

Cellular "spring cleaning." Brain sharpness rises.

24–36 HOURS: DEEP REPAIR

- **Fuel Source:** Ketones high, stable.
- **Growth Hormone:** 3–5× baseline.
- **Autophagy:** Intensifies, especially in the liver & immune cells.
- **Stem Cell Activation:** Begins in some tissues.

NARRATIVE:

A firefighter named James, who tries a 24-hour fast once a week, describes it as "a reset button." By dinner the next day, hunger is less gnawing than expected — he feels strangely light, focused, and calm.

36–48 HOURS: IMMUNE RENEWAL

- **Ketones:** Peak stability, fueling the brain and muscles.
- **Inflammation:** Significant drop.
- **Immune Cells:** Old, damaged ones cleared; stem cells recruited.
- **Gut Microbiome:** Shifts toward bacteria that thrive on fiber and fasting.

BEYOND 48–72 HOURS: REGENERATION

- **Stem Cells:** Begin repopulating the immune system.

- **IGF-1 (growth signal):** Drops → longevity signaling pathways (FOXO, AMPK) activate.

- **Autophagy:** Deep cellular renewal across tissues.

- **Mood:** Many report calm, meditative clarity.

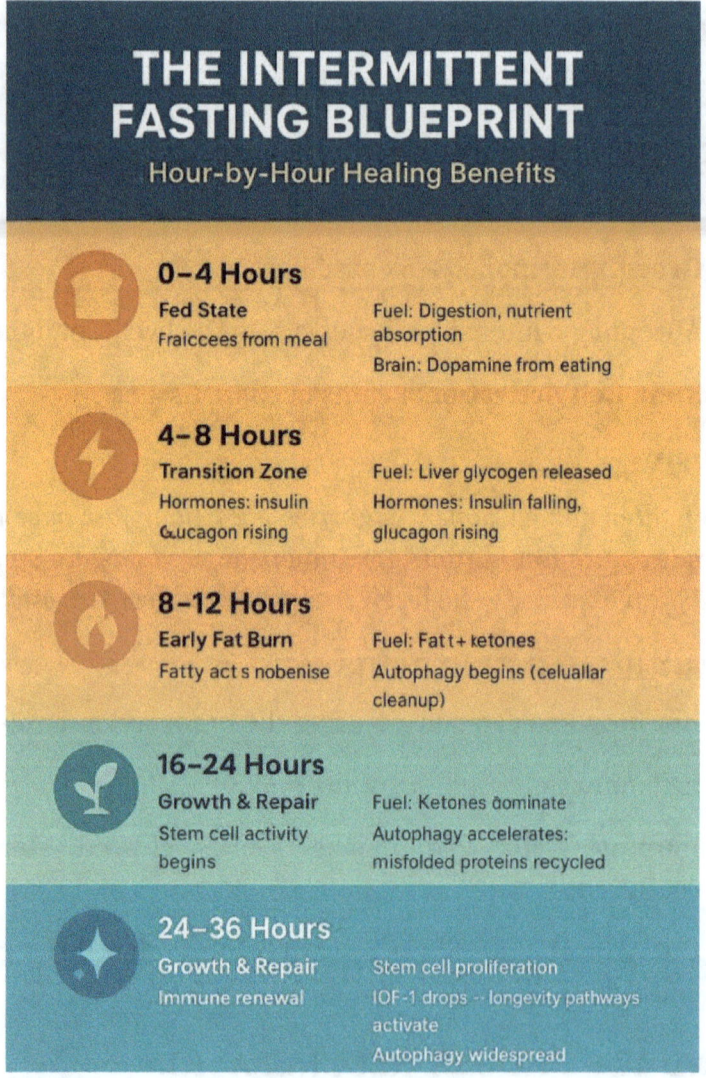

THE INTERMITTENT FASTING BLUEPRINT
Hour-by-Hour Healing Benefits

0–4 Hours
Fed State
Fraiccees from meal

Fuel: Digestion, nutrient absorption
Brain: Dopamine from eating

4–8 Hours
Transition Zone
Hormones: insulin
Glucagon rising

Fuel: Liver glycogen released
Hormones: Insulin falling, glucagon rising

8–12 Hours
Early Fat Burn
Fatty act s nobenise

Fuel: Fat t+ ketones
Autophagy begins (celuallar cleanup)

16–24 Hours
Growth & Repair
Stem cell activity begins

Fuel: Ketones ðominate
Autophagy accelerates: misfolded proteins recycled

24–36 Hours
Growth & Repair
Immune renewal

Stem cell proliferation
IOF-1 drops -- longevity pathways activate
Autophagy widespread

HORMONAL PATHWAYS OF FASTING

1. **Insulin** ↓ → unlocks fat burning, improves sensitivity.

2. **Glucagon** ↑ → mobilizes energy stores.

3. **Growth Hormone** ↑ → protects muscle, promotes fat loss.

4. **Cortisol (balanced)** → ensures blood sugar remains steady, though chronic stress alters this.

5. **Ghrelin (hunger hormone):** Comes in waves, doesn't linearly rise — adapts with practice.

6. **Leptin:** Long-term regulator of fullness; fasting resets sensitivity.

PATIENT NARRATIVES

- **Maria (teacher):** Used to graze all day. With fasting, she finds hunger comes in waves — and passes. Afternoon clarity replaces crashes.

- **James (firefighter):** Fast 24 hours once a week. Calls it his "reset day" to sharpen focus before a heavy shift.

- **Anita (busy mom):** Found that a 16:8 fasting window helped her curb late-night stress eating. Sleep improved, and bloating disappeared.

KEY MESSAGE

Fasting is not starvation. It is **programmed biology** — a rhythm encoded by millions of years of feast and famine.

When you stop eating, your body doesn't panic — it **remembers.**

PART 3 — FASTING & HORMONES: MALE VS. FEMALE WINDOWS

TWO VERY DIFFERENT MORNINGS

Picture this.

It is 10:30 AM in New York. James is a 42-year-old software engineer who hasn't eaten since dinner the previous night. He's working through some code and drunk on black coffee, deep into deep work. Mentally, he feels like a laser beam. Energy? A nice even keel. He loves his 16:8 intermittent fast, stating he has "never felt better."

On the other side of town, Maria, 39, a high school teacher, is attempting the same thing. She skips breakfast because her favorite podcast said that "breakfast is optional." Instead of laser focus, Maria can't stop feeling light-headed. She's irritable. Her cravings are zigzagging. By the end of the school day, Maria finds herself buried face-first into the teacher's lounge snacks, asking herself: How could James fast for hours without a problem, yet I feel like I am losing my mind?

The answer is not willpower. It's biology.

THE HORMONAL ORCHESTRA

Fasting interacts with hormones, and hormones aren't identical between men and women. The broad strokes of metabolism are the same, but the details — estrogen, progesterone, testosterone, insulin sensitivity, cortisol rhythms — make the fasting experience fundamentally different.

Think of fasting as a "signal." Your body interprets that signal through the hormonal system. Men and women often *hear* different music from the same signal.

MEN: TESTOSTERONE, GROWTH HORMONE, AND METABOLIC STABILITY

- **Testosterone & fasting:** In men, intermittent fasting tends to support testosterone indirectly by reducing visceral fat and improving insulin sensitivity. Less fat = less conversion of testosterone into estrogen via aromatase.

- **Growth hormone boost:** Studies (Ho et al., 1988; Weltman et al., 1992) show fasting increases growth hormone 2–5× in men, especially during 16–24 hr windows. This protects muscle mass and supports fat mobilization.

- **Metabolic robustness:** Men's bodies generally have more stable reserves of glycogen and muscle and tolerate longer fasting windows without hormonal disruption.

OPTIMAL WINDOW FOR MEN:

- **16:8 or 18:6 protocols** are typically well-tolerated.

- Extended fasts (24–36 hrs) can be done safely when guided and with refeeding protocols.

WOMEN: ESTROGEN, PROGESTERONE, AND SENSITIVITY TO ENERGY DEFICIT

Here's where it gets nuanced.

- **Estrogen:** Enhances insulin sensitivity, supports metabolic flexibility. During certain phases of the menstrual cycle (follicular phase, pre-ovulation), fasting can feel empowering — steady energy, focus, and appetite control.

- **Progesterone:** Rises in the luteal phase (post-ovulation). This increases metabolic rate and appetite. Fasting aggressively during this time often backfires, leading to binge–restrict cycles.

- **Cortisol interplay:** Women's HPA axis (stress system) is more sensitive to energy deprivation. Prolonged fasting can amplify cortisol, disrupting thyroid hormones and menstrual cycles.

- **Fertility signaling:** From an evolutionary standpoint, women's bodies are biologically designed to be more sensitive to "famine signals." Chronic under-fueling can lead to hypothalamic amenorrhea (loss of cycle).

OPTIMAL WINDOW FOR WOMEN:

- **12–14 hr overnight fasts** are safe and effective for most.

- **Cycle-syncing approach:**

  - **Follicular phase (Day 1–14):** Can stretch to 14–16 hrs fasting if energy is good.

  - **Luteal phase (Day 15–28):** Keep windows shorter (12–13 hrs), prioritize nourishment.

- **Perimenopause & menopause:** Women may tolerate 14–16 hr windows more consistently, since estrogen/progesterone fluctuations smooth out.

THE SCIENCE: MALE VS. FEMALE FASTING RESPONSES

1. Cortisol sensitivity

a. Study (O'Reilly et al., *J Clin Endocrinol Metab*, 2014): Women show greater cortisol spikes during fasting stress compared to men.

b. Translation: A "16:8" that feels fine for James might leave Maria wired and tired.

3. Reproductive health

a. Animal studies: Females are more likely to show disrupted reproductive cycles under fasting than males (Cameron et al., *Endocrinology*, 1991).

b. Humans: Women with low body fat or high stress are more vulnerable to cycle disruption.

4. Glucose regulation

a. Heilbronn et al., *Am J Clin Nutr*, 2005: Alternate-day fasting improved insulin sensitivity in men, but worsened glucose tolerance in some women.

5. Long-term adaptation

a. Men: Improved fat oxidation, testosterone stability, and reduced insulin resistance.

b. Women: Benefits are real (improved insulin sensitivity, reduced inflammation), but only when fasting respects hormonal rhythm.

MINI-STORIES

- **James (42):** Feels energized on 18:6. Testosterone levels improved after losing belly fat. His doctor notes a better lipid panel.

- **Maria (39):** After trying to copy James, she had irregular cycles and worsened cravings. When she switched to a **14 hr fast in the follicular phase / 12 hr in the luteal**, she regained energy and consistency.

- **Sarah (52, menopausal):** With stable hormones, she thrives on a 16:8, losing weight steadily and feeling sharper.

PRACTICAL GUIDELINES: FASTING BY GENDER

FOR MEN

☑ Start with 14:10, progress to 16:8 or 18:6.

☑ Extended fasts (24 hrs) 1×/week can enhance growth hormone.

☑ Combine fasting with resistance training to preserve testosterone.

☑ Avoid over-relying on caffeine to mask hunger.

FOR WOMEN

☑ Start with 12:12, only extend if energy remains steady.

☑ Sync fasting with menstrual phases.

☑ Prioritize protein/fiber in the feeding window to reduce rebound cravings.

☑ Perimenopause/menopause: 14–16 hr windows are effective, but don't push into chronic calorie restriction.

QUICK-REFERENCE BOX

FASTING WINDOWS BY GENDER

- **Men:** 16–18 hrs, flexible; extended fasts possible.

- **Women:** 12–14 hrs baseline, cycle-sync if premenopausal.

- **Golden rule:** Fasting should feel energizing, not draining.

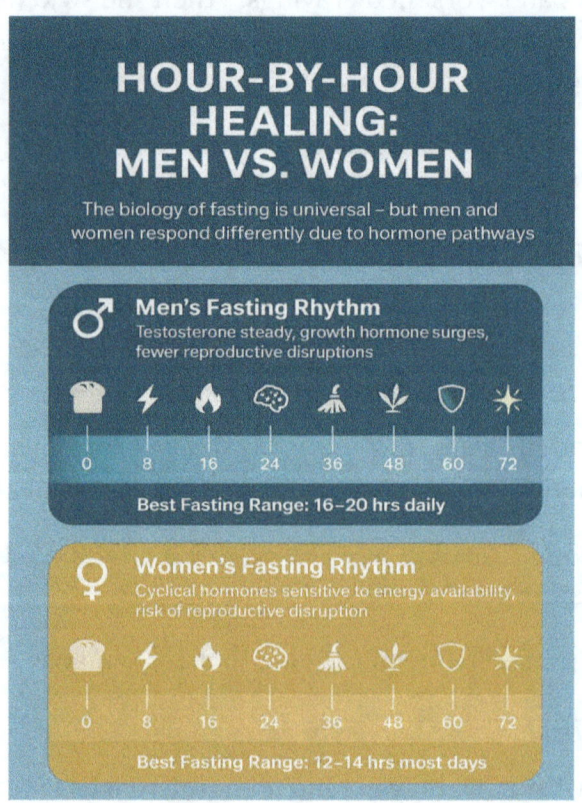

PART 4: THE HEALING MECHANISMS — AUTOPHAGY, INFLAMMATION, LONGEVITY PATHWAYS

THE BODY'S HIDDEN REPAIR CREW

Envision stepping into a big, dark factory. Machines are humming, conveyor belts are creaking, and workers in oil-stained uniforms dart around between stations. Some fix broken pieces, others turn scrap metal into usable steel, and others sweep whatever toxic garbage is on the floor. At first glance, this factory looks chaotic. Upon closer inspection, you can see a beat, a system of order and renewal that keeps the entire structure alive.

This factory is your body, and the night shift, the one that does the most substantial repair work in your body, only shows up when you are not eating.

For most of human history, fasting wasn't a trending wellness practice; it was a biological matter of life and death. Life periods of scarcity meant the body created a set of survival tools and repair systems that kick into gear when the calories stop flowing in. Modern science has now uncovered what ancient rhythms knew instinctively: fasting flips powerful switches inside us; autophagy, inflammation control, and longevity pathways that we cannot access in a constantly fed state.

Let's explore these healing systems one at a time.

SECTION 1: AUTOPHAGY — THE CELLULAR HOUSEKEEPER

The word *autophagy* comes from the Greek roots *auto* (self) and *phagein* (to eat) — literally "self-eating." It sounds grim, but this process is the single most important cleanup system your cells have.

When you fast, insulin drops and nutrient-sensing pathways shift. This signals cells to begin dismantling broken proteins, damaged mitochondria, and cellular junk. Like Marie Kondo for your biology, autophagy doesn't just clear clutter — it recycles it into new, usable parts.

SCIENCE SPOTLIGHT:

- Yoshinori Ohsumi won the 2016 Nobel Prize for discovering the molecular machinery of autophagy.

- In animal studies, fasting-induced autophagy delays aging, improves brain resilience, and protects against neurodegeneration.

- Autophagy is particularly powerful in the brain. It helps recycle misfolded proteins like beta-amyloid (linked to Alzheimer's) and tau tangles (linked to dementia).

NARRATIVE CASE STUDY:

Maria, our teacher from earlier chapters, once described her brain as "fogged over" every afternoon. When she tried her first 16-hour fast, she was surprised — not by the hunger, but by the clarity. She described it as "like someone opened the blinds in a dark room." That's autophagy working in real time — clearing waste, creating efficiency, sharpening focus.

ACTION PRIMER:

- Autophagy begins around 12–16 hours into fasting but accelerates with longer fasts (20–24 hours).

- It's enhanced by exercise, especially fasted workouts.

- Sleep strengthens autophagy in the brain — the "glymphatic system" flushes toxins overnight.

SECTION 2: INFLAMMATION — THE FIRE WITHIN

Chronic inflammation is the hidden accelerant behind most modern diseases — obesity, diabetes, heart disease, cancer, and depression. Think of it as a low-grade fire smoldering in your tissues, damaging blood vessels, impairing insulin signaling, and exhausting the immune system.

Fasting is one of the body's natural fire extinguishers.

HOW IT WORKS:

- When insulin falls and ketones rise, inflammatory signaling molecules like IL-6 and TNF-alpha decline.

- Ketones themselves (especially beta-hydroxybutyrate, BHB) act as signaling molecules that *block the* NLRP3 *inflammasome* — a major driver of chronic inflammation.

- Immune cells reset. Old, hyperactive cells are cleared through autophagy, while new ones emerge during refeeding.

SCIENCE SPOTLIGHT:

- A study in *Cell Metabolism* (2014) showed intermittent fasting reduced pro-inflammatory monocytes in humans.

- Research in *Nature Medicine* (2019) found that BHB, produced during fasting, suppresses inflammation in the brain and may protect against neurodegeneration.

- Clinical trials show fasting-mimicking diets improve markers of inflammation and immune aging in people with metabolic syndrome.

NARRATIVE CASE STUDY:

John, a 52-year-old accountant, lived on takeout lunches and ibuprofen for his knee pain. After 30 days of time-restricted eating (12 p.m. to 8 p.m.), he reported less pain, clearer energy, and — to his surprise — fewer headaches. His doctor noted drops in CRP (C-reactive protein), a blood marker of inflammation. John didn't just lose weight; he cooled the fire.

ACTION PRIMER:

- Even 16:8 fasting windows improve inflammatory markers within weeks.

- Pair fasting with anti-inflammatory foods on eating days — omega-3s, polyphenols, colorful vegetables.

- Avoid breaking fasts with ultra-processed foods — they reignite inflammation immediately.

SECTION 3: LONGEVITY PATHWAYS — TURNING ON THE SURVIVAL SWITCHES

Every cell in your body has sensors that respond to nutrients. When you're constantly eating, especially high-sugar foods, those sensors stay flipped to "growth mode." This is fine in youth, but constant growth signaling accelerates aging and disease later in life.

Fasting flips the switch from *growth* to *repair*.

THE THREE MAJOR PATHWAYS:

1. MTOR (Mechanistic Target of Rapamycin):

a. Growth-promoting pathway that's beneficial in bursts (muscle building), but harmful if always "on."

b. Fasting suppresses mTOR, allowing autophagy and repair.

2. AMPK (AMP-Activated Protein Kinase):

a. Energy sensor of the cell.

b. Activated by fasting, AMPK increases fat burning, improves insulin sensitivity, and boosts mitochondrial biogenesis.

3. Sirtuins (Longevity Genes):

a. Proteins that regulate DNA repair, inflammation, and metabolism.

b. Fasting and ketones activate sirtuins, similar to calorie restriction — linked to longer lifespan in animals.

SCIENCE SPOTLIGHT:

- Studies in yeast, worms, and mice show intermittent fasting extends lifespan by 30–40%.

- In primates, calorie restriction slows aging, reduces cancer, and improves metabolic health.

- Human studies (like the CALERIE trial) suggest fasting improves longevity biomarkers even without major weight loss.

NARRATIVE CASE STUDY:

Anika, a 44-year-old runner, wasn't fasting for weight loss. She wanted to age well. "I don't care about abs," she said. "I care about seeing my grandkids." Her lab work after six months of alternate-day fasting showed improved insulin sensitivity, lower triglycerides, and increased HDL cholesterol. She wasn't just running marathons — she was running a cellular longevity program.

ACTION PRIMER:

- 16:8 windows give a taste of longevity activation.

- Occasional longer fasts (24–36 hours) deepen sirtuin and AMPK signaling.

- Pair refeeding with nutrient-dense whole foods — this "rebuild" phase is as important as the fast.

SECTION 4: THE CONVERGENCE — FASTING AS BIOLOGICAL SYMPHONY

What's striking is how these pathways don't work in isolation. Autophagy, inflammation reduction, and longevity signaling weave together like instruments in a symphony:

- **Autophagy** cleans up cellular junk.

- **Inflammation control** prevents tissue damage.

- **Longevity pathways** rebuild resilience.

Together, they create an inner environment of renewal and efficiency — one that can't be accessed in a state of constant eating.

SECTION 5: ACTION STEP BOX — "SWITCHING ON THE REPAIR CREW"

☑ Fast long enough (12–16 hrs) to trigger autophagy.

☑ Use fasting windows to reduce inflammation, not fuel it (avoid junk refeed).

☑ Think of fasting as rhythm, not punishment — alternate growth (feeding) with repair (fasting).

☑ Consider occasional extended fasts (24–36 hrs) for longevity pathways.

☑ Sleep, exercise, and whole foods amplify the effects.

Your body is not a machine that runs until it breaks. It is a self-healing, self-repairing ecosystem. But just like the factory floor, the cleanup crew can't do their work if the conveyor belts never stop.

Fasting is not about deprivation. It's about making space for repair, renewal, and resilience. It is the forgotten superpower hidden inside your biology — and once you unlock it, the body you live in begins to feel timeless.

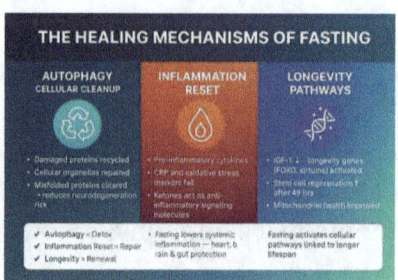

PART 5 — THE CRAVINGS CODE + FASTING: WHY IT WORKS

Maria always awoke and believed she was starving. By 9:30 a.m., her stomach growled, her hands shook, and her brain would beg for a muffin or sugary latte. She believed it was hunger. However, when she tried her first intermittent fast, she was shocked to realize the "hangry" storm never came. Here is what that looked like: after a few days of fasting, the desperation around mid-morning went away. She was able to think straight, her energy leveled off, and ultimately realized she was chasing cravings, not true hunger.

This is really the point that fasting begins, to rewire the cravings code. Not only does it provide discipline, but it also rewires the pattern of your hunger hormones.

THE SCIENCE: HUNGER IS A RHYTHM, NOT A CONSTANT

Your body runs on predictable patterns. Hunger is no exception.

- **Ghrelin (The Hunger Hormone):**
  Often called the "meal initiator," ghrelin doesn't rise endlessly the longer you go without food. Instead, it pulses in waves, typically at the times you usually eat. Skip breakfast? That 8 a.m. spike eventually fades. By 10 a.m., your body is calm again.

- **Adaptation to Fasting:**
  Studies show that after just a few days of fasting, ghrelin levels decrease overall, and the hunger spikes grow smaller and more manageable (Cummings et al., *Journal of Clinical Endocrinology & Metabolism*, 2004).

- **Why You Don't Get Hungrier Forever:**
  Contrary to the myth, hunger isn't a balloon filling up with pressure. It's a tide, rising and falling, reset daily by your eating schedule. Fasting simply shifts the tide to align with biology instead of cravings.

MYTH-BUSTING: CRAVINGS VS. HUNGER

Many people confuse cravings with hunger. Here's how fasting helps separate them:

- **Cravings:** Emotional, specific ("I need chocolate"), urgent, often triggered by stress or boredom.

- **True Hunger:** Physical, general ("I could eat anything"), grows slowly, tied to the body's real need for fuel.

Fasting exposes the difference. By extending the gap between meals, you experience the fading of cravings while still accessing steady energy through fat metabolism. That clarity makes it easier to say, *"I don't actually need that muffin, I just wanted the dopamine hit."*

CASE VIGNETTE: MARIA'S SHIFT

Before fasting, Maria's mornings were ruled by sugar cycles. The muffin at 9:30 led to a blood sugar spike, followed by a crash at 11:00. By noon, she was tired, cranky, and craving lunch.

After three weeks of a 16:8 fasting window:

- **Week 1:** She felt hunger pangs at 9:30 but learned to ride them out with water and tea.

- **Week 2:** The pangs faded. Her energy at 11:00 was stable, her mind clearer.

- **Week 3:** She laughed at her old "hangry" self. She could now distinguish real hunger (which came later, slower, and without the panic) from old dopamine-driven cravings.

Fasting didn't make her hungrier—it freed her from the cravings loop.

WHY FASTING RETRAINS THE BRAIN

- **Dopamine Reset:** Processed foods hijack reward circuits. Fasting breaks constant stimulation, restoring sensitivity.

- **Insulin Control:** Lower insulin during fasting prevents sugar crashes, a common trigger for "false hunger."

- **Ketones as Fuel:** Once the body produces ketones, the brain runs on a steady, non-crash energy source. Studies show ketones reduce appetite and enhance mental clarity (Stubbs et al., *Obesity Reviews*, 2018).

ACTION PRIMER: HOW TO REWIRE HUNGER

1. **Ride the Wave:** When hunger hits, wait 20 minutes. If it fades, it was a craving. If it grows steadily, it's real hunger.

2. **Hydration First:** Drink water or tea when the pangs start—often thirst disguises itself as hunger.

3. **Protein Anchor:** Break your fast with protein + fiber to reduce rebound cravings.

4. **Track the Pattern:** Journal when your hunger arrives each day. Notice how it shifts and shrinks over 1–2 weeks of fasting.

QUICK-REFERENCE BOX:

☑ FASTING ISN'T STARVATION—IT'S SEPARATION.

It separates cravings from hunger, noise from signal, and teaches your body to thrive on rhythm, not impulse.

PART 6 — FASTING FRAMEWORKS (PRACTICAL OPTIONS)

THE MENU OF PAUSES

Imagine this, you step into a café—but instead of coffee and croissants, there is a menu of "fasting windows", each like a flavor and rhythm you can try on like a suit. Some are light and intermittent, while others are more therapeutic and structured.

That's what fasting frameworks are, not rigid systems you adhere to, but rather tools—different doors into the same biological house.

The beauty of fasting is that it's not "one-size-fits-all." The right framework depends on your lifestyle, your goals, and sometimes even your gender and stage of life. The key is learning the spectrum—from gentle to intensive—and experimenting with the rhythm that makes you thrive.

1. TIME-RESTRICTED EATING (TRE): EATING WITH THE SUN

THE RHYTHM:

- **12:12 (Gentle Entry):** Eat during a 12-hour window, fast for 12 hours. For example, 7 a.m.–7 p.m. eating, then nothing until the next morning.

- **16:8 (Popular Reset):** Eat during an 8-hour window, fast for 16 hours. A common version: 12 p.m.–8 p.m. eating, then fast until noon the next day.

- **18:6 (Deeper Fat-Burn):** Eat in a 6-hour window, fast for 18.

THE SCIENCE:

- TRE aligns eating with the circadian rhythm. Studies show restricting food to daylight hours improves insulin sensitivity and reduces nighttime glucose spikes (*Cell Metabolism*, 2018).

- Even **12:12** is powerful for beginners. It cuts out late-night eating, the most damaging feeding pattern for metabolic health.

- **16:8** consistently lowers body weight and blood pressure in trials without calorie counting (Gabel et al., *Nutrition and Healthy Aging*, 2018).

NARRATIVE VIGNETTE:

Take *Ravi*, a night owl coder. He started with 12:12, simply stopping late-night snacking. His sleep improved within a week. By month two, he shifted to 16:8. His productivity soared—he described it as "debugging my brain with fasting."

2. THE 24-HOUR RESET

THE RHYTHM:

- One or two times a week, skip two consecutive meals, for example, dinner-to-dinner or lunch-to-lunch.

THE SCIENCE:

- **Autophagy Activation:** After ~24 hours, the recycling program in your cells ramps up.

- **Insulin Reset:** Insulin levels drop significantly, boosting fat-burning and cellular repair.

- Trials show that alternate-day fasting or 24-hour fasts improve cardiovascular markers and reduce inflammation (*Annual Review of Nutrition*, 2017).

NARRATIVE VIGNETTE:

Maria used this method after her 16:8 routine. Every Sunday, she would finish dinner at 6 p.m. and not eat again until the next evening. Mondays became her clearest, most energized workdays. "It feels like I'm running on clean fuel," she said.

3. THE 5:2 APPROACH

THE RHYTHM:

- Eat normally 5 days a week. On two non-consecutive days, reduce calories (usually 500–600).

THE SCIENCE:

- Developed by Dr. Michael Mosley, this style has shown consistent benefits in weight management, insulin sensitivity, and cholesterol.

- Easier adherence for people who dislike daily fasting.

- Clinical studies show 5:2 lowers fasting glucose and triglycerides even without weight loss (*British Journal of Nutrition*, 2013).

NARRATIVE VIGNETTE:

Clara, a nurse working long shifts, couldn't do strict daily windows. But she found 5:2 perfect—on her quieter days off, she'd do a light soup and salad day. Her blood sugar improved, and she loved the flexibility.

4. THE FASTING-MIMICKING DIET (FMD)

THE RHYTHM:

- Created by Dr. Valter Longo, FMD is a 5-day low-calorie, plant-based protocol (~800–1,100 calories/day).

- Done once every 1–3 months under guidance.

THE SCIENCE:

- FMD induces fasting-like effects while still providing food.

- Shown to promote stem cell regeneration, reduce IGF-1 (growth signals linked to cancer risk), and extend healthspan in animal and human studies (*Science Translational Medicine*, 2017).

- Especially valuable for people hesitant about water-only fasting.

George, a 58-year-old teacher, tried FMD quarterly. He described it as "resetting my hardware." His cholesterol dropped 20 points in 6 months, and his doctor reduced his blood pressure medication.

5. EXTENDED FASTS (36–72 HOURS+)

THE RHYTHM:

- Rare, supervised, longer fasts where you go beyond 36 hours.

THE SCIENCE:

- **36 hours:** Immune cell renewal accelerates.

- **48–72 hours:** Stem cell activation peaks, deep autophagy occurs.

- Clinical trials suggest longer fasts can reset chemotherapy tolerance, improve autoimmune markers, and enhance metabolic flexibility (*Cell Stem Cell*, 2014).

Caution: Should be supervised by a medical professional or an expert, especially for those on medications, with diabetes, or with chronic conditions.

NARRATIVE VIGNETTE:

Sarah, struggling with autoimmune flares, did 48-hour supervised fasts every few months. "It was hard, but it felt like hitting a reset button on my body's inflammation."

MATCHING FRAMEWORKS TO LIFESTYLE

- **Beginner / Stressed Parent:** Start with **12:12** → lowest barrier, highest sleep benefit.

- **Busy Professional: 16:8** for focus + energy.

- **Weight Loss / Metabolic Reset: 18:6** or occasional **24-hour fasts**.

- **Shift Workers:** 5:2 may work best—flexibility around unpredictable schedules.

- **Longevity Seekers:** Periodic **FMD** or supervised **extended fasts**.

ACTION STEPS: CHOOSING YOUR FASTING FIT

1. **Start Small:** Master 12:12 before 16:8.

2. **Sync With Life:** Match your window to work, family, and social rhythms.

3. **Honor Gender Differences:** Women may thrive more with 12:12 or 14:10; men tolerate deeper fasting windows.

4. **Consistency > Intensity:** A sustainable 14:10 beats a short-lived 18:6.

5. **Experiment, Don't Obsess:** Treat it like testing operating systems. Your body will tell you when the rhythm is right.

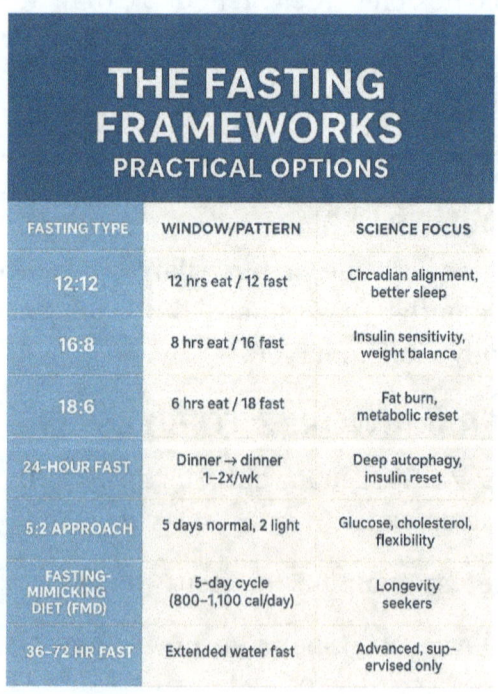

THE FASTING FRAMEWORKS
PRACTICAL OPTIONS

FASTING TYPE	WINDOW/PATTERN	SCIENCE FOCUS
12:12	12 hrs eat / 12 fast	Circadian alignment, better sleep
16:8	8 hrs eat / 16 fast	Insulin sensitivity, weight balance
18:6	6 hrs eat / 18 fast	Fat burn, metabolic reset
24-HOUR FAST	Dinner → dinner 1–2x/wk	Deep autophagy, insulin reset
5:2 APPROACH	5 days normal, 2 light	Glucose, cholesterol, flexibility
FASTING-MIMICKING DIET (FMD)	5-day cycle (800–1,100 cal/day)	Longevity seekers
36–72 HR FAST	Extended water fast	Advanced, supervised only

PART 7 — COMMON MYTHS + PITFALLS

Picture Maria again. She's been reading about fasting for weeks. The headlines promise glowing skin, fat loss, and sharper focus. But in the back of her mind, an old story whispers: *"If I don't eat, I'll starve... I'll ruin my metabolism."*

That whisper isn't Maria's fault. It's the cultural script most of us inherited. For decades, we were told:

- "Breakfast is the most important meal of the day."

- "Never skip meals."

- "Eat six times a day to keep your metabolism from crashing."

The irony? None of these slogans came from human biology. Most came from food companies eager to sell more cereal, snack bars, and packaged "mini-meals." Science, on the other hand, has been quietly rewriting the script.

MYTH 1: FASTING = STARVATION

The truth: Starvation is involuntary, fasting is intentional. Starvation breaks the body down; fasting activates repair.

When you fast, your body isn't panicking — it's switching programs.

- **Hormones adjust:** Insulin drops, glucagon rises, and growth hormone increases to protect muscle.

- **Metabolism doesn't shut down:** A meta-analysis in the *American Journal of Clinical Nutrition* (2016) found resting metabolic rate often rises slightly during short-term fasting due to increased norepinephrine.

- **Energy shifts:** You tap stored glycogen, then fat — the way humans survived countless winters.

Starvation is depletion. Fasting is an adaptation.

MYTH 2: FASTING SLOWS METABOLISM

This fear is deeply ingrained, but science paints the opposite picture.

- **Study spotlight:** Heilbronn et al. (2005) found that alternate-day fasting increased norepinephrine and preserved resting metabolic rate.

- **Evolutionary lens:** If metabolism "shut down" after skipping meals, our ancestors would have collapsed before finding food. Instead, fasting sparks alertness, sharper focus, and physical drive — exactly the traits needed for Thriving.

What really slows metabolism? Chronic underfeeding combined with nutrient deficiency (think crash diets). Fasting, paired with nutrient-dense meals, enhances metabolic resilience.

PITFALL 1: OVEREATING THE "JUNK WINDOW"

Fasting is powerful — but it's not a magic shield against ultra-processed foods.

WHAT HAPPENS WHEN SOMEONE FASTS ALL DAY, THEN BREAKS THEIR FAST WITH CHIPS, SODA, AND FAST FOOD?

- Insulin spikes harder after long restriction.

- The gut microbiome misses its chance to rebuild.

- Inflammation re-flares.

Solution: Break the fast like you're fueling a recovery system, not rewarding deprivation.

☑ Protein + fiber + healthy fats (eggs + vegetables, lentils + olive oil, salmon + greens).

✗ Processed sugar bombs that undo the repair work.

PITFALL 2: IGNORING HYDRATION & ELECTROLYTES

When insulin drops, the kidneys release sodium and water — this is why many people lose water weight quickly in early fasting. But it also means dehydration and electrolyte imbalance can sneak in.

Signs: Headaches, fatigue, dizziness, muscle cramps.

Fix:

- Drink water consistently.

- Add electrolytes (salt, potassium, magnesium) if fasting beyond 16 hours.

- Herbal teas and black coffee are supportive allies.

Hydration isn't optional. It's the lubrication that keeps fasting smooth.

PITFALL 3: USING FASTING AS PUNISHMENT

Perhaps the most dangerous trap: turning fasting into a whip of shame.

For many, food is tied to guilt. Fasting then becomes a way to "undo" indulgence:

- Ate cake last night → punish with a 24-hour fast.

- Overate at dinner → "I'll starve myself tomorrow."

But biology doesn't reward shame. Stress hormones rise, digestion falters, and cravings rebound harder. The cycle deepens.

REFRAME:

Fasting isn't a punishment. It's permission — permission to rest your system, permission to reset, permission to heal.

PATIENT STORY: MARIA'S SHIFT

Maria began with the wrong mindset. After overeating pizza, she'd fast out of guilt, feeling punished and weak. But when she learned the science — that fasting is cellular restoration, not penance — everything changed.

She stopped "making up" for indulgences and started scheduling fasting windows to support her energy, her sleep, her focus. She hydrated; she broke fasts with protein-rich meals. The result? Food no longer felt like a battle. It felt like rhythm.

QUICK-REFERENCE BOX

THE FASTING MYTHS & PITFALLS RESET

- ☑ **Fasting ≠ starvation** → It's programmed into your biology.

- ☑ **Metabolism doesn't slow** → Hormones spark alertness and repair.

- ✖ **Don't binge the "junk window"** → Break fast with nutrient-rich meals.

- ☑ **Hydrate + electrolytes matter** → Especially past 16 hours.

- ✖ **Don't punish yourself** → Fasting is healing, not atonement.

Key takeaway: The difference between healing and harm isn't fasting itself — it's how you frame, fuel, and flow with it.

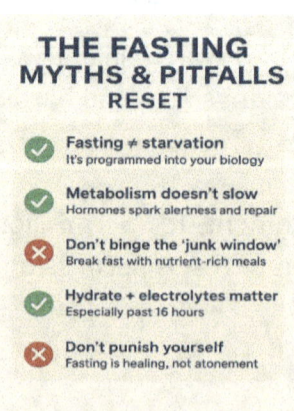

SAFE FASTING ELECTROLYTE MIX (PER 1 LITRE OF WATER)

- **Sodium chloride (sea salt or pink salt):** 1 tsp (≈ 2,300 mg sodium)

- **Potassium chloride ("NoSalt" / potassium salt):** ¼ tsp (≈ 900–1,000 mg potassium)

- **Magnesium (powdered citrate, glycinate, or drops):** 200–400 mg

- **Optional cayenne:** pinch (⅛ tsp) for appetite suppression & circulation (avoid if you get stomach irritation)

- **Optional lemon/lime juice:** squeeze for taste + vitamin C

Mix well and sip slowly throughout the day.

WHY THIS FORMULA WORKS

1. **Sodium (2,300 mg):** Restores the salt lost through fasting-induced diuresis and prevents dizziness, fatigue, and low blood pressure.

2. **Potassium (1,000 mg):** Supports nerve, heart, and muscle function without reaching dangerous levels. This is within the daily recommended intake and well below risky supplement doses.

3. **Magnesium (200–400 mg):** Crucial for muscle relaxation, energy metabolism, and preventing cramps. Magnesium is often overlooked but essential.

4. **Cayenne (tiny pinch):** May reduce hunger and boost thermogenesis slightly, but in safe amounts.

5. **Citrus juice:** Adds flavor, alkalinity, and antioxidants without breaking your fast in a meaningful way (under ~5 kcal).

☑ HOW TO USE DURING FASTING

- Drink 1–2 litres per day while on long-term intermittent or extended fasting.

- Sip slowly over hours — don't chug, to avoid overwhelming your stomach.

- Pair with **plain water** as needed for extra hydration.

- On prolonged fasts (>48 hours), prioritize **rest and hydration,** and consult a doctor if you have kidney, heart, or blood pressure issues.

⚠ SAFETY NOTES

- **Don't exceed 1 tsp potassium salt/day** unless under medical supervision.

- If you take **blood pressure meds, diuretics, or have kidney issues**, talk to a doctor before supplementing potassium or magnesium.

- Stop immediately if you feel heart palpitations, weakness, or numbness.

PART 8 — ACTION STARTER: YOUR FASTING DAY BLUEPRINT

Think of this as your **training wheels for fasting**—a one-day template that brings all the science you've absorbed into a lived rhythm. Not extreme, not punishing, but a structured way to taste what your body has been designed to do: cycle between nourishment and renewal.

MORNING: AWAKENING WITHOUT FOOD

- **Timeline:** Wake → 3–4 hours

- **What happens biologically:**

- o Insulin stays low, keeping your fat-burning switch on.

- o Cortisol peaks naturally (your body's built-in "get-up hormone"), sharpening focus.

- o Growth hormone pulses protect muscle.

- **Practice:**

  - o **Hydrate first thing.** Water, black coffee, or green tea.

  - o **Light movement.** Walk outside for sunlight or a few mobility stretches.

  - o **Breath reset.** Two minutes of slow exhale breathing to calm cortisol surges.

- **Mindset mantra:** "This is energy, not emptiness."

MIDDAY: THE FIRST MEAL WINDOW

- **Timeline:** 11 AM–1 PM (depending on your fasting schedule, e.g., 16:8)

- **What happens biologically:**

  - o Digestive enzymes re-engage.

  - o Insulin rises gently, ready to shuttle nutrients.

  - o Cells become more insulin-sensitive → less glucose spillover, more efficient storage.

- **Practice:**

  - o Breakfast with **protein + fiber** (e.g., eggs, lentils, salmon, leafy greens).

  - o Avoid sugary "crash foods" (pastries, soda) that spike glucose and undo the reset.

  - o Eat mindfully: chew slowly, savor, pause halfway.

- **Mindset mantra:** "Food is signal, not just calories."

AFTERNOON: METABOLIC FLOW

- **Timeline:** 1 PM–6 PM

- **What happens biologically:**

  o Glucose stabilizes.

  o Hunger hormone **ghrelin** adapts downward—you feel steady rather than ravenous.

  o Micro-autophagy continues between meals.

- **Practice:**

  o Take a **movement snack**: walk after meals, stretch, or bodyweight push-ups/squats.

  o Hydrate again. Add electrolytes (pinch of sea salt + lemon in water).

  o If hungry, opt for a **fast-friendly snack**: nuts, Greek yogurt, or fermented foods.

- **Mindset mantra:** "Movement multiplies fasting's effects."

EVENING: THE SECOND MEAL

- **Timeline:** 6–8 PM (last eating window)

- **What happens biologically:**

  o Insulin rises briefly, then tapers into the night.

  o The body prepares for a growth hormone surge during sleep.

  o Fasting clock resets for another cycle.

- **Practice:**

- o Keep dinner **lighter and earlier.** Focus on lean protein, veggies, and healthy fats.

- o Avoid heavy starches, alcohol, or late sugar bombs → they block deep sleep benefits.

- o Gentle wind-down ritual: walk outside, stretch, sip calming tea.

- **Mindset mantra:** "Rest is the final nutrient."

NIGHT: THE RESET WINDOW

- **Timeline:** 9 PM–morning
- **What happens biologically:**
  - o Sleep + fasting overlap = maximum repair.
  - o Melatonin rises, cortisol falls.
  - o Autophagy deepens; the brain clears waste via the glymphatic system.
- **Practice:**
  - o No late-night snacking.
  - o Tech off 1 hour before bed.
  - o Gratitude journaling → proven to lower stress and aid sleep quality.
- **Mindset mantra:** "Tomorrow's energy is built tonight."

QUICK-REFERENCE CHECKLIST

☑ Hydrate often (water, black coffee, tea, electrolytes).

☑ Anchor the day with protein + fiber meals.

☑ Move lightly before and after meals.

☑ Stop eating 2–3 hours before bed.

☑ Treat fasting as a rhythm, not a restriction.

"One day of fasting is one day of renewal. Each cycle is a message to your body: repair, restore, and rise stronger.

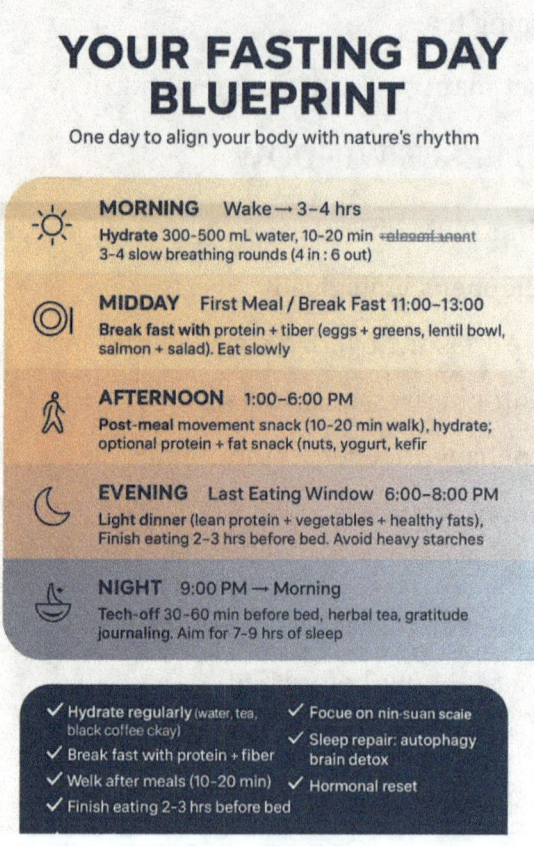

YOUR FASTING DAY BLUEPRINT
One day to align your body with nature's rhythm

MORNING Wake → 3–4 hrs
Hydrate 300–500 mL water, 10–20 min ̶e̶l̶e̶e̶e̶l̶ ̶e̶n̶e̶n̶t̶
3–4 slow breathing rounds (4 in : 6 out)

MIDDAY First Meal / Break Fast 11:00–13:00
Break fast with protein + fiber (eggs + greens, lentil bowl, salmon + salad). Eat slowly

AFTERNOON 1:00–6:00 PM
Post-meal movement snack (10–20 min walk), hydrate; optional protein + fat snack (nuts, yogurt, kefir

EVENING Last Eating Window 6:00–8:00 PM
Light dinner (lean protein + vegetables + healthy fats), Finish eating 2–3 hrs before bed. Avoid heavy starches

NIGHT 9:00 PM → Morning
Tech-off 30–60 min before bed, herbal tea, gratitude journaling. Aim for 7–9 hrs of sleep

✓ Hydrate regularly (water, tea, black coffee ckay)
✓ Break fast with protein + fiber
✓ Welk after meals (10–20 min)
✓ Finish eating 2–3 hrs before bed
✓ Focue on nin-suan scaie
✓ Sleep repair: autophagy brain detox
✓ Hormonal reset

POST-FASTING REFEEDING PROTOCOL

◇ **After Intermittent Fasting (16–24 hrs)**

Goal: ease digestion, but can return to normal foods fairly quickly.

1. **Start with:** 1–2 cups warm bone broth (with marrow if available).

2. **Wait 20-30 minutes** → let electrolytes and amino acids settle.

3. **First meal:** lean protein (chicken, fish, eggs) + cooked vegetables + healthy fat (olive oil, avocado).

4. **Avoid:** ultra-processed carbs/sugar (spike hunger + crash).

◇ **After a 48-72 hr Fast**

Goal: reintroduce food gently and prevent bloating or stomach upset.

1. **Start with:** bone broth (1-2 cups). Add a little marrow fat if tolerated.

2. **Small snack 1-2 hrs later:**

   o Steamed or lightly cooked vegetables (zucchini, spinach, carrots).

   o Small portion of protein (poached egg, ½ chicken breast, or fish).

3. **Second meal (later that day):**

   o Broth-based soup with veggies + shredded chicken or fish.

   o Add fermented food (sauerkraut, kimchi) for gut microbiome support.

4. **Next day:** return to balanced whole-food meals (protein + veggies + healthy fats).

◇ **After Extended Fasts (4+ days)**

Goal: minimize risk of refeeding syndrome (electrolyte imbalance) and restart digestion gradually.

Day 1:

- **Morning**: 1–2 cups bone broth (with a pinch of extra salt or potassium if needed).

- **Midday:** diluted vegetable soup or blended vegetable broth (easy on the gut).

- **Evening:** soft protein (scrambled egg, poached fish, or a small portion of chicken). Pair with cooked non-starchy vegetables.

Day 2:

- Continue bone broth between meals.

- Add more solid protein (chicken, salmon, beef stew meat).

- Add healthy fats (avocado, olive oil, marrow).

- Start reintroducing carbs carefully (sweet potato, squash, or fruit).

Day 3+:

- Transition to a normal balanced diet: lean protein, vegetables, healthy fats, whole-food carbs.

- Avoid large binges — digestion and insulin sensitivity are still adjusting.

⚠ SAFETY & SPECIAL NOTES

- **Electrolytes are critical.** Sodium, potassium, magnesium, and phosphate can dip dangerously after extended fasts (refeeding syndrome risk). Bone broth covers sodium well, but consider electrolyte supplementation if fasting >4 days.

- **Chew thoroughly** and eat slowly to reduce stomach shock.

- **Portion control:** Start small — the first meal should be about **25–30% of a normal meal** and increase gradually.

- **Avoid alcohol, processed sugar, and very fatty meals** immediately after fasting — these overwhelm the liver and gut.

Bone broth with marrow is an excellent refeeding starter: it hydrates, restores electrolytes, delivers gentle amino acids and fats, and soothes the digestive system. From there, layering in soft proteins, cooked vegetables, and eventually healthy carbs ensures a safe, nourishing transition back to regular eating.

PART 9 — JOYFUL FASTING: BLUE ZONE & CULTURAL WISDOM

Picture a serene village located in Sardinia. The Church bells have just struck, dinner is done, and families come together in a cutout on an open courtyard. They share laughter, conversations, wine, and allow hours to pass before silence takes over the night. No late-night munchies, no bright fluorescent 24-hour stores with neon chips and candy. Their bodies are resting in alignment with the night - fasting in nature but not calling it fasting.

Now, envision a Buddhist monastery at dawn. The monks wake quietly, meditate, then share their one main meal before noon. They fast for the rest of the day, and their fast is not deprivation; it's devotion. Their energies are invested in stillness, clarity, and service.

Or consider Ramadan: millions around the world breaking their fast with dates and water, meals framed by prayers, family, and gratitude. Fasting here is not just biological — it is communal, spiritual, a reminder that the body is resilient and that hunger can be transformed into empathy.

THE ANCIENT PULSE WE FORGOT

Across traditions, fasting has always been about more than calories. It was rhythm. It was wisdom passed from generations who intuitively understood what modern science now proves: that the body heals when it rests from constant eating.

- **Lent** created periods of abstinence — fish replacing meat, simple meals replacing indulgence.

- **Yom Kippur** invites stillness and reflection through fasting.

- **Hara Hachi Bu** in Okinawa teaches: "Eat until you are 80% full." This practice naturally extends the fasting window and lowers chronic disease risk.

These weren't "biohacks." They were cultural operating systems, embedding fasting into identity, rituals, and community.

BLUE ZONES: FASTING WITHOUT LABELS

When researchers studied **Blue Zones** — the regions of the world where people live the longest, healthiest lives — they found fasting quietly woven into daily life:

- **Sardinia:** Dinner is early, often before sunset. The rest of the night is spent fasting until morning.

- **Okinawa:** Smaller portions, long gaps between meals, the cultural mantra of *hara hachi bu.*

- **Ikaria (Greece):** Periodic fasting is aligned with the Orthodox Christian calendar, over 200 days of the year.

- **Loma Linda (California):** Many Seventh-Day Adventists practice 12–16-hour fasts simply as part of spiritual discipline.

What links them is not rigidity, but joy. Meals are shared, not counted. Fasts are rhythms, not punishments. They fast **with life, not against it.**

SCIENCE MEETS TRADITION

Today, research confirms what these traditions have carried for centuries:

- **Fasting communities report lower chronic illness rates.** (Blue Zone studies show reduced cardiovascular disease, diabetes, and cancer.)

- **Periodic religious fasts reduce inflammation markers.** (Trepanowski & Bloomer, *Nutrition Journal*, 2010.)

- **Eating with restraint and gratitude changes brain chemistry.** Hormones like ghrelin (the hunger signal) not only regulate appetite but also enhance neuroplasticity — sharpening the mind during fasts.

THE JOY OF SHARED RESTRAINT

What these cultures reveal is that fasting becomes sustainable when it's not just about *you*. When families, friends, or communities fast together, the cravings lose their bite. Food transforms from a constant demand into a moment of meaning.

This is where modern fasting often fails: when it is stripped of joy and community, reduced to an app timer and calorie math. But when reframed — as Sardinian families do with laughter, as monks do with stillness, as Blue Zone elders do with wisdom — fasting becomes not just sustainable, but beautiful.

ACTION STARTER BOX: BRINGING JOY BACK TO FASTING

☑ Share one fast-breaking meal each week with others (family, friends, or community).
☑ Try "hara hachi bu" — stop at 80% full, notice the difference.
☑ Reframe fasting from "restriction" to "ritual."
☑ Anchor your fast in gratitude: write down one thing you gained, not lost.

If fasting is the ancient rhythm, **then the challenge of our era is reclaiming it in a modern world of abundance.** The next step: building frameworks to practice fasting in daily life without guilt or confusion — bringing science and wisdom together into a living blueprint.

The story of fasting is not about skipping meals. It is not about willpower, punishment, or restriction. It is about **remembering**.

Remembering that your body evolved in a world of rhythms — cycles of feast and famine, light and dark, activity and rest. For most of human history, we thrived not because we ate constantly, but because we didn't. Each pause gave our cells a chance to recalibrate, to sweep away debris, to spark renewal.

Today, with refrigerators humming at midnight and snacks within arm's reach at every moment, we live in a world of constant "on." Fasting, then, is not a fad — it is a **recalibration**. It is the act of reclaiming an ancient rhythm we never should have abandoned.

Think of it this way:

- Every hour you go without food is not emptiness, but a message.
- Every pause is not a deprivation, but communication.
- You are telling your cells: **Heal. Repair. Thrive.**

And they listen.

Mitochondria reset. Inflammation cools. Hormones synchronize. Your body receives the signal that it is not under siege but in control — resilient, adaptable, alive.

When you begin to view fasting not as a struggle but as a **language**, you realize something profound: you are in constant dialogue with your biology. Each fast is a phrase, each pause a paragraph, each cycle a chapter in the story of your renewal.

THE BRIDGE FORWARD

But here's the truth: fasting is only one half of the ancient rhythm. Just as day requires night, and inhale requires exhale, fasting requires its counterpart: **deep recovery**.

Because you don't grow stronger while you push — you grow stronger while you restore. Muscles heal in rest. Brains consolidate in sleep. Hormones recalibrate when you finally turn off the world and surrender to the dark.

That's where we go next.

In the next chapter, we explore **Recovery as Renewal** — why rest is not idleness but an anabolic signal. And then, the keystone: **The Sleep Prescription** — your body's nighttime pharmacy, the single most potent performance enhancer and healer you already own.

Fasting taught us the power of the pause. Now, we'll learn how recovery makes every movement, every fast, every effort count.

CHAPTER 10:

RECOVERY AS RENEWAL — YOUR BODY'S FORGOTTEN MODE OF HEALING

PART 1 — THE FORGOTTEN MODE OF HEALING

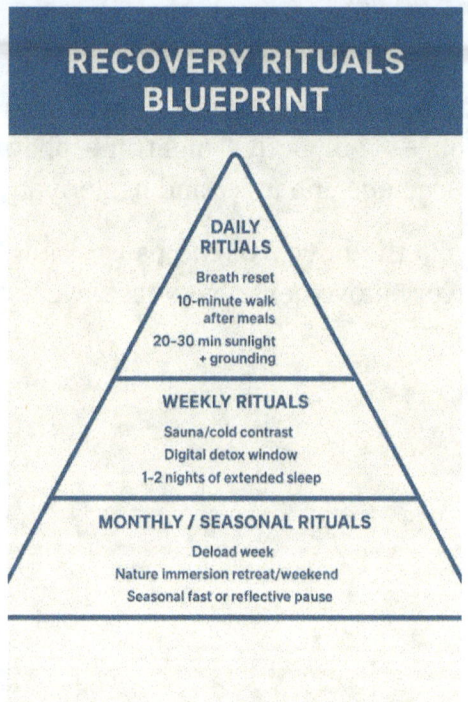

THE MODERN GRIND

Alarm screams at 6:00 a.m. Your cell phone lights up with the emails, messages, and notifications you received overnight. Coffee first, no breakfast, time to commute. By mid-morning, you're fueled by caffeine and cortisol. Lunch? At my desk, at a glowing screen. The afternoon slump hits, but there is no pause: just another latte, another meeting, another fire to put out. The evening arrives with exhaustion, but the brain is still buzzing. Instead of winding down, you scroll blue-lit screens until midnight and collapse into broken sleep.

And do it all again tomorrow.

This is the modern cycle - always on, always being stimulated. The cultural script states that to rest is to be lazy, to recover is to be weak, and to slow down is to fall behind. Productivity is worshipped, exhaustion is worn like a badge of honor.

But biology doesn't buy into hustle culture. Your body has its own script, written over millions of years through evolution. It holds onto a truth we have forgotten - growth and repair do not happen in the grind. They happen in recovery.

NATURE'S RHYTHMS

Look outside: nature does not run at full throttle all of the time. The forest has seasons. The ocean has tides. Animals have cycles of hunt and rest, exertion and stillness. A lion does not sprint all day - it bursts with ferocity, then will rest still for hours while conserving energy and repairing.

Even the tiniest organisms on Earth follow rhythms. There are small circadian clocks, ticking with the rise and set of the sun. Our cells are the same. They expect not only movement and nourishment, but also deep renewal.

The paradox of human health is this: We have extended our capacity to "do more" but have shortened our willingness for "being still." Our biology is ancient, but our lifestyles are artificial - and that mismatch produces fatigue, inflammation, burnout, and dysfunction.

THE ANCIENT HEALING MODE

Here's the hidden truth: your body has two operating systems.

- **Sympathetic Mode** → "fight or flight." This is the system modern life keeps switched on: fast heart rate, high cortisol, muscles primed for action. Essential in danger. Destructive when chronic.

- **Parasympathetic Mode** → "rest and digest." This is the forgotten system, the one that heals you. It slows the heart, deepens the breath, digests food, rebuilds muscle, clears inflammation, and even repairs the brain during sleep.

Every meaningful repair of your tissues, your nervous system, your hormones—happens when parasympathetic tone dominates. Yet most of us never enter it fully. We stay locked in sympathetic overdrive, mistaking fatigue for weakness, masking it with caffeine or willpower.

This is why "recovery" isn't optional. It's not indulgence. It's the very foundation of resilience, longevity, and joy.

MARIA'S CRASH

Maria was a 42-year-old project manager, mother of two, weekend warrior athlete with some level of healthy pride in "pushing through." 4 gym sessions a week. 11+ hour workdays. Late-night emails to catch up. Her mantra was - I'll sleep when I'm dead.

But her body fought back. Fatigue deepened. Her workouts plateaued; instead, her muscles ached for days. She added weight to her waist, even with clean eating. Her sleep became fragmented and shallow. Her doctor flagged her rising blood pressure and fasting glucose.

What happened? Maria was not broken. She was under-recovered. Her sympathetic system was dominating her physiology, and the repair mechanisms her body needed were never switched on. When we added recovery rituals—earlier sleep, parasympathetic breath resets, gentle movement on "rest" days—her biomarkers improved, her energy returned, and her performance increased. She relearned what athletes know and professionals forget: performance = work + recovery.

THE HIDDEN CURRENCY OF RECOVERY

Let's go deeper. Every rep in the gym creates micro-tears in muscle fibers. Every stressful work meeting sends cortisol into your bloodstream. Every late night makes your brain draw from its credit, skipping the glymphatic wash that clears toxic protein buildup. These are not problems in themselves—they are signals for adaptation.

Adaptation only happens through recovery. Muscles get stronger only with rest. The nervous system rewires only in deep sleep. The immune system restores balance only in parasympathetic mode. If you never recover, the load builds up, and the body no longer adapts. In fact, it breaks.

Think of recovery as a secret bank account. Stress spends from it. Recovery replenishes it. Most of us are overdrafting our recovery time daily, living in the red until we burn out, get sick, or an injury forces us into addressing it.

SCIENCE OF THE FORGOTTEN MODE

Research confirms what our bodies already know:

- **HRV (Heart Rate Variability)** is a biomarker of recovery. High HRV = balanced autonomic system, resilience. Low HRV = sympathetic overdrive, poor adaptation.

- **Sleep studies** show that deep slow-wave sleep is when growth hormone surges, tissues repair, and memory consolidates.

- **Immune research** reveals that parasympathetic activity lowers inflammatory cytokines, while chronic sympathetic activity drives systemic inflammation.

- **Performance science** in athletes proves that recovery days improve long-term progress more than overtraining.

Recovery is not passive. It is an *active biological state*. It is where the magic happens.

THE FORGOTTEN CULTURAL WISDOM

Long before HRV monitors and sleep labs, ancient cultures built recovery into daily life. Siestas in Mediterranean villages. Tea rituals in Asia. Sabbath rests in religious traditions. Even hunter-gatherers, who worked intensely during hunts, spent long hours in rest, community, and low-level activity.

We didn't invent recovery science. We forgot it.

Here's the truth: you don't get stronger during stress. You get stronger during recovery.

And in this chapter, we reclaim recovery as your body's forgotten superpower—the mode of healing that grind culture stole from you, but that your biology has been waiting for you to remember.

PART 2 — THE PHYSIOLOGY OF RECOVERY: NERVOUS SYSTEM BALANCE, HRV, REPAIR SCIENCE

TWO SYSTEMS, ONE BODY

Imagine driving a car with two gears: one for acceleration, one for braking and repair. Both are essential. But what if you only pressed the gas? Eventually, the engine overheats, the brakes rust, and the car breaks down.

Your body works the same way. The "gas" is your **sympathetic nervous system**—the fight-or-flight engine. The "brake and repair" is your **parasympathetic nervous system**—the rest-and-digest mode. Together, they form the **autonomic nervous system (ANS)**, your hidden operating system that runs 24/7.

- **Sympathetic mode** prepares you for action: dilates pupils, accelerates heart rate, releases glucose into the bloodstream, spikes cortisol.

- **Parasympathetic mode** restores you: lowers heart rate, increases digestion, enhances nutrient absorption, and boosts immune repair.

Neither system is "good" or "bad." Both are necessary. The problem is imbalance. Modern life overstimulates the sympathetic mode and starves parasympathetic recovery.

THE PHYSIOLOGY OF IMBALANCE

Research shows that chronic sympathetic dominance—living always "on"—leads to:

- Elevated **cortisol**, which in short bursts sharpens you, but chronically erodes muscle, weakens immunity, and raises belly fat.

- Suppressed **digestion**, contributing to reflux, bloating, IBS, and nutrient malabsorption.

- Reduced **immune surveillance**, increasing vulnerability to infections and even cancer risk.

- Lowered **HRV (Heart Rate Variability)** is a signal that your system is rigid and less adaptable to stress.

Think of HRV as the *music* of your nervous system. A healthy, resilient system plays with rhythm and variation. A stressed, rigid system beats like a monotone drum—predictable, unyielding, fragile.

JAMES, THE CORPORATE SPRINTER

James, 35, a tech executive, was an avid Apple Watch wearer. His resting heart rate was totally normal, but his HRV—once robust in his 20s—was tanking. He woke up exhausted after 8 hours of sleep. His digestion was off, and his mood was anxious.

When we layered HRV tracking with lifestyle changes—midday breath resets, shorter intense workouts accompanied by yoga, and early sleep—his HRV bounced back to normal within a few weeks. He had energy again. The numbers matched what his body already knew: recovery was missing.

THE REPAIR PATHWAYS INSIDE YOU

When parasympathetic mode dominates, a symphony of repair switches on:

1. **Cardiac Repair:**

   a. HRV rises, signaling vagus nerve strength.

   b. Blood pressure normalizes.

   c. Endothelial function (the lining of blood vessels) improves, lowering the risk of cardiovascular disease.

2. **Hormonal Balance:**

   d. Cortisol levels drop to baseline.

   e. Growth hormone surges during deep sleep, repairing tissues and aiding fat metabolism.

   f. Sex hormones (testosterone, estrogen, progesterone) balance, improving fertility and mood.

3. **Digestive Recovery:**

   g. Saliva enzymes flow.

   h. Stomach acid and bile increase, allowing better protein and fat digestion.

   i. Gut motility normalizes, reducing IBS symptoms.

4. **Immune Reboot:**

j. Parasympathetic tone reduces pro-inflammatory cytokines (IL-6, TNF-alpha).

k. Natural killer cells strengthen surveillance against viral and tumor cells.

l. Tissue repair accelerates at wound sites.

5. **Neural Repair:**

m. During deep sleep, the glymphatic system clears beta-amyloid and tau proteins from the brain, which are linked to dementia.

n. BDNF (Brain-Derived Neurotrophic Factor) rises, helping neurons grow and rewire.

RESEARCH SNIPPETS

- **HRV Studies:** Athletes with higher HRV recover faster and perform better under pressure. (Stanlcy ct al., *Sports Med*, 2013).

- **Cortisol Rhythm Research:** Healthy cortisol peaks in the morning, declines by evening. Chronic stress flattens this curve, predicting burnout. (Miller et al., PNAS, 2007).

- **Sleep + Growth Hormone:** Nearly 70% of daily growth hormone pulses occur during deep slow-wave sleep. (Van Cauter et al., *J Clin Endocrinol Metab*, 2000).

- **Vagus Nerve + Immunity:** Electrical vagus stimulation reduces inflammation in autoimmune diseases by activating the cholinergic anti-inflammatory pathway. (Tracey, *Nature Rev Immunology*, 2009).

THE ATHLETE'S SECRET

High-performance athletes recognize that it is in recovery where performance is built. They take naps in between training. They track their HRV every day. They alternate hard training days with active recovery. They utilize sauna, ice baths, and mobility flows. Why? Because stress alone does not make you stronger, stress plus recovery does.

The sad reality is that non-athletes—people working long hours, juggling families, battling stress —need recovery just as much if not more. Yet they're denied it by culture and habit.

THE NURSE ON NIGHT SHIFT

Lydia, a 29-year-old ICU nurse, worked rotating shifts. Her HRV was consistently low, and she struggled with anxiety and irregular cycles. We built micro-recovery into her schedule:

- 10-minute sunlight walks after shifts.

- Noise-canceling naps mid-afternoon.

- A digital wind-down ritual before sleep, even if her bedtime shifted.

Her HRV rose, her cycles normalized, and her mood stabilized. Recovery isn't about quitting—it's about weaving repair into chaos.

RECOVERY AS ADAPTATION CURRENCY

Think of recovery as **adaptation currency**. Every stressor—workout, deadline, emotional fight—spends from your balance. Recovery deposits back.

- If deposits > withdrawals → growth, resilience, vitality.

- If withdrawals > deposits → burnout, breakdown, illness.

Your biology isn't asking you to stop stressing. It's asking you to *recover as much as you stress*. That balance is the gateway to longevity.

All recovery roads eventually converge on one foundation: **sleep**. Sleep is the ultimate parasympathetic state, the nightly reboot that repairs tissues, restores hormones, rewires the brain, and recharges your soul.

And in the next part, we'll unlock sleep as your body's forgotten pharmacy—the recovery prescription nature wrote into your DNA.

PART 3 — SLEEP AS FOUNDATION: YOUR BODY'S FORGOTTEN PHARMACY

THE WORLD THAT NEVER SLEEPS

It's 2:37 a.m. Saturday morning. Somewhere, a phone goes off on a nightstand. A blue light touches a sleepy face. A half-written email is open. A streaming show rolls directly into the next episode. The city outside hums on—restaurants are still "open" and glowing screens clutter every apartment.

Modernity has obliterated night. Yet biology has not caught up.

Inside every cell's nucleus, clocks are still ticking. Genes oscillate on 24-hour rhythms signaling when to repair DNA, release hormones, digest food, or bolster the immune system. But when sleep is inhibited, prevented, or broken, those clocks misfire. The body gets out of sync, like an orchestra where every instrument plays in a different key.

SLEEP IS NOT PASSIVE

We often think of sleep as "doing nothing." But inside, it's the busiest time of your day. Sleep is your body's **pharmacy, repair shop, and reset button.**

- In your **brain**, waste is flushed out through a special network.

- In your **muscles**, microtears are repaired with growth hormone.

- In your **immune system**, antibodies strengthen, and inflammation drops.

- In your **endocrine system**, cortisol resets, leptin and ghrelin recalibrate appetite, and sex hormones pulse.

You don't sleep to rest. You sleep to **heal**.

THE ARCHITECTURE OF SLEEP

Sleep is not one monolithic block but a **cycle of stages**, repeating roughly every 90 minutes.

1. **NREM Stage 1 & 2 (Light Sleep):** Transition phases. Heart rate slows, body temperature drops, external awareness fades.

2. **NREM Stage 3 (Deep Slow-Wave Sleep):** The body's repair shop. Growth hormone peaks, immune cells restore tissue, and glucose metabolism recalibrates.

3. **REM Sleep (Dream Sleep):** The brain's therapy session. Emotional memories are processed, creativity enhanced, and problem-solving sharpened.

A healthy night delivers 4–6 complete cycles. Deprivation of any stage sabotages repair.

THE GLYMPHATIC REVELATION

For centuries, scientists wondered: how does the brain clear waste without a lymphatic system? The answer emerged in 2013: the **glymphatic system**.

At night, especially during **deep sleep**, brain cells shrink by up to 60%, creating channels for cerebrospinal fluid to wash through. This flushes out **beta-amyloid and tau proteins**, whose accumulation is linked to Alzheimer's.

Think of it as your brain's nightly dishwasher cycle. Skip sleep, and dirty dishes pile up. Chronic sleep debt is now considered a risk factor not just for dementia, but also for depression, anxiety, and metabolic disease.

MELATONIN, CORTISOL, AND THE CLOCKWORK INSIDE

Sleep is choreographed by a hormonal symphony.

- **Melatonin:** Released by the pineal gland as darkness falls. It signals the body to cool, slow, and prepare for rest. Blue light from screens suppresses melatonin, tricking the body into "daytime mode."

- **Cortisol:** Peaks in the morning, helping you wake. Should decline steadily into the evening. Chronic stress flattens this curve, leaving cortisol too high at night (insomnia) or too low in the morning (grogginess).

- **Growth Hormone:** Secreted in pulses during slow-wave sleep, repairing tissues and burning fat.

- **Leptin + Ghrelin:** Appetite hormones recalibrate at night. Sleep loss drives ghrelin up (hunger) and leptin down (satiety), fueling cravings.

Your hormones are like musicians in an orchestra. Sleep is the conductor keeping them in sync. Without it, chaos.

MARIA'S MIDNIGHT STRUGGLE

Maria, the patient we have tracked in the previous chapters, experienced a relapse of depression. This time, she was not eating excessively or avoiding movement—she was sleeping 5–6 broken hours each night.

Her HRV dropped, her cravings went up, and her mood dipped. After implementing a "digital sunset" (screens off one hour before bed, soft lamp lights, herbal tea), her sleep was extended to 7.5 hours. Her morning cortisol curve returned to normal. In a matter of weeks, her energy and emotional resilience were regained.

THE COST OF SLEEP DEBT

Research paints the picture starkly:

- One week of 6 hours/night → gene expression shifts, upregulating inflammation pathways and downregulating immunity. (PNAS, 2013).

- Two nights of poor sleep → insulin resistance rises, mimicking prediabetes. (*Lancet*, 1999).

- Chronic sleep debt → doubles risk of depression and anxiety. (JAMA *Psychiatry*, 2017).

- Short sleep duration (<6 hrs) → 12% higher risk of premature death. (*Sleep*, 2010).

Sleep is not optional. It is a daily survival drug.

SLEEP ACROSS THE NIGHT — A REPAIR TIMELINE

- **10 p.m.–12 a.m.:** Growth hormone surges, muscle + tissue repair begins.

- **12 a.m.–3 a.m.:** Deep slow-wave sleep, immune cells restore balance, and the glymphatic system is active.

- **3 a.m.–6 a.m.:** REM dominates—emotional memory processing, creativity, dreaming.

- **6 a.m.–8 a.m.:** Cortisol rises, melatonin falls, body prepares for waking.

Missing the early part of the night (pre-midnight) costs you **deep sleep repair**. Missing the later part (pre-dawn) costs you **emotional processing**.

THE ATHLETE AND THE EXECUTIVE

High-performing athletes protect their sleep like it's gold. Roger Federer claims to sleep around 12 hours when in training blocks.

LeBron James, 10-12. Why? They understand that skill practice and strength training hardly matter without a sleep-driven consolidation and recovery period.

On the other hand, executives brag about "only getting by on four hours of sleep." Meanwhile, their decision-making, creativity, and emotional regulation plummet. Research shows 24 hours of wakefulness reduces cognition as much as a blood alcohol content of .10% - at that level, you are legally drunk.

Now, who is really performing?

DESIGNING FOR SLEEP RECOVERY

You cannot "force" sleep. You can only create the conditions for biology to take over. Recovery-focused sleep hygiene is about **signals**:

- **Light:** Morning sunlight sets circadian clocks. Evening darkness protects melatonin.

- **Temperature:** Cooler environments (~65°F / 18°C) deepen sleep.

- **Routine:** Going to bed/waking at consistent times anchors the circadian rhythm.

- **Digital Sunset:** Screens off 1 hr before bed, or blue-light filters if unavoidable.

- **Wind-Down Rituals:** Journaling, stretching, reading fiction, and herbal teas.

THE FORGOTTEN FOUNDATION

Nutrition matters. Movement matters. Stress management matters. But without sleep, they're building on sand. Sleep is not the third pillar of health—it is the **foundation on which nutrition, movement, and stress resilience stand.**

When you sleep, your body doesn't rest. It **rewires, rebalances, and renews.**

THE NIGHTLY REPAIR TIMELINE

10–12 PM	Growth hormone surge Muscle + tissue repair
12–3 AM	Deep sleep Immune restoration
3–6 AM	REM sleep Emotional processing
6–8 AM	Cortisol rise Waking preparation

PART 4 — BEYOND SLEEP: ACTIVE RECOVERY

Sleep is the foundation, yes...but recovery doesn't stop when we wake up.

Your body carries its need for restoration throughout every waking hour, and there are cultural practices from ages past that daily utilize heat, cold, movement, and pause to achieve that. These are the active recovery levers - mechanisms of extending recovery beyond the bed to support the nervous system and tissue to reset into balance, repair, and resilience.

1. THE FORGOTTEN WISDOM OF CONTRAST THERAPY

Think of an ancient Finnish village in winter. There is waist-deep snow and a frozen lake nearby. Huddled inside a wooden hut is a family in a smoke sauna. Sweat drips off the skin as heat elevates heart rate, dilates blood vessels, and triggers the release of heat shock proteins- Molecular guardians that repair damaged proteins and protect cells. And then, without hesitation, the family steps outside and plunges their bodies into ice-cold water. There are gasps, laughs, and then an adrenaline rush.

This is not torture or Punishment- this is restoration.

And as the 21st century honors- current science confirms what these ancient cultures knew so well: alternating heat and cold jolts the cardiovascular system like an elastic band, increasing vascular flexibility. Sauna sessions can lower all-cause mortality risk by up to 40% (Laukkanen et al., JAMA Intern Med, 2015). Cold plunges activate brown fat, spike norepinephrine (a natural antidepressant), and enhance vagal tone. The body learns adaptability—the essence of resilience.

2. MICRO-RESTORATIONS IN MOTION

Recovery isn't always grand rituals—it's also the small pauses woven into a day.

A 5-minute mobility flow between Zoom calls. A 20-minute nap that resets the hippocampus, restoring learning capacity. Even a short stretch break lowers allostatic load—the "wear and tear" of stress hormones on the body.

Science calls these "micro-recoveries." They seem trivial, yet research shows they compound. A study in *Occupational Health* found that employees who took brief restorative breaks every 90 minutes had **higher HRV, lower fatigue, and improved focus** compared to those who "powered through." The truth? Recovery is not passive—it's actively practiced.

3. BREATHWORK AS RECOVERY IN REAL TIME

Your breath is a steering wheel for your nervous system. Slow exhales activate the parasympathetic branch, dropping heart rate, lowering blood pressure, and increasing HRV. Techniques like "box breathing" (inhale 4s, hold 4s, exhale 4s, hold 4s) or resonance breathing (5.5 breaths per minute) are proven to rebalance the autonomic system.

This is recovery you can do anywhere—on the train, between meetings, even standing in line. Unlike sleep, you don't have to wait for night. Each breath pattern is a switch you can flip toward renewal.

4. THE REVIVAL POWER OF NAPS

In Mediterranean cultures, the **siesta** is not laziness—it's biology aligned with the circadian dip in alertness after lunch. Modern studies confirm the nap's potency: a 20–30-minute nap boosts alertness and memory consolidation. Longer 90-minute naps can mimic a full sleep cycle, aiding emotional regulation. NASA tested naps for pilots and found **a 34% improvement in performance and 100% increase in alertness**.

The catch: naps are best earlier in the day, or they interfere with nighttime sleep. Done right, they're a turbocharger for the recovery system.

5. NUTRITION AS A RECOVERY LEVER

Recovery is not only what you rest from—it's also what you refuel with.

After stress, movement, or fasting, the body craves building blocks: amino acids for muscle repair, polyphenols for inflammation control, and electrolytes for cellular balance.

- **Polyphenol-rich foods** (berries, green tea, turmeric) lower inflammatory cytokines.

- **Magnesium** restores calm by supporting over 300 enzymatic reactions, including ATP synthesis and GABA regulation.

- **Collagen + vitamin C** rebuild connective tissues stressed during movement.

Think of nutrition here not as "fuel" but as "construction material" for the repair crew inside you.

6. NATURE AS AN ACTIVE RECOVERY SPACE

Not all recovery happens indoors. Forest bathing (shinrin-yoku in Japan) reduces cortisol by up to 16% after only 20 minutes in greenery (Park et al., *Environ Health Prev Med*). Sunlight not only anchors circadian rhythms but also stimulates nitric oxide release from the skin—improving vascular function.

Nature amplifies all the other levers: you breathe differently, your nervous system shifts, your heart rate slows, and your body remembers its evolutionary baseline—calm alertness.

MARIA'S RESET RITUAL

Maria, who has followed us through stress, food, and fasting, finds active recovery in small doses. After months of depletion, she introduces one ritual: 10 minutes of stretches in the evening with dim light, a warm shower, and 2 minutes of cold rinse. Within weeks, her sleep gets deeper. Her daytime heart rate variability (HRV) scores increase. More importantly, she feels "reset", her body no longer buzzing with unprocessed stress.

She finds recovery is not a once-per-year vacation, but a once-per-day rhythm.

Active recovery shows us that rest is not the absence of activity; it is the presence of activity. Whether it is breath, heat, cold, stillness, or nourishment. Sleep is one foundation, and all of the above are the scaffolding that make your sleep strong. When you take recovery as a living practice, you begin to move towards thriving in the natural cycles of stress and renewal of your biology as opposed to surviving through the grind of a busy life.

ACTIVE RECOVERY LEVERS

 **CONTRAST THERAPY**
Heat and cold exposure

 **MICRO-RESTORATIONS**
Naps, mobility, stretching

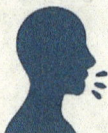 **BREATH WORK**
Slows heart rate, calms nerves

 **NUTRITION**
Anti-inflammatory, nutrient-rich

 **NATURE**
Forest bathing, sunlight

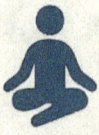 **MICRO-BREAKS**
Short rest, reset, refocus

PART 5 — STRESS + RECOVERY SYNERGY

You've heard the mantra: "No *pain, no gain.*" But in truth, the body's mantra is quieter, wiser: "*Stress me, then let me heal.*"

The paradox of resilience is this: the stress is not what makes you stronger. It's the **recovery window** afterward—the time when tissues rebuild, hormones reset, and the nervous system rebalances. Without that sacred interval, stress doesn't forge strength—it chisels cracks.

OVERTRAINING SYNDROME: WHEN STRESS BECOMES POISON

In sports science, it has a name: **overtraining syndrome.** At first, the symptoms are subtle: lingering soreness, mood dips, restless sleep. Then comes the hormonal unraveling—cortisol stays locked in the *on* position, testosterone drops, thyroid hormones wobble.

- The immune system falters; colds linger.

- Motivation evaporates.

- Injuries creep in where muscles and joints once felt bulletproof.

And it's not limited to athletes. Overtraining syndrome has a modern twin: **life overtraining.**

- Double-shot espressos for deadlines.

- High-intensity workouts squeezed between back-to-back Zoom calls.

- Late-night   scrolling   instead   of   sleep.
  It's the same biology at work—stress input stacked without a recovery buffer.

CORTISOL + THE RECOVERY WINDOW

Cortisol is not the villain—it's your built-in survival fuel. A morning spike of cortisol wakes you, primes your brain, and mobilizes glucose. But it was never meant to be left humming at midnight, grinding your body into erosion.

What brings cortisol back to baseline?

- **Parasympathetic reset**: Slow breaths, sunlight, laughter, or sleep trigger the "rest-and-digest" nervous system.

- **Glycogen + repair**: During recovery, muscles refill energy stores, and microtears stitch stronger.

- **Immune balance**: Anti-inflammatory cytokines rise, calming the storm.

When that window is skipped, stress hormones remain elevated. Day bleeds into night. Fatigue becomes the background music of life.

THE RESILIENCE PARADOX

You don't grow stronger during stress. You grow stronger *after the stress* if recovery is allowed. That's the paradox at the heart of training, learning, even living.

- Lift weights: stress the muscle. Growth comes in sleep.

- Study hard: stress the neurons. Memory consolidates in rest.

- Face setbacks: stress the psyche. Wisdom arises in reflection.

Every adaptation is **post-stress biology**. Miss the recovery, and all you collect is breakdown.

SCIENCE IN FOCUS

- Studies in elite endurance athletes show that those with **inadequate recovery windows** have suppressed NK-cell activity, the very immune soldiers that fend off viruses.

- Research on military trainees during "hell week" reveals hormone profiles resembling clinical depression: cortisol up, serotonin down, thyroid sluggish.

- Longitudinal data: Athletes who prioritized sleep and active recovery had **50% fewer injuries** across a season compared to those who trained harder but slept less.

THE PLATEAU BREAKER

Consider Jenna, an extremely dedicated CrossFitter. She trained twice a day – woke up before dawn for a WOD (workout of the day), then hit the gym after hours for lifting. She survived on black coffee and protein shakes and wore signs of fatigue like a badge of honor. She just continued grinding. Then one day, her lifts plateaued, she became fatigued, and then developed nagging tendon pain.

It wasn't until her coach intervened that they dialed things back:

o   Training has been reduced to 5 days a week

o   The Coach added mobility sessions, contrast showers, and a hard and fast rule of 8 hours of sleep.

o   A full day off also became a non-negotiable.

Would you believe, in just two months, she started making gains in the gym. Her tendon pain went away. Her body was not lazy; it was just waiting for permission to heal.

THE TAKEAWAY

Recovery isn't weakness. It's the **hidden half of strength.** Stress opens the door, but recovery builds the house.

When you honor the synergy—stress applied, recovery allowed— you transform burnout into resilience, plateaus into breakthroughs, and life into a sustainable rhythm.

PART 6 — ACTION STARTER: RECOVERY RITUALS BLUEPRINT

If stress is the ignition that creates resilience, then recovery is the oxygen that keeps the fire burning. Without oxygen, the fire goes out. Without recovery, the body fails.

Recovery is not just sleep or rest days; recovery is a structured rhythm, purposely layered into daily, weekly, and seasonal life. Think of recovery not as pampering, but preparation for longevity.

The Recovery Pyramid

Think of a pyramid. At the bottom are daily rituals—small, mandatory, sacred action that keeps your nervous system aligned. In the middle zone are weekly rituals, antidotal resets that replenish reserves. At the top are seasonal rituals, infrequent but resetting rituals that reboot your biology for the long game.

DAILY RITUALS: MICRO-RESTORATIONS

These are the anchors that tell your body, *"You're safe, you can repair."*

- **Breath Reset (Parasympathetic Switch)**
  Just 2 minutes of slow exhale-focused breathing lowers heart rate, signals vagal tone, and flips you out of fight-or-flight.
  Science note: HRV (heart rate variability) improves measurably after just a few cycles of slow breathing.

- **10-Minute Walk After Meals**
  A humble walk does double duty: it blunts post-meal glucose spikes *and* calms the nervous system.
  Science note: Postprandial walking reduces insulin demand by up to 30%.

- **20–30 Minutes of Sunlight + Grounding**
  Morning light sets your circadian clock, boosting cortisol appropriately early while priming melatonin for the evening. Barefoot grounding on earth may reduce inflammatory markers.
  Science note: Sunlight-driven vitamin D + circadian entrainment correlate with longer telomeres (longevity marker).

WEEKLY RITUALS: DEEPER RECOVERY

Think of these as your **system-wide tune-ups.**

- **Sauna/Cold Contrast**
  Alternating heat and cold is hormetic training for your vascular and nervous system.
  Science note: Finnish sauna use 4–7 times a week is linked to ~40% lower cardiovascular mortality.

- **Digital Detox Window**
  Pick one evening per week: no phone, no notifications. Create a "neural quiet hour" to reset overstimulated circuits.

- **1–2 Nights of Extended Sleep**
  Catch-up sleep isn't a myth—it's a recovery tool. Extending sleep by even one hour boosts immune response and improves cognitive performance.

MONTHLY / SEASONAL RITUALS: DEEP RECALIBRATION

These are the rare, high-impact practices that help you **zoom out of the daily grind** and remind your body what renewal feels like.

- **Deload Week (Exercise Taper)**
  Every 6–8 weeks, intentionally reduce exercise volume/intensity by 40–50%. Muscles recover, joints reset, and the nervous system restores.
  Science note: Athletes who deload cyclically show greater long-term strength gains than those who never back off.

- **Nature Immersion Retreat / Weekend**
  A full weekend unplugged in nature lowers cortisol, restores creativity, and enhances immune activity (NK cells spike for up to a week after forest bathing).

- **Seasonal Fast or Reflective Pause**
  Whether a short water fast, spiritual practice, or simply a digital sabbatical, seasonal rituals act as metabolic and psychological "hard resets."

SCIENCE ANCHOR: RECOVERY = LONGEVITY

Blue Zone cultures know this secret—Sardinians nap midday. Okinawans weave in communal downtime. Adventists protect Sabbath rest. Their lives are not built on endless productivity, but on **intentional cycles of pause.**

The lesson: longevity is not earned through relentless grind, but through **strategic oscillation between stress and rest.**

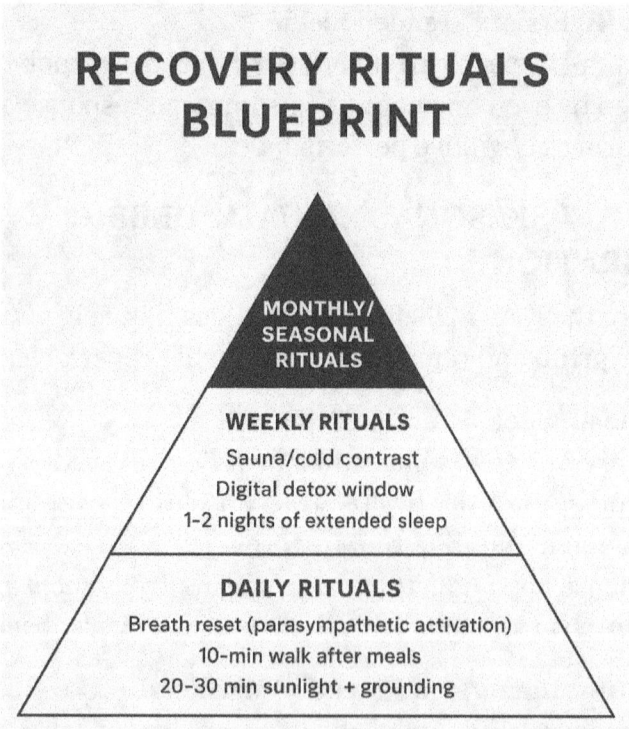

RECOVERY RITUALS BLUEPRINT

MONTHLY/ SEASONAL RITUALS

WEEKLY RITUALS
Sauna/cold contrast
Digital detox window
1-2 nights of extended sleep

DAILY RITUALS
Breath reset (parasympathetic activation)
10-min walk after meals
20-30 min sunlight + grounding

Takeaway: Recovery is not the opposite of productivity—it's the foundation of it. Every ritual is a micro-message to your biology: "*You are safe. You can heal. You can thrive.*

SLEEP AS THE ULTIMATE RECOVERY PRESCRIPTION

Recovery is not merely resting—it's rejuvenation. In the absence of recovery, resilience is built on sand and inevitably begins to crumble. With recovery, growth multiplies; resilience can only accumulate. Muscles fuse back stronger, the nervous system recalibrates, and the mind rediscovers clarity.

But here's the more profound truth: all recovery rituals are fundamentally revolving around one gravitational pull: sleep. Breathwork, sunlight, sauna, nature—those are the satellites, while sleep is the planet.

Visualize recovery as a garden. Stress is planting - breaking up the soil, dropping new seedlings. Recovery is the rich soil that keeps those seedlings alive. And sleep? Sleep is the waterfall of sustenance flowing right to the root, plant, seed, system. Without water, the soil crumbles. Without sleep, recovery rituals will do very little to none of recovery.

Thus, why do elite athletes care more about their sleep than their training volume? This is why memory, immunity, metabolism, and emotional stability all rely on nightly sleep cycles; This is why the next chapter is the most important thing we've discussed in this book, probably even more than every other chapter.

Because if recovery is the soil of progress, then sleep is the water—the nightly flood that feeds every inch of your being.

We will turn the page and enter Chapter 11: The Sleep Prescription—a deep dive into your most powerful, most ignored medicine cabinet inside your body. Night after night, your brain detoxes, your hormones reset, and your biology heals.

Sleep is not rest. Sleep is medicine.

PART IV

THE RESTORATION OF MIND AND MEANING

CHAPTER 11:

THE SLEEP PRESCRIPTION

YOUR BODY'S NIGHTTIME PHARMACY

PART 1: THE FORGOTTEN PILL

Imagine this:

A surgeon has just finished a 12-hour shift; she is exhausted, red-eyed, and shaky. She is drinking vending-machine coffee to keep her scalpel from shaking. In another place, a startup founder is scrolling Slack at 2 a.m., looking at his screen bathed in blue light while his body begs for sleep. A new mother is nursing her infant at 3 a.m., heart racing, cortisol firing, wondering if she will sleep at all before dawn.

Now, consider a different world of experience.

A desert tribe where firelight fades with the stars, people going into deep sleep as the Milky Way rises. The next morning, when they wake with the sun, they are energized and grounded (sometimes literally lying on the ground), in sync with the rhythm of the earth.

The experience is polar. In one experience, sleep is a luxury and optional – it is a fluffy pillow for the weak. In another, it is recognized as a biological law, as non-negotiable as air or water.

THE HIDDEN PRESCRIPTION

Here's the truth science has finally caught up to: **Sleep is not rest. Sleep is repair.**

Every night, while you think you are doing "nothing," your brain is flushing out toxins through the glymphatic system, your immune army is reorganizing, your hormones are recalibrating, and your DNA is repairing. Skip or skimp on it, and the consequences are merciless:

- **One night of 4–5 hours of sleep**: insulin sensitivity crashes by up to 30% (the metabolic profile of prediabetes in a single day).

- **One week of poor sleep**: testosterone drops, cortisol skyrockets, immunity plummets.

- **One month of chronic deprivation**: mood disorders flare, memory fragments, Alzheimer's risk pathways ignite.

And yet — the opposite is just as dramatic. Give the body **real, deep, consistent sleep**, and it will return the favor: sharper focus, younger biology, improved resilience, even protection from chronic disease.

Sleep is not just the body's downtime. **It is the most powerful prescription you'll never get from a pharmacy.**

We live in a culture that worships productivity but steals from its own future to fuel the present. "I'll sleep when I'm dead," people joke, not realizing the irony: skipping sleep is the fastest way to speed that up.

Meanwhile, the "sleep economy" has exploded — pills, apps, devices, mattresses promising miracles. But here's the irony: **sleep is free, natural, coded into your biology.** You don't need a gadget to unlock it — you need to reclaim the rhythms that your body has known for millennia.

The narrative of this chapter is simple but urgent:

- If recovery is the soil for growth, then sleep is the water.

- It's the ultimate recovery prescription, the one that heals every organ, every system, every cell.

- And yet, it's the one most of us have forgotten how to use.

BRIDGE INTO SCIENCE

In the next sections, we'll open the curtain on what actually happens during sleep: the cycles, the brain waves, the nightly glymphatic wash, the hormonal symphony that recalibrates metabolism, mood, and immunity.

But before we step into the science, pause and consider this: What if the single greatest act of self-care, longevity, and resilience isn't another supplement or workout — but **choosing to turn off the light, let go, and sleep?**

PART 2 — THE ARCHITECTURE OF SLEEP: CYCLES, STAGES, AND BRAIN REPAIR

THE HIDDEN BLUEPRINT OF THE NIGHT

For the majority of people, sleep looks like a light switch: on or off. You're awake, and then you're asleep. But inside your brain and body, the night is an elaborate opera, synchronicities in phases, each taking on its own distinctive part.

Sleep is not a passive endeavor. Rather, it is an active, cycling architecture — a repeating rhythm of electrical patterns, hormonal pulses, and cellular housekeeping.

Think of it as a **four-act play** that repeats 4–6 times a night, each cycle lasting about 90 minutes:

1. **Light Sleep (N1 & N2)** – The gateway. The body begins to shift gears.

2. **Deep Sleep (N3)** – The restoration chamber. Growth, repair, and memory encoding.

3. **REM (Rapid Eye Movement)** – The dream theater. Emotional regulation, learning, and creativity.

Like a well-designed training program, **you need all phases**. Skipping one is like skipping leg day every week — you pay the price.

STAGE 1: LIGHT SLEEP (N1 & N2)

Duration: 5–10 minutes (N1), then 30–60 minutes (N2) in early cycles.

- Your brain waves slow, moving from alert beta rhythms toward calmer theta waves.

- Heart rate and breathing begin to drop. Muscles twitch, sometimes giving that familiar "falling" sensation.

- In **N2**, your brain unleashes *sleep spindles* — rapid bursts of activity thought to stabilize memories and cut off external sensory input, protecting sleep.

- **K-complexes**, big spikes in electrical activity, act like "night sentries," keeping you asleep despite noises.

💡 **Why it matters:** Light sleep is the brain's "transition zone," a rehearsal before the real repair work. It primes the nervous system and acts as a shield, giving the deeper stages room to work.

STAGE 2: DEEP SLEEP (N3)

Duration: 20–40 minutes per cycle, heaviest in the first half of the night.

This is the **holy grail** of physical repair.

- Brain waves slow to **delta rhythms**, the slowest and deepest.

- Growth hormone surges — fueling tissue repair, muscle recovery, bone density, and fat metabolism.

- Immune cells reprogram, targeting infection and inflammation.

- The **glymphatic system** (a recently discovered brain cleansing mechanism) kicks on: cerebrospinal fluid washes through neural pathways, flushing out toxins like beta-amyloid, the protein linked to Alzheimer's.

- Blood pressure dips, heart rate steadies — giving your cardiovascular system a nightly reset.

💡 **Why it matters:** Miss deep sleep and you miss the body's *construction crew*. Chronic deprivation here links directly to obesity, type 2 diabetes, immune suppression, and accelerated aging.

STAGE 3: REM SLEEP

Duration: 10 minutes in early cycles, stretching to 60+ minutes in later cycles.

This is the mind's repair zone.

- Brain waves shift to a pattern similar to wakefulness, but the body is paralyzed by *atonia* (so you don't act out your dreams).

- Emotional circuits (amygdala, hippocampus) fire intensely. REM is where your brain processes trauma, stabilizes mood, and integrates emotional memory.

- Dopamine and acetylcholine surge, sharpening learning and creativity.

- Researchers call REM "overnight therapy." In PTSD patients, impaired REM correlates with trauma flashbacks and emotional instability.

💡 **Why it matters:** Miss REM and you miss your **psychological healing**. You'll feel irritable, anxious, and less resilient. It's not just dreams — it's emotional regulation.

THE CYCLICAL DANCE

Each night, you cycle through **light** → **deep** → **REM** about 4–6 times. But the proportions shift:

- Early night = **more deep sleep**, less REM.

- Late night = **more REM**, less deep sleep.

This is why a midnight bedtime cuts disproportionately into deep sleep (physical repair), while a 5 a.m. wake-up cuts disproportionately into REM (emotional healing).

💡 **Science anchor:** Sleep scientist Matthew Walker puts it plainly — **"If you're not sleeping 7–9 hours, you're shortchanging one or both halves of the night's therapy."**

BRAIN REPAIR IN ACTION

What actually happens inside your brain during these cycles is breathtaking:

- **Memory filing:** The hippocampus (short-term memory bank) "downloads" to the neocortex (long-term storage). Without this, new learning doesn't stick.

- **Neuroplasticity:** Synaptic pruning removes weak connections, while important ones strengthen — like editing the brain's hard drive.

- **Detox:** The glymphatic wash removes waste 60% more efficiently in deep sleep than in wakefulness.

- **Hormone orchestration:** Melatonin, cortisol, leptin, ghrelin, growth hormone — all pulse on their nightly schedule. Disturb them, and metabolism spirals out of sync.

WHY ARCHITECTURE MATTERS

Sleep is not a luxury. It is an **orchestrated recovery sequence** — a nightly software update for your brain and body. Miss a night, and it's like skipping a backup. Miss weeks or months, and you're running corrupted files.

This is why even small changes — delaying bedtime, chronic stress, blue light exposure — wreak havoc. They don't just reduce sleep *time*; they **disrupt the very architecture**.

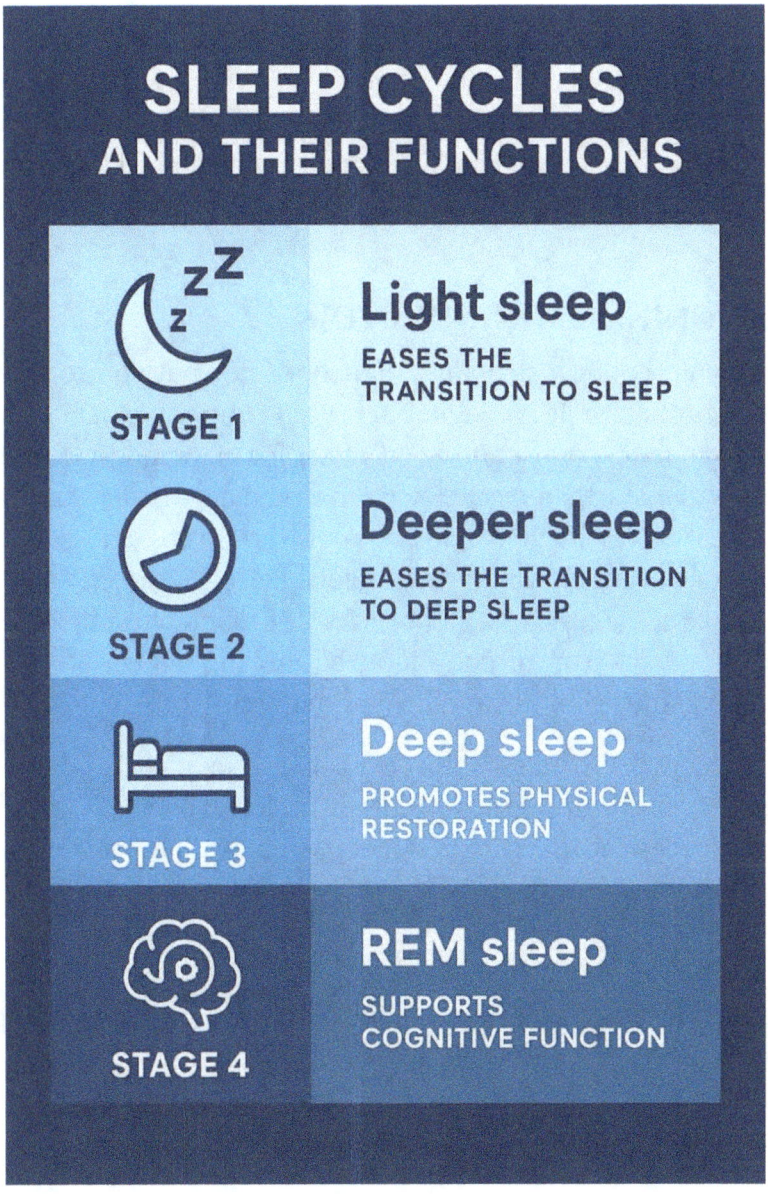

SLEEP CYCLES
AND THEIR FUNCTIONS

STAGE 1 — Light sleep
EASES THE TRANSITION TO SLEEP

STAGE 2 — Deeper sleep
EASES THE TRANSITION TO DEEP SLEEP

STAGE 3 — Deep sleep
PROMOTES PHYSICAL RESTORATION

STAGE 4 — REM sleep
SUPPORTS COGNITIVE FUNCTION

PART 3 — HORMONES IN THE NIGHT: THE SLEEP SYMPHONY

Picture this: An Amazing orchestra sitting in a quiet, dark concert hall. The musicians lift their bows, stretch their strings, and start clearing their throats. First is the silence, the hush as we wait with anticipation. Then, at the right moment, the conductor lifts his baton, and the first note resounds.

That's what happens in our body every night, when the sun is falling. Your internal orchestra begins its symphony, a closely coordinated choreography of hormones, rising and falling, signaling to each cell to renew, to heal, to reset, or to remain on emergency alert.

MELATONIN: THE CONDUCTOR

Melatonin is not a sleeping pill. It does not put you to sleep—it cues the orchestra. It is a signal, secreted from the pineal gland, as the sunlight fades, to your body, "It's time for night mode." Melatonin release is the starter's pistol for your circadian rhythm. Lights out, your digestion slows, your body temperature drops, and your heart rate starts to slow down. In the modern world of screens and late-night text messages, it is a chore for the conductor to be heard against the backdrop of continuously blinking lights, like blasting heavy metal music, in the middle of a symphony.

Science note: Studies show even a single night of late-night screen exposure suppresses melatonin release by up to 50%. That delay cascades into fragmented sleep, weaker immune repair, and foggy mornings.

CORTISOL: THE DRUMMER

Cortisol plays the role of an engine during the day—cortisol spikes at sunrise, wakes you up, mobilizes glucose, and sharpens your focus. At night, cortisol should drop and quiet the tempo, so slower and more attentive instruments can join in.

When stress lingers—a deadline, the late-night news, scary thoughts—the drummer never stops. Cortisol levels remain high, blocking you from going into deep sleep, keeping your body in a subtle fight-or-flight mode. Instead of restoration, your system spends the night in guarded vigilance.

Science note: Chronic night-time cortisol elevation is linked to a higher risk of depression, belly fat accumulation, and insulin resistance.

GROWTH HORMONE & TESTOSTERONE: THE BUILDERS

When you finally sink into deep, slow-wave sleep, the anabolic musicians step onto the stage. Growth hormone pulses repairing micro-tears in muscle, reinforcing bones, and mobilizing fat for fuel. In men and women, testosterone release follows, reinforcing tissue recovery, energy balance, and mood resilience.

Miss deep sleep, and these builders never fully report to work. You wake unrefreshed, weaker, and more vulnerable to stress.

Science note: Up to 70% of daily growth hormone is secreted during the first deep sleep cycles. Losing that is like skipping payroll for your body's repair crew.

LEPTIN & GHRELIN: THE APPETITE DUO

Leptin, secreted by fat cells, is the satiety signal: *"You've had enough."* Ghrelin, secreted by the stomach, is hunger's call: *"Feed me."*

In healthy sleep, leptin rises at night, calming hunger and stabilizing energy. Ghrelin dips, letting your body focus on repair. But when sleep is cut short, the script flips. Leptin drops, ghrelin surges—your orchestra is hijacked. The result? Morning cravings for sugar, processed carbs, and comfort foods.

Science note: After just 5 nights of 4–5 hours of sleep, ghrelin levels increase by 28%, leptin falls by 18%—a perfect storm for weight gain.

INSULIN SENSITIVITY: THE SILENT STRING SECTION

During deep sleep, cells become more insulin-sensitive—meaning glucose is handled efficiently, energy is replenished, and inflammation stays low. But cutting sleep short, insulin sensitivity drops by as much as 30% overnight. Your cells resist the signal, glucose lingers in the blood, and the stage is set for prediabetes and metabolic dysfunction.

MARIA'S STORY: THE LATE-NIGHT GLOW

Our previous patient, Maria, thought that her late-night scrolling was harmless – just a way to "unwind" after a long and difficult day. But the morning told a different story. She woke up groggy and unfocused, irritable and craving muffins and lattes. By mid-morning, she was already "hangry" with a bagel, and by evening, felt guilty.

Her sleep tracker read something that her hormones knew all too well: delayed melatonin, elevated cortisol, reduced deep sleep. Within weeks of bringing back a nighttime wind-down (phone off at 9 pm, herbal tea, dim lights), her cravings disappeared. She was automatically reaching for protein and fiber foods in the morning, in a good mood, with decent energy. The orchestra was back in harmony.

KEY TAKEAWAY:

Sleep is not passive. It is a nightly hormonal symphony. Every note—melatonin's cue, cortisol's descent, growth hormone's surge, leptin's rise—must be played in rhythm. Miss the symphony, and the next day's performance falters. Protect the concert hall, dim the lights, and let the music play.

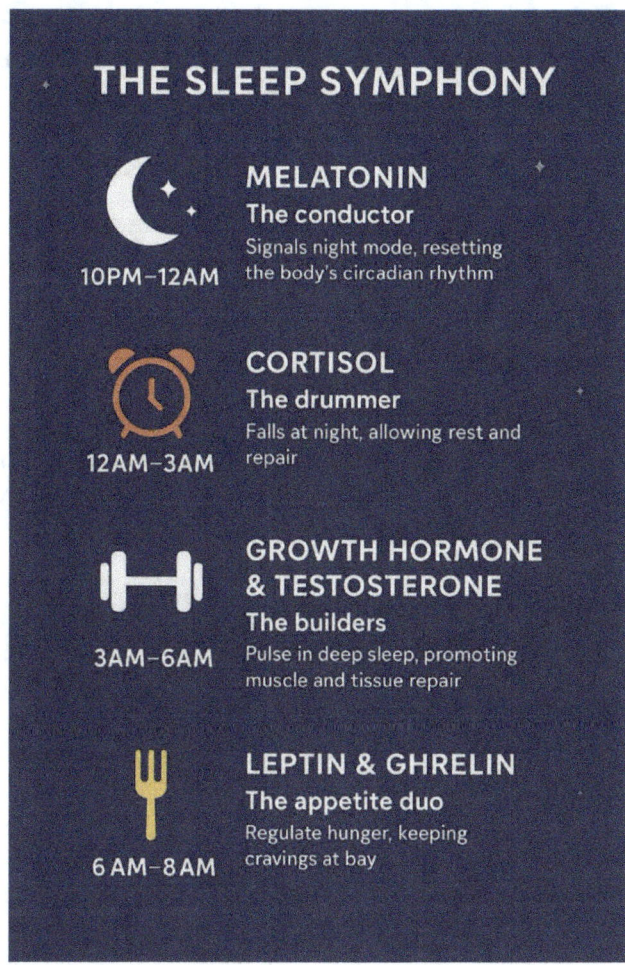

THE SLEEP SYMPHONY

MELATONIN
The conductor
Signals night mode, resetting the body's circadian rhythm
10PM–12AM

CORTISOL
The drummer
Falls at night, allowing rest and repair
12AM–3AM

GROWTH HORMONE & TESTOSTERONE
The builders
Pulse in deep sleep, promoting muscle and tissue repair
3AM–6AM

LEPTIN & GHRELIN
The appetite duo
Regulate hunger, keeping cravings at bay
6 AM–8AM

PART 4 — SLEEP + MOOD + MICROBIOME

Imagine this: a shift worker walking home again at 5:00 a.m. The city is asleep, but its mind is activated. They fall into bed, curtains shut, but sleep is broken up. By noon, they wake up tired, looking for sugary, heavy foods, bloated in their stomach and heavy in their mind. Over weeks and months, this continues. It feels like they are moving through molasses. Their digestion and their mental acuity are gradually reduced to nothing.

This is not just "being tired." This is an entire ecosystem being thrown off balance – the gut, the mind, and the holistic dance of the microbiome.

THE GUT-BRAIN-SLEEP AXIS

Sleep is not only for the mind — it's for the microbes too. Inside your gut lives an entire metropolis of bacteria, fungi, and other organisms. These microbes run on rhythms, just like your body does. They "wake up" and "rest" according to light, food, and sleep cycles.

When you cut sleep short or scatter it across odd hours, you don't just throw off your brain clock — you also throw off your gut's circadian rhythm. Studies show:

- **Two nights of only 4 hours sleep** can already **reduce microbiome diversity** — meaning fewer protective species and more opportunistic ones.

- This imbalance raises intestinal permeability ("leaky gut"), fueling systemic inflammation.

- Inflammation crosses into the brain, where it blunts mood-regulating neurotransmitters like serotonin and dopamine.

No wonder poor sleep feels like both a gut ache and a mood storm.

THE MOOD CONNECTION

The gut produces nearly **90% of the body's serotonin**, the molecule that stabilizes mood. But serotonin output depends on a balanced microbiome — and a balanced microbiome depends on adequate, consistent sleep.

Lose sleep → lose microbial balance → serotonin dips → depression and anxiety risk rise.

It's a vicious loop:

- Sleep loss → gut dysbiosis → inflammation → poor neurotransmitter regulation.

- Poor mood → more late-night scrolling, alcohol, or stress snacking → even less sleep.

CORTISOL, INFLAMMATION, AND THE MICROBIOME

Chronic sleep loss keeps **cortisol** elevated. Cortisol, when constantly high, changes the microbiome's population: beneficial species decline, while inflammatory microbes expand.

This "inflammatory bloom" worsens insulin resistance, drives sugar cravings, and creates the very metabolic storm we've been tracing throughout this book.

THE SHIFT WORKER'S STORY

Let's come back to our shift worker — we'll call him James.

Initially, his late-night shifts just made him "sort of tired." But within months, digestion worsened. Gas, bloating, irregular bowel movements. Soon after: irritability, sugar binges, and a creeping sadness he couldn't shake.

When James finally went to the doctor, he was diagnosed with early-stage insulin resistance, inflammation (lab results showed elevated inflammatory markers), and low microbial diversity in the gut. His body wasn't wrecked — it was begging for a rhythm.

By restructuring his schedule, incorporating small rituals (consistent sleep window even on non-work days, early sunlight exposure, probiotics, and earlier night-time fasting), James eventually restructured his gut-brain axis. Within three months, more energy, moods stabilized, and digestion was normal!

WHAT WE LEARNED

Sleep is not passive. Sleep is an active reset of the gut ecosystem. When you do not sleep, you not only become tired — you're also inflamed, hormonally imbalanced, and emotionally drained.

The gut and the brain are always communicating, and sleep is the moderator of that conversation.

To protect your mood and metabolism, you must protect your sleep.

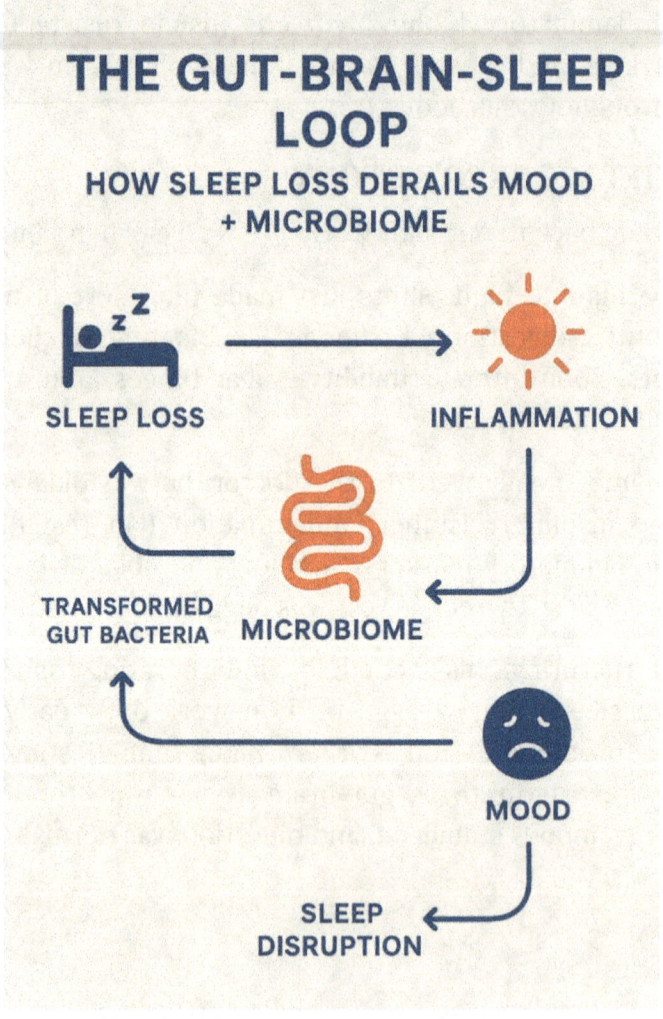

THE GUT-BRAIN-SLEEP LOOP

HOW SLEEP LOSS DERAILS MOOD + MICROBIOME

SLEEP LOSS

INFLAMMATION

TRANSFORMED GUT BACTERIA

MICROBIOME

MOOD

SLEEP DISRUPTION

PART 5 — MODERN SLEEP DISRUPTORS

Every night, think of sleep as a cathedral your body constructs. The foundation layers, as we quietly fall into dusk, the inner scaffolding builds as melatonin tells us it's time for dark, and by the time we reach midnight, deep-restorative processes are chiseling new stone, renovating the very architecture of our cellular structure.

In the hustle of the modern world, most people do not access this sacred place in an untouched manner. Instead, we bring neon floodlights, cups of over-sweetened coffee we finish long after they should be gone, illuminated screens that convince our brain it's still high noon, and stresses that follow us to bed like a bill to be paid. Therefore, our nightly cathedral crumbles before the roof can be finished.

Let's break down the biggest saboteurs of restorative sleep, modern nuisances that dismantle the very process designed to repair us.

1. BLUE LIGHT + TECH → MELATONIN SUPPRESSION

The smartphone has become the new bedside candle. But its glow is not the warm flicker of firelight—it's a blast of blue-spectrum light tuned to mimic the midday sun.

Your pineal gland, the master switch for melatonin release, reads this light as a command: *"Stay awake. Daytime isn't over."* Melatonin, the chemical nightfall signal, is suppressed. The entire cascade of sleep readiness—drop in core temperature, slowing heart rate, release of growth hormone—gets delayed.

- **Science Snapshot:** Research shows that just 2 hours of blue light exposure before bed can delay melatonin production by *up to 90 minutes*. That means a midnight Netflix binge is like telling your biology it's still 10 p.m.—even if the clock says 1 a.m.

- **Narrative:** Maria, our patient, noticed she couldn't fall asleep until after midnight despite "feeling tired." Her habit? A nightly scroll through Instagram in bed. When she swapped her phone for a book under warm light, she fell asleep 45 minutes earlier, waking refreshed instead of foggy.

2. CAFFEINE & ALCOHOL → CHEMICAL IMPOSTERS

Caffeine is a clever saboteur. It doesn't give you energy—it *blocks the signal of fatigue*. Specifically, it plugs into adenosine receptors, the ones responsible for telling your brain, "You're tired now." But caffeine has a half-life of 6–8 hours, meaning that a 3 p.m. latte could still be active at 9 or 10 p.m., quietly stealing deep sleep.

Alcohol, on the other hand, feels like a sedative—it makes you drowsy and helps "knock you out." But that's not sleep; that's unconsciousness—alcohol fragments REM, the dream-rich phase responsible for emotional regulation and memory. You may fall asleep faster, but you wake up unrefreshed, dehydrated, and hormonally disrupted.

- **Science Snapshot:** A single evening drink can suppress REM sleep by 20–40%. Combine that with caffeine in the afternoon, and you've essentially dismantled both halves of the sleep cycle: deep restorative and dream-rich REM.

3. STRESS (RACING MIND) → HYPERAROUSAL

Sleep is the art of letting go. But in our productivity-obsessed culture, bedtime often becomes an extension of the day: replaying emails, rehearsing conversations, tallying tomorrow's to-do list.

This keeps the sympathetic nervous system (fight-or-flight) switched on. Cortisol, which should be dipping at night, stays elevated. The brain races, the body thrums, and sleep becomes something you chase rather than something that arrives.

- **Science Snapshot:** Elevated evening cortisol not only delays sleep onset but reduces slow-wave sleep—the phase responsible for growth hormone release and tissue repair.

- **Narrative:** One executive described her nights as "lying in bed with my laptop in my head." She was exhausted but wired. Once she implemented a "worry journal" ritual—offloading tasks to paper an hour before bed—her body finally got the signal it was safe to downshift.

4. NOISE + ENVIRONMENT → HIDDEN MICRO-AWAKENINGS

Even when you think you've slept through the night, your environment might be quietly fracturing your rest. Traffic noise, a partner's snoring, even a phone vibrating on the nightstand can cause *micro-arousals*—brief awakenings too short to notice but enough to pull you out of deep sleep.

Temperature also matters. The body naturally cools by 1–2°F during sleep. If your room is too hot, this cooling can't occur, and deep sleep is disrupted.

- **Science Snapshot:** In a landmark study, people sleeping in noisy urban environments had 25% less deep sleep than those in quiet rooms—even if they reported "sleeping fine."

THE METABOLIC FALLOUT: SLEEP RESTRICTION AS PREDIABETES

Sleep is not just about energy—it's metabolic currency. Chronic restriction of even 1–2 hours per night begins to show up in bloodwork within days.

- **Research Spotlight:** After just one week of 5 hours per night, healthy adults in a controlled study showed *prediabetic levels of insulin resistance.* Their cells couldn't process glucose efficiently, mirroring the metabolic dysfunction of type 2 diabetes.

This is why short sleep isn't just a personal choice—it's a public health crisis. We are walking around metabolically older than we are, not from overeating alone, but from undersleeping.

NARRATIVE: THE ENTREPRENEUR'S COLLAPSE

A young tech entrepreneur boasted about his 4-hour night's sleep: "Sleep is for the weak". At some point, he powered on adrenaline and ambition. But in under two years, health collapsed: oppressive weight gain, never-ending colds, brain fog, and ultimately, depression. His labs showed chronic cortisol elevation, low testosterone, and pre-diabetes.

Only after he rebuilt his sleep - blue-light blockers, caffeine cutoffs after 3 pm, meditation, and strict 7-hour confines - did he see biomarkers improve. Not only did he get energy back - he got his creativity back.

Key Point: The modern world is rigged against sleep. From screens to stimulants to hyperactive minds - every force is geared to postpone, fragment, or diminish the one process evolution perfected for renewal. Protecting sleep is like defending the cathedral from intruders.

PART 6 — THE SLEEP PRESCRIPTION PROTOCOL

If recovery is the soil, and sleep is the nightly water, then the protocol is the gardener's guide—the rituals and the conditions that ensure that your biology's most powerful healer has the space to function.

Modern sleep medicine is discovering what ancient traditions always knew: sleep is not something you force; it is something you elicit. The appropriate cues, the appropriate rhythms, the right environment—these are the means to open the doors through which sleep naturally comes in.

Let's build your prescription.

1. EVENING RITUALS: DIM THE DAY, INVITE THE NIGHT

The body is not a switch. It's a dimmer.

Just as dusk in nature slowly turns down the lights, your nervous system needs gentle cues that it's time to transition.

- **Light dimming:** Lower overhead lights 1–2 hours before bed. Use lamps, amber bulbs, or candlelight. Melatonin release depends on this darkness signal.

- **Digital sunset:** No screens for 60 minutes before sleep. The blue light suppresses melatonin; the mental stimulation hijacks attention.

- **Calming cues:** Herbal tea, a warm shower, light stretching, journaling. These are not indulgences—they are parasympathetic activators, telling your nervous system it is safe to downshift.

NARRATIVE:

Following a late night of grading papers, one teacher began a simple practice: "sleep tea" at 9 p.m., phone in a different room, and reading a novel under warm light. Within 2 weeks, she was going to bed an hour earlier and waking up refreshed with an energy she hadn't felt in years.

2. DAYTIME ANCHORS: SETTING THE STAGE BEFORE BED

Sleep begins in the morning. What you do during the day sets up how your night unfolds.

- **Morning sunlight:** Within 30 minutes of waking, step outside for 5–10 minutes of natural light. This anchors the circadian rhythm, increases serotonin (the melatonin precursor), and sharpens alertness.

- **Exercise:** Regular movement promotes deeper slow-wave sleep, but avoid high-intensity training within 2–3 hours of bed.

- **Caffeine cutoff:** Stop caffeine 6–8 hours before bedtime. Its half-life means even a 2 p.m. coffee can linger into the night.

- **Stress release:** Build mini-restorations throughout the day (breath resets, walks, breaks). A wired system doesn't suddenly "switch off" at bedtime.

3. SCIENCE SPOTLIGHT: BEHAVIOR BEATS PILLS

Cognitive Behavioral Therapy for Insomnia (CBT-I)—which is essentially structured behavioral and environmental interventions—has consistently outperformed many prescription sleep medications in long-term trials. Unlike pills, these changes don't just sedate the brain; they restore the natural architecture of sleep cycles.

- Sleep drugs often suppress REM or slow-wave sleep.

- Behavioral protocols preserve the full symphony: deep sleep, REM, and cycling transitions.

☑ **Key Takeaway:** Sleep is not a luxury or a side quest. It's the most powerful *daily medicine* your body knows. Rituals, environment, timing, and daytime anchors are the four pillars of your Sleep Prescription Protocol.

PART 7 — SLEEP ENHANCERS (BEYOND THE BASICS)

If sleep is the body's pharmacy, then the fundamentals, rituals, light, and environment are the dispensing bottle. However, there are also enhancers: little strategic boosters that can deepen, prolong, and fine-tune your night-time repair. They are not quick hacks or silver bullets. They are evidence-based "boosters" which have now accumulated on top of the fundamentals. Be advised that you can upgrade decent sleep to transformative sleep.

1. HEAT & COLD: MANIPULATING BODY TEMPERATURE

Your core body temperature naturally dips as you enter sleep. This drop is one of the strongest triggers for the onset of slow-wave sleep. By working *with* this biology, you can accelerate the process.

- **Sauna before bed:** Paradoxically, heating your body with a sauna or a hot shower actually enhances sleep. Why? After heat exposure, your body activates cooling mechanisms, producing a more dramatic drop in core temperature once you step out. This "thermal rebound" signals the body: sleep time.

- **Cold exposure:** Cold plunges earlier in the day can build resilience and stress tolerance, but too close to bedtime may be overstimulating. If used at night, keep it gentle—like a cool shower.

- **Science:** A meta-analysis (Haghayegh et al., Sleep Med Rev, 2019) found that passive body heating (hot bath, shower, or sauna) 1–2 hours before bed significantly improved sleep quality and shortened sleep onset.

2. NUTRIENT ALLIES: NATURAL COMPOUNDS THAT NUDGE SLEEP

The supplement aisle is crowded, but only a few compounds carry solid evidence for enhancing sleep quality without sedation.

- **Magnesium (glycinate or threonate):** Supports GABA activity, calming the nervous system. Low magnesium is associated with restless sleep.

- **Glycine:** An amino acid that lowers core body temperature and shortens time to sleep onset (Inagawa et al., Sleep Biol Rhythms, 2006).

- **Tart cherry:** A natural source of melatonin and anti-inflammatory compounds. Clinical trials show tart cherry juice can improve sleep duration and efficiency, especially in older adults.

- **Rule of thumb:** Supplements enhance what you've already prepared with good sleep hygiene. They are not substitutes for the fundamentals.

3. BREATHWORK & VAGUS ACTIVATION: TURNING OFF THE STRESS SWITCH

The enemy of sleep is hyperarousal—the "racing mind" that keeps cortisol elevated at night. Activating the vagus nerve before bed flips the nervous system into parasympathetic mode.

- **Breathing practices:** Try 4-7-8 breathing (inhale 4 sec, hold 7, exhale 8) or slow diaphragmatic breathing.

- **Humming, chanting, or gentle singing:** Vibrations stimulate the vagus nerve.

- **Body scan meditation:** Redirects the mind's spotlight from mental chatter to physical sensations, reducing pre-sleep rumination.

- **Science:** Research on heart rate variability (HRV) shows that vagal activation before sleep correlates with faster onset and deeper restorative sleep cycles.

4. CHRONOTYPES: THE BIOLOGY OF LARKS AND OWLS

Not everyone's "ideal sleep window" is identical. Genetic chronotypes shape whether you're a morning lark or a night owl.

- **Morning larks:** Naturally alert early, sleep earlier. Best to align with sunrise and protect evening wind-down.

- **Night owls:** Naturally alert later, but vulnerable in a society structured for early mornings. Consistency, morning light exposure, and gradual shifting of bedtime can help re-anchor rhythms.

- **Takeaway:** Honor your biology when possible, but use light as the master cue to adapt gently.

5. NAPS: THE DOUBLE-EDGED SWORD

A nap is not weakness—it's recovery in miniature. But like medicine, dosage and timing matter.

- **Power naps (10–20 minutes):** Boost alertness and memory without entering deep sleep, so you avoid grogginess.

- **Long naps (90 minutes):** Allow a full sleep cycle, useful for sleep-deprived individuals.

- **The danger zone:** 30–60 minutes puts you in deep sleep but wakes you before REM, producing grogginess (sleep inertia).

- **Timing rule:** Nap before 3 p.m. to avoid interfering with nighttime sleep drive.

- **Science:** NASA studies show short naps dramatically improve cognitive performance and alertness—used widely for astronauts and pilots.

☑ **Key Takeaway:**

The fundamentals of sleep are non-negotiable. But once they are set, these enhancers—temperature rituals, nutrient allies, vagus activation, chronotype alignment, and strategic napping—act like amplifiers, refining your sleep into a true nightly superpower.

5 SLEEP ENHANCERS BEYOND THE BASICS

 **HEAT & COLD**
Sauna before bed

 **NUTRIENT ALLIES**
Magnesium, glycine, tart cherry

 **BREATHWORK**
Vagus activation

 **CHRONOTYPES**
Lark vs. owl

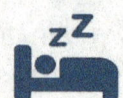 **NAPS**
Power nap, long nap

PART 8 — ACTION STARTER: THE SLEEP RESET DAY

Think of this as your **24-hour rehearsal for better nights**. Not a forever program, not a strict regimen—just one clean slate where you align with your body clock and remind your biology how good deep, effortless sleep feels.

The goal isn't perfection. It's rhythm. You're teaching your cells: *this is how we rest, this is how we renew.*

MORNING (SUNRISE → MIDDAY)

ANCHOR YOUR CIRCADIAN CLOCK.

- ☺ **Sunlight:** Within 30–60 minutes of waking, step outside. Natural light hits your retina, signals your suprachiasmatic nucleus (the brain's master clock), and starts the countdown for melatonin release ~14 hours later.

- 🚶 **Movement:** A brisk walk or light mobility session. You're pairing light + motion, the same cues ancient bodies used to know "day has begun."

- ☕ **Caffeine window:** Enjoy coffee or tea—but keep it **before 10 a.m.** (Caffeine has a half-life of 6–8 hours; late cups quietly rob deep sleep).

☑ *Quick science:* Morning light boosts serotonin, the raw material for tonight's melatonin.

MIDDAY (12 P.M. → 3 P.M)

KEEP STRESS LOW, DIGESTION STEADY.

- 🍽 **Balanced lunch:** Avoid ultra-processed carbs that spike insulin and crash energy. Go for protein + fiber + healthy fats.

- 🧘 **Stress breaks:** 5-minute breath reset or short walk between tasks. Cortisol naturally dips early afternoon; don't fight it with sugar bombs or energy drinks.

- **Caffeine cutoff:** Draw the line by 2 p.m. at the latest.

Quick science: Protecting cortisol's natural rhythm keeps melatonin's nighttime rise smooth.

EVENING (6 P.M. → 9 P.M)

SIGNAL SAFETY + SLOWING DOWN.

- **Light dinner:** Eat 2–3 hours before bed. Heavy meals keep digestion buzzing when repair should begin.

- **Digital sunset:** Dim overhead lights, switch to warm lamps, and set devices to night mode. Bright blue light at night suppresses melatonin like a biological false dawn.

- **Wind-down ritual:** Options: warm shower (temp drop after = sleep cue), journaling, stretching, or reading real paper.

Quick science: Body temperature drop and melatonin rise act like the twin gears of sleep onset.

NIGHT (9 P.M. → 10:30 P.M)

PROTECT YOUR SLEEP CAVE.

- **Environment:** Cool (65–68°F / 18–20°C), dark (blackout curtains or mask), and quiet (earplugs or white noise if needed).

- **No late-night scroll:** Phone light, notifications, and mental stimulation tell your brain *day isn't over yet.*

- **Consistent timing:** Aim for a stable sleep window. Go to bed within the same 30-minute band nightly.

Quick science: Consistency strengthens circadian rhythm, like adding fresh layers to a groove in your brain's timekeeping system.

Quick-Reference Checklist

- ☑ Morning sunlight + movement.
- ☑ Caffeine cutoff by early afternoon.
- ☑ Digital sunset + calming evening ritual.
- ☑ Light dinner, heavy on protein + veggies.

☑ Bedroom = cool, dark, quiet cave.

☑ Consistent bedtime within a fixed window.

Big takeaway: A **single Sleep Reset Day** can show you what fully aligned rest feels like. Once you experience the difference—morning energy, sharper mood, fewer cravings—you'll want to repeat, refine, and make it your personal prescription.

PART 9 — QUICK-REFERENCE CHECKLIST: THE SLEEP LAWS

These aren't hacks. They're the non-negotiables—the biological guardrails your body depends on. Master these, and sleep transforms from fragile to foundational.

☑ DARKNESS IS MEDICINE.

Your brain interprets light as time. Evening darkness is not just the absence of day—it's the signal for melatonin to rise and repair to begin.

☑ CONSISTENCY BEATS DURATION.

Seven hours at the same time every night is more restorative than nine hours scattered across shifting bedtimes. Rhythm is the real nutrient.

☑ SLEEP IS RECOVERY, NOT LUXURY.

Deep rest is not optional downtime. It is the nightly operating system update, repairing tissues, consolidating memory, and resetting hormones.

☑ PROTECT DEEP SLEEP → PROTECT REPAIR.

The first half of the night is dominated by slow-wave sleep. That's when growth hormone pulses, autophagy clears debris, and your immune system fortifies. Guard it fiercely.

☑ SLEEP DEBT IS REAL—AND ONLY SLEEP REPAYS IT.

You can't hack your way out of missed rest. Stimulants mask fatigue, naps help, but true recovery comes only when you repay in full, cycle by cycle.

✦ These laws aren't rules to follow once. They're truths to live by. Build your nights on them, and you build resilience, repair, and longevity.

THE SLEEP LAWS

✓ **Darkness is medicine.**
Your brain interprets light as time. Evening darkness is not just the absence of day—it's the signal for melatonin to rise and repair to begin.

✓ **Consistency beats duration.**
Seven hours at the same time every night is more restorative than nine hours scattered across shifting bedtimes. Rhythm is the real nutrient.

✓ **Sleep is recovery, not luxury.**
Deep rest is not optional downtime. It is the nightly operating system update, repairing tssues, consolidating memory, and resetting hormones.

✓ **Protect deep sleep → protect repair.**
The first half of the night is dominated by slow-wave sleep. That's when growth hormone pulses, autophagy clears debris, and your immune system fortifies. Guard it fiercely.

✓ **Sleep debt is real—and only sleep repays it.**
You can't hack your way out of missed rest. Stimulants mask fatigue, naps help, but true recovery comes only when you repay in full,

Sleep is not downtime. It isn't wasted hours. It is not the thing you sacrifice to squeeze more into your day.

Sleep is active renewal; every time you close your eyes at night, and your conscious mind wanders off, your body goes into repair mode. Neurons are washed clean. Muscles knit back together. Hormones are recalibrated. Your microbiome resets. Your immune system gets re-equipped.

Think of it like this - every time you sleep, your body initiates the most sophisticated operating system upgrade. If you forego sleep, you forego the essential patch to fix your weaknesses, enhance your performance, and regulate your emotions. Would you decline to upgrade your phone if it kept giving you update signals and crashes constantly? Then why do we deny the nightly update that prevents human breakdown?

We live in a culture that idolizes the grind at the expense of a restful night. The truth? Resilience is not built up in the hours we work hardest. It's built up in the hours we rest.

Sleep is not a luxury. It's the foundation.

And the most liberating thing? You already own the most powerful medicine in the world. You do not have to purchase, inject, or download it. It is readily available each night, in the dark; it is available, surplus, and immensely transformative.

"Every sleep pause is not wasted life, but multiplied life. Every night provides the opportunity for us to be rewoven, restored, and reborn. When you protect your sleep, you are protecting the future of who you will become."

If sleep is the soil of our growth and nourishment, then emotional resilience is the root system that maintains our upright balance when the storms of life shake us. In the next chapter, we will learn to train the hidden core of your emotional life, how to bend without breaking, reset under pressure, and build an inner stability as reliable as the heart that beats inside you.

CHAPTER 12:

EMOTIONAL RESILIENCE: TRAINING YOUR INNER CORE

PART 1: THE BOUNCE-BACK BLUEPRINT

It always begins with the storm.

For Maria, the storm was the call that changed her world forever: her job was gone. She had given her all - early mornings, late nights, as well as the weekends. In return, she received a 30-minute meeting and a polite "we're restructuring." The floor just dropped out from beneath her.

At first, Maria felt what anyone would feel: shock, fear, and that awful, empty feeling in her stomach. The human body is made to respond to a threat; for her, the threat showed up as an email (not a tiger). Heart racing, cortisol pumping, and the sleep was gone. The nights were long and filled with "What now? What if I fail?" loops.

But here's what made her story remarkable - it wasn't her end.

After riding waves of panic, something else emerged. A voice she had forgotten about long ago surfaced. She recalled her grandmother saying, "An oak tree that stands tall, does not fight against the wind - it bends with it." Gradually, she recognized that this was a painful event, AND in that painful event was a concealed training ground.

Within a few months, Maria started to rebuild. She made some new plans, got some support, and did breathing resets every day when she started to panic. Every time she was knocked down by self-doubt, she learned how to get up quicker. She did not avoid stress - she figured out how to encounter stress differently.

This is resilience. Not an absence of struggle, but an ability to bend without breaking. To fall and get back up.

And here is the scientific part: resilience isn't luck, or genetics, or reserved for the naturally "tough." It is a trainable system inside you. Just as your muscles grow stronger when you lift weights, your emotional core strengthens when it is challenged—if you give it the right conditions to adapt.

Oh, and don't confuse resilience with a trait. It is a practice. A physiological skill set. A living shield.

Picture two soldiers fighting on the same battlefield. One soldier has trained with live fire drills, the other soldier has only read about combat. Which one performs better when under stress? It is the same with your nervous system. If you train it, stress is not a wrecking ball; it is a forging process.

"The storms of life will roll in. The point is not whether you will fall—it is whether you will rise. Your hidden core is emotional resilience, and like all cores, it can be trained."

PART 2 — STRESS INOCULATION: HORMESIS, ADAPTATION

There is a paradox at the heart of all living things: those forces that threaten us are simultaneously the forces that shape us.

Think about fire. When it gets out of control, it can wipe a forest clean. But in small, controlled burns, it can clean out dead wood, fertilize the soil, and allow other growth to thrive. The same goes for stress. Too much, and it can burn out the body and mind. But the correct amount? It breeds resilience.

This is called hormesis; from the Greek word hormáein, "to set in motion." It's the biological truth that small, manageable doses of stress do not weaken us; instead, they awaken us.

THE BIOLOGY OF THE STRESS DOSE

Inside your body, every stressor—whether it's a cold shower, a 20-minute run, or the jolt of public speaking—follows the same biological script.

1. **Trigger:** Stress activates the **HPA axis** (hypothalamic-pituitary–adrenal system). Cortisol rises, adrenaline primes your body for action.

2. **Response:** Heart rate increases, glucose floods the bloodstream, and immune cells sharpen their vigilance.

3. **Recovery:** Once the challenge ends, the parasympathetic system—the "rest-and-digest" arm—activates. Cortisol falls, insulin restores balance, tissues repair.

If you live here—in the cycle of challenge and recovery—your system gets stronger. Your stress curve sharpens, but your recovery curve deepens.

But if the challenge never ends—if you're in constant fight-or-flight without the chance to repair—the body stops adapting and starts breaking.

That's the difference between hormesis and harm.

EVERYDAY STRESS INOCULATION

You already know these practices intuitively:

- **Exercise:** A 30-minute run is a micro-stress. The heart works harder, and muscles tear microscopically. In recovery, capillaries grow, mitochondria multiply, and strength increases. Without this stress, the body grows weaker.

- **Cold Exposure:** Immersing in cold water spikes norepinephrine and cortisol—but when practiced intermittently, it reduces baseline inflammation and boosts resilience.

- **Heat (Sauna):** The heat stress of sauna elevates heart rate, induces heat shock proteins that repair cellular damage, and lowers long-term cardiovascular risk.

Even **fasting**—the subject of Chapter 9—is a form of hormesis. Short-term stress of food absence flips on repair pathways, activating autophagy and insulin sensitivity.

The pattern is the same: **dose → stress → adaptation.**

THE RESILIENCE CURVE

Imagine a curve shaped like a hill.

- On the left: **too little stress**. The body weakens. Muscles atrophy, the mind grows fragile, the immune system dulls. This is underload.

- In the middle: **optimal stress**. The sweet spot where challenge meets adaptation. Here resilience grows, capacity expands, confidence deepens.

- On the right: **too much stress**. Burnout, breakdown, collapse.

Resilience is built in the middle zone—the training ground where stress isn't overwhelming, but it's real enough to force adaptation.

FROM SOLDIERS TO STUDENTS: TRAINING STRESS

The U.S. military knows this truth well. Elite forces undergo what's called **stress inoculation training (SIT)**. Recruits are deliberately exposed to high-pressure environments—loud noises, chaotic decision-making drills, sleep restriction—under safe supervision.

Why? Because when the real stress comes, their nervous systems don't panic. They've already rehearsed. Their bodies recognize the cortisol surge, their breath control kicks in, and their focus narrows instead of shattering.

But stress inoculation isn't just for soldiers.

- A **college student** giving class presentations. Each talk feels terrifying at first, but over time, the rapid heartbeats stop feeling like danger and start feeling like readiness.

- A **new parent** learning to calm a crying baby at 3 am. The stress never disappears—but over months, the nervous system adapts, shifting from panic to practiced patience.

- A **cancer survivor** is enduring rounds of chemotherapy. Each cycle leaves scars, but each cycle also trains a deeper capacity for persistence, for finding light in dark hours.

These are resilience gyms. Life provides the weights.

THE SCIENCE OF HORMESIS

EXERCISE HORMESIS:

- Studies show that a single bout of aerobic exercise temporarily increases oxidative stress. Yet in response, the body upregulates antioxidant enzymes (SOD, catalase), strengthening long-term defenses.

- Resistance training causes microtears in muscle fibers, releasing inflammatory cytokines. But in recovery, growth factors (IGF-1, mTOR) repair tissue stronger than before.

THERMAL STRESS:

- Finnish studies on sauna use show a 50% reduced risk of sudden cardiac death in regular users. The heat stress induces **heat shock proteins (HSPs)**—molecular guardians that refold damaged proteins and protect neurons.

PSYCHOLOGICAL STRESS INOCULATION:

- Research on **exposure therapy** in anxiety disorders reveals that controlled, repeated exposure to feared stimuli reduces long-term stress responses. Each exposure recalibrates the amygdala, teaching the brain: "This is survivable."

In every case, the curve is the same. Small doses → temporary stress → adaptive repair.

MARIA'S NEXT LESSON

Remember Maria, who lost her job? She discovered hormesis without even realizing it.

At first, she avoided stress altogether. She turned down interviews, skipped social gatherings, and retreated into her apartment. She told herself she was "recovering," but what she was really doing was atrophying her resilience.

Then, one day, a mentor invited her to volunteer at a community event. It terrified her. "I don't have the energy," she thought. "I can't handle the crowd." But she went anyway.

In the first hour, her anxiety surged. Heart pounding, palms sweating, she almost walked out. But she stayed. And by the end of the day, something inside her shifted. She realized that challenge hadn't broken her—it had stretched her.

The next week, she said yes to an interview. Then a networking call. Each stressor, uncomfortable but survivable, became her inoculation. Slowly, she was retraining her nervous system, like a vaccine for life's chaos.

THE RESILIENCE EQUATION

Here's the core formula of this chapter:

Stress + Recovery = Strength

- Without stress, no growth.
- Without recovery, no repair.

- With both resilience.

This is the paradox modern life misunderstands. Grind culture glorifies stress without recovery. Comfort culture glorifies recovery without challenge. Resilience is built in the **dance between the two.**

PRACTICAL STRESS INOCULATION TOOLS

1. **Cold Showers, Warm Hearts**

   o   Begin with 30 seconds of cold water. Cortisol spikes—but norepinephrine rises too, sharpening alertness. Over days, the discomfort shrinks. The brain learns: "This is survivable."

2. **Public Speaking Reps**

   o   Toastmasters, teaching, or even leading a team meeting. Each repetition inoculates against the fear of judgment.

3. **Exercise as Training Stress**

   o   Resistance training and aerobic bursts are controlled physical stress. Start with tolerable loads; let your nervous system adapt.

4. **Mindful Micro-Stress**

   o   Deliberately expose yourself to small discomforts: taking stairs, fasting for a meal, sitting in silence. These are miniature resilience reps.

5. **Recovery Is Non-Negotiable**

   o   Every stressor must be followed by a deliberate recovery window. This is where resilience is cemented.

Stress isn't your enemy—it's your sculptor. Like the controlled fire in the forest, it burns away the weak and clears space for the strong.

But here's the catch: resilience only grows when you lean into stress at the right dose, then step back to let your body and mind repair.

KEY TAKEAWAY:

"Every controlled discomfort is a deposit into your resilience bank. Each challenge rehearses your comeback. The storms don't shrink—but you grow larger."

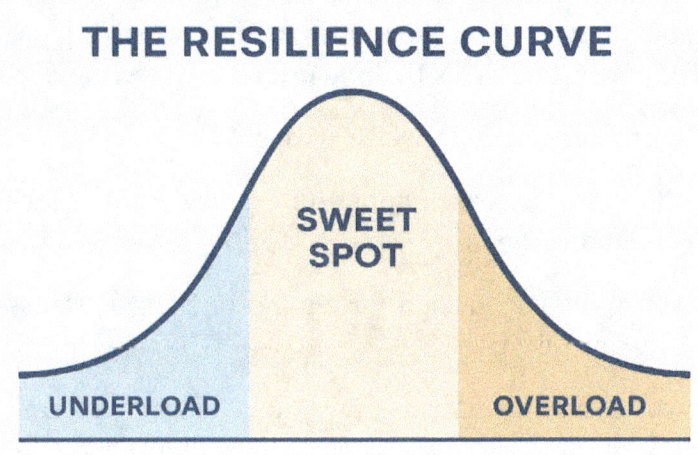

PART 3 — EMOTIONAL EATING VS. EMOTIONAL REGULATION

It's midnight. Maria stands in front of her refrigerator, feeling the pale blue light. The day was awful - deadlines, conflicts, and continuous digital distractions. Her heart is still pounding. She doesn't feel physically hungry - she just had dinner two hours ago. But there is an awful hollowness in her chest.

Her hand hovers over a container of leftover cake. She is not grabbing for calories - she is grasping for comfort, for relief, for distraction from the tensions pirouetting in her nervous system.

This is not about food. It is about regulation.

And this matter is hardly isolated. For millions, food is the most available strategy to relieve stress, anxiety, or loneliness. But the conundrum is this - what seems like soothing/filling in the moment, is often nourishing the stress cycle in the long run.

To exit, we must see all emotional eating for what it is: a nervous system seeking safety.

SECTION 1: WHY WE EAT OUR EMOTIONS

Science shows that stress doesn't just shape behavior — it literally alters **metabolism, hunger hormones, and brain wiring.** Emotional eating is not a weakness; it's **biology intersecting with psychology.**

1. **Stress Hormones Drive Cravings**

   - Cortisol increases appetite, especially for calorie-dense "comfort foods."

   - Evolutionary design: in famine or danger, stress + food meant survival.

   - Modern mismatch: now the "danger" is emails, not predators, and the food is a bag of chips, not wild tubers.

2. **Neurochemistry of Soothing**

   - Sugar, refined carbs, and fatty foods release **dopamine** in the brain's reward pathways.

   - They temporarily boost **serotonin**, creating a fleeting calm.

   - Emotional eating is less about filling the stomach, more about **hacking brain chemistry** to self-soothe.

3. **Childhood Conditioning**

   - Many of us learned early: "Don't cry, here's a cookie."

   - Food becomes coded as comfort, celebration, or distraction.

- These scripts run unconsciously unless we rewrite them.

Key insight: Emotional eating isn't about hunger. It's about unmet emotional needs being temporarily patched with calories.

SECTION 2: THE AFTERMATH — WHY IT BACKFIRES

While emotional eating provides short-term relief, it often sets off a **biological and psychological backlash.**

- **Blood Sugar Rollercoaster:**
  Refined carbs spike glucose → insulin surge → crash → irritability and more cravings.
  Maria's midnight cake doesn't calm her nervous system — it jolts it like a faulty rollercoaster track.

- **Shame Cycle:**
  After emotional eating comes guilt ("Why did I do that again?").
  Guilt itself is a stressor → more cortisol › more vulnerability to cravings.
  This creates the **stress–craving–shame spiral.**

- **Sleep Disruption:**
  Late-night eating interferes with melatonin and growth hormone release, leaving the body less restored.
  Next day: more stress sensitivity + less resilience.

Over time, emotional eating erodes both metabolic and emotional stability.

SECTION 3: EMOTIONAL REGULATION — THE UPGRADE

If emotional eating is a patch, **emotional regulation** is a full system upgrade. It's the difference between silencing a fire alarm by pulling out the batteries (temporary) vs. putting out the fire (restorative).

What is emotional regulation?

It's the ability to notice, process, and respond to emotions in adaptive ways, without needing to numb, escape, or suppress them.

Core skills include:

4. **Awareness (Name it to tame it):**
   Neuroscientist Daniel Siegel's research shows that simply labeling emotions ("I feel anxious") activates the prefrontal cortex, calming the amygdala's alarm.

5. **Pause + Space Creation:**
   A 90-second window exists between an emotional trigger and an automatic reaction. Learning to create space allows choice instead of compulsion.

6. **Body-Based Regulation:**

7. Breathwork (lengthened exhale = vagus nerve activation).

8. Movement (walk, stretch, shake → discharges stress chemistry).

9. Sensory grounding (touching textures, noticing sounds).

10. **Rewiring Reward Pathways:**
    Just as food temporarily releases dopamine, so do alternatives: journaling, calling a friend, stepping outside, and creative play. These healthier dopamine hits build **resilient wiring** over time.

SECTION 4: SCIENCE SPOTLIGHT — THE GUT-BRAIN-EMOTION LOOP

Recent studies reveal that emotional eating isn't just "in your head" — it's also in your **gut microbiome.**

- **Stress → Microbiome Imbalance:**
  Cortisol disrupts gut flora balance. Dysbiosis alters

cravings, often toward sugary foods that feed the wrong microbes.

- **Microbiome → Brain Signals:**
  Gut bacteria produce neurotransmitters (serotonin, GABA). When the gut is imbalanced, emotional regulation falters.

- **Sleep & Emotion Connection:**
  Two nights of sleep loss reduce microbiome diversity → higher inflammation → amplified stress reactivity → emotional eating is more likely.

This creates a **feedback loop**: stress → microbiome disruption → cravings → worse sleep → more stress.

Emotional regulation, then, isn't just mental—it's **cellular, hormonal, and microbial.**

SECTION 5: CASE VIGNETTES

1. Maria — Breaking the Midnight Cycle

Maria began journaling when she experienced late-night cravings. She realized her "hunger" was actually loneliness after stressful days at work. After a while, she replaced raiding the cake stand with tea + 10 minutes of breathwork, and her cravings faded.

James — Rage at the Work Desk

James would snack anytime his inbox spiked. He had an epiphany when he created a "walk trigger": each time he got stressed, he'd stand up and go for a walk around the block. Food stopped being his distractor.

Leah — Healing from the Childhood Script

Leah grew up in a family where sweets meant love. As an adult, every time she felt unworthy, she would binge eat. She learned to intentionally validate her emotions and use friends for support through therapy. Food stopped being her go-to comfort.

Lesson: Each person's emotional eating pattern hides a deeper emotional or nervous system need. When the real need is addressed, the food grip loosens.

SECTION 6: PRACTICAL FRAMEWORK — "PAUSE, NAME, NOURISH"

A simple 3-step system to pivot from emotional eating → emotional regulation:

1. **Pause:**
   When the craving strikes, pause for 90 seconds. Don't say no, just delay.

2. **Name:**
   Ask: "What am I actually feeling?" (bored, stressed, lonely, anxious). Label it.

3. **Nourish:**
   Choose a regulation tool that addresses the need:

   o   Stressed → breathwork.

   o   Lonely → call a friend.

   o   Anxious → grounding exercise.

   o   Tired → rest or nap.

If still hungry after regulation, eat intentionally, not compulsively.

SECTION 7: THE BIGGER PICTURE

Emotional eating is a symptom of a deeper disconnection — between mind and body, stress and recovery, biology and awareness. When we restore **emotional regulation**, we not only transform eating but also unlock **resilience, clarity, and freedom.**

Emotions are waves. Emotional eating tries to hold the ocean still with your hands. Emotional regulation teaches you to surf.

PART 4 — NERVOUS SYSTEM TOOLS: BREATH, VAGAL TONE, MINDFULNESS

THE HIDDEN LEVER INSIDE YOU

Imagine this: You stand on a stage ready to speak, and your palms are sweating, your chest is tightening, and your heart is racing as if you are being chased by a lion. No lion is there — just a room of people.

What you might be experiencing isn't weakness, but rather the fight-or-flight part of your nervous system. And here's the secret most of us were never taught about: you can learn to flip the switch.

Your body has a built-in control panel for resilience. It's not in a pill or supplement - it's in your breath, your vagus nerve, and your ability to anchor awareness.

This section is about giving you the tools to train your nervous system like a muscle, so it bends under stress instead of breaking.

SECTION 1: THE NERVOUS SYSTEM'S TWO GEARS

Your autonomic nervous system has two primary modes:

1. **Sympathetic (Fight-or-Flight):**

   - Heart rate ↑

   - Cortisol ↑

   - Muscles primed, digestion paused

   - Designed for short sprints of survival

2. **Parasympathetic (Rest-and-Repair):**

   - Heart rate ↓

   - Digestion & immunity restored

   - Hormonal balance recalibrates

- Mode of healing, growth, and creativity

Resilience is not the absence of stress — it's the ability to shift gears.

When stress ends, your system should slide back into parasympathetic balance. But in modern life, many of us get stuck in "sympathetic overdrive."

The tools below are like clutch pedals, helping you downshift.

SECTION 2: BREATH — THE REMOTE CONTROL OF THE NERVOUS SYSTEM

Breathing is the only system in the body that is both **automatic** and **voluntary.** That makes it a direct access point to shift state.

- **Science of the Exhale:**
  Inhale = mild sympathetic activation (heart rate rises).
  Exhale = parasympathetic activation (heart rate lowers).
  By lengthening the exhale, you activate the vagus nerve — your body's "calm command."

- **Protocols to Train Calm:**

  1. **Box Breathing (4-4-4-4):** Inhale 4, hold 4, exhale 4, hold 4. Used by Navy SEALs under pressure.

  2. **Physiological Sigh (double inhale + long exhale):** Stanford research shows it rapidly lowers stress.

  3. **Coherence Breathing (5.5 in / 5.5 out):** Balances heart rate variability (HRV), improving emotional regulation.

Vignette:

Maria (from earlier chapters) replaced late-night stress snacking with a 5-minute breath reset. Her cravings shrank not because she had more willpower, but because her nervous system was calm enough to choose differently.

SECTION 3: VAGAL TONE — STRENGTHENING YOUR INNER BRAKE

The **vagus nerve** is the longest cranial nerve, running from the brainstem to the gut. It regulates the heart, digestion, and inflammation. Think of it as your **resilience brake.**

- **High vagal tone:** quicker recovery after stress, better emotional regulation.

- **Low vagal tone:** anxiety, inflammation, poor recovery.

WAYS TO TRAIN VAGAL TONE:

1. **Cold Exposure:** Splashing face with cold water or brief cold showers stimulates the vagus nerve.

2. **Humming, Chanting, Singing:** Vibrations stimulate vagal pathways in the throat.

3. **Gargling:** Simple, daily vagal exercise.

4. **Slow Breathing (esp. extended exhale):** Direct vagal activation.

Science Spotlight:

Research shows vagal nerve stimulation reduces symptoms of depression, PTSD, and inflammatory conditions. Daily practices act like "natural vagal stimulators."

SECTION 4: MINDFULNESS — TRAINING THE WITNESS

Mindfulness is not about emptying the mind. It's about shifting from **being inside the storm** to **watching the storm.**

- **Science:**

  o Regular mindfulness reduces amygdala reactivity (the fear center).

- o Increases prefrontal cortex activity (executive control, regulation).

- o Enhances HRV, showing nervous system balance.

- **Practices:**

  - o **Micro-Mindfulness:** 1-minute check-ins ("What do I feel in my body right now?").

  - o **Anchoring Attention:** Focus on breath, a sound, or a body sensation.

  - o **Expanding Awareness:** Noticing thoughts as passing clouds rather than commands.

Vignette:

James, the finance professional, practiced 3 minutes of mindfulness before checking his email. His stress-driven snacking plummeted. Why? Because he stopped reacting blindly to his nervous system's alarms.

SECTION 5: THE SCIENCE OF HRV — YOUR RESILIENCE SCORECARD

Heart Rate Variability (HRV): the tiny differences in time between each heartbeat.

- **High HRV:** flexible, adaptive nervous system.

- **Low HRV:** rigid, stressed system stuck in survival mode.

HRV is a biomarker of resilience, linked to:

- Emotional regulation capacity

- Reduced anxiety & depression risk

- Longevity

HOW TO RAISE HRV:

- Regular breathwork

- Consistent sleep

- Physical activity (without overtraining)

- Nature exposure

Tracking HRV (via wearable tech) gives feedback: Did your nervous system recover, or are you running on stress debt?

SECTION 6: PUTTING IT TOGETHER — THE RESILIENCE TOOLBOX

DAILY PRACTICES TO REGULATE THE NERVOUS SYSTEM:

- 5 minutes of breathwork (exhale-focused).

- Brief cold splash or humming for vagal tone.

- 1–2 micro-mindfulness pauses during the day.

- Nature + sunlight exposure to anchor circadian rhythm.

- Evening ritual to signal parasympathetic entry.

This is not about "one more task." These are **tools to rewire your body's stress-response system,** transforming how you meet life's challenges.

Your nervous system is like a piano. Stress plays the high notes; recovery plays the low. Emotional resilience is not avoiding the high notes — it's learning to play the full range with harmony.

THE NERVOUS SYSTEM TOOLBOX

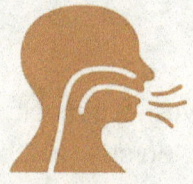

BREATH

Slow, deep breathing engages the parasympathetic nervous system

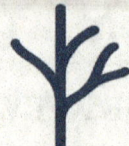

VAGUS

Stimulate the vagus nerve to increase resiliency

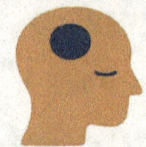

MINDFULNESS

Bring awareness to the present moment

PART 5 — THE RESILIENCE PRESCRIPTION

One of the best ways to think about resilience is as a muscle. Like all muscles, it weakens if you don't use it, it gets tired and requires rest if you overuse it, but it grows stronger when stressed and then given the right conditions to recover. We make a great mistake in modern culture when we believe that resilience is something you either have or don't. Research shows it's a trainable competency. And it has precise doses, rituals, and methods, like a prescription.

THE FORMULA FOR EMOTIONAL RESILIENCE

Resilience emerges from three interconnected domains:

1. **Physiology (the body):** nervous system balance, hormones, sleep, and gut-brain health.

2. **Cognition (the mind):** how you frame stress, interpret events, and self-talk under pressure.

3. **Connection (the social fabric):** who you turn to, the quality of your relationships, and the cultural rituals that remind you you're not alone.

Skip one domain and the structure wobbles. Build all three and you create what psychologists call *psychological hardiness*—a shield against burnout and a scaffold for growth.

1. THE BODY: ANCHORING PHYSIOLOGY FIRST

Resilience begins in the nervous system, not in willpower.

- **Daily Recovery Windows:** Micro-rest periods during the day—five deep breaths, a 10-minute walk—reset cortisol.

- **Sleep as Non-Negotiable:** HRV studies show emotional regulation plummets after a single night of poor sleep. You don't "power through"—you unravel.

- **Fuel and Mood:** Blood sugar crashes mimic anxiety. Stable meals = stable moods.

Think of physiology as the foundation. Without it, cognitive strategies feel like pushing against a locked door.

2. THE MIND: STRESS REFRAMING

Cognitive reappraisal—the scientific term for reframing—changes the biological impact of stress.

- **Threat vs. Challenge:** The same event (presentation, exam, conflict) spikes cortisol differently depending on your mindset. See it as a challenge → adrenaline fuels focus. See it as a threat → cortisol erodes performance.

- **The Navy SEAL Lesson:** Operators are taught to break overwhelming missions into "chunks" (reach that tree line, then the next). This keeps the brain in present-focused problem-solving rather than panic spirals.

- **Language Audit:** Replace "I can't handle this" with "This is hard, but I've handled hard before." This rewires stress appraisal at a neural level.

3. THE SOCIAL SHIELD: WHY RESILIENCE IS CONTAGIOUS

Humans regulate stress socially. Isolation amplifies it. Community dampens it.

- **Oxytocin Buffer:** Connection—eye contact, a hug, supportive words—lowers cortisol within minutes.

- **Blue Zone Wisdom:** Communities that prioritize shared meals, rituals, and intergenerational bonds show resilience into old age.

- **Case Study:** After natural disasters, those with stronger community ties recover faster—financially, emotionally, and biologically.

THE PRESCRIPTION PYRAMID

If resilience were a doctor's prescription, it might look like this:

- **Base layer (daily rituals):** Sleep, movement, breath resets, balanced meals.

- **Middle layer (mental training):** Journaling, reframing stress, mindfulness practices.

- **Top layer (connection):** Weekly check-ins with friends, shared meals, acts of service.

You don't need perfection—just consistency. Each small act is like a pill in a larger prescription, compounding its effect.

THE CROSSROADS MOMENT

David is a 42-year-old firefighter. In his mind, resilience was never to bend. After years of night shift, skipped meals, and "toughing it out", he broke down with anxiety attacks, a short temper at home, and exhaustion that no amount of sleep could resolve. His turning point was not about more grit—his prescription was daily recovery walks, reframing stress as service, and regular communal dinners with his teammates. His heart rate variability improved, stabilized moods returned, and resilience was restored—not by gritting it out, but by powering down at the right time.

THE TAKEAWAY

Resilience isn't a gift of birth. It's a skill, a rhythm, a prescription you refill daily.

The hardest part isn't starting—it's believing you're worth the care it requires.

And here's the paradox: The more you invest in recovery and connection, the more capacity you gain to face storms. Resilience is not built in the moment of crisis; it is prepared in the quiet rituals of everyday life.

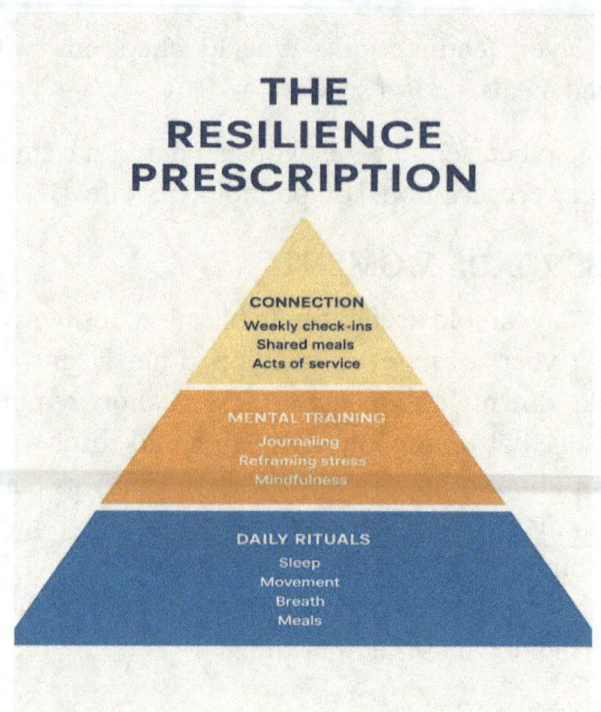

THE RESILIENCE PRESCRIPTION

CONNECTION
Weekly check-ins
Shared meals
Acts of service

MENTAL TRAINING
Journaling
Reframing stress
Mindfulness

DAILY RITUALS
Sleep
Movement
Breath
Meals

ACTION STARTER: DAILY RESILIENCE RITUALS

Resilience isn't something you "find" in a crisis—it's something you **train every day in micro-moments**, the way muscles strengthen with steady use. The good news? You don't need hours of meditation retreats or week-long digital detoxes to rewire your inner core. The nervous system is plastic, adaptable, and hungry for **tiny, repeated cues of safety and recovery**.

Think of these rituals as **emotional micro-workouts**. Each one takes just minutes, but together they build a foundation that makes you harder to break, quicker to reset, and stronger in the face of stress.

📷 MORNING: ANCHOR YOUR DAY

- **60-second breath reset:** Before coffee, three slow inhales and long exhales. Signals safety to your nervous system.

- **Sunlight + posture check:** Step outside, stand tall. Light on your eyes sets cortisol rhythm; upright stance communicates confidence to brain circuits.

- **Intention note:** One sentence: *"Today I choose calm in challenge."*

Science anchor: Early light stabilizes circadian rhythm; intentional priming lowers amygdala reactivity.

◷ MIDDAY: INTERRUPT THE STRESS SPIRAL

- **5-minute movement snack:** Walk, stretch, or shake it out. Moves cortisol out of the bloodstream.

- **Micro-gratitude jot:** Write one thing going well. Shifts the brain from threat mode to possibility mode.

- **Breath cue:** 4-7-8 or box breathing for 1 minute.

Science anchor: Pattern interrupts + gratitude shown to lower inflammatory markers and increase HRV.

🛌 EVENING: DOWNSHIFT THE SYSTEM

- **Digital sunset:** Turn off notifications 1 hour before bed. Reduces mental hyperarousal.

- **Wind-down ritual:** Tea, warm shower, gentle yoga. Repeated cues teach the brain: *"It's safe to rest now."*

- **Reflection close:** Quick journal: *"Where did I bend, not break, today?"*

Science anchor: Evening rituals increase sleep quality; reflection builds self-efficacy, a resilience amplifier.

⚡ MICRO-RITUALS (ANYTIME, ANYWHERE)

- **The exhale rescue:** One slow exhale lengthened beyond inhale. Calms the vagus nerve in 10 seconds.

- **The pause button:** Notice when your mind is racing, whisper *"Noticing is enough."*

- **The smile trigger:** Even a fake smile sends feedback to the brain that tension is lowering.

☑ QUICK-REFERENCE CHECKLIST: DAILY RESILIENCE RITUALS

- Anchor mornings with light + intention.

- Break stress loops with breath + gratitude.

- Downshift evenings with ritual, not distraction.

- Use micro-tools anytime the wave of stress hits.

Resilience isn't built in grand gestures—it's **stacked in small, repeated choices**. Each pause, each breath, each reset is like laying bricks in the fortress of your nervous system. Do this daily, and life's storms stop feeling like destruction—they start feeling like training.

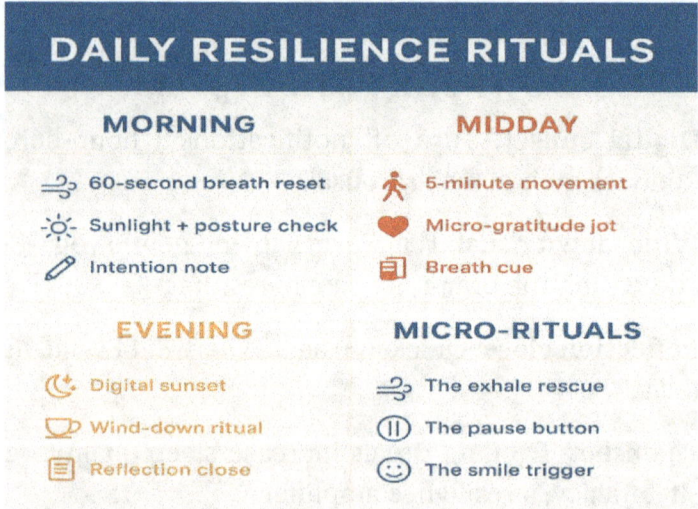

DAILY RESILIENCE RITUALS

MORNING
- 60-second breath reset
- Sunlight + posture check
- Intention note

MIDDAY
- 5-minute movement
- Micro-gratitude jot
- Breath cue

EVENING
- Digital sunset
- Wind-down ritual
- Reflection close

MICRO-RITUALS
- The exhale rescue
- The pause button
- The smile trigger

Resilience is not a fixed trait; it's a muscle, a living system, and a program that updates each time you experience stress and choose your response. You have seen that stress inoculates, that cravings can be redirected, that the nervous system can be rewired through breath, vagal activation, and mindfulness. But all of that—every prescription and ritual—comes down to one fact: resilience begins with you and the stories you tell yourself.

Your mind runs in loops, and your nervous system listens. If your loop sounds like, "I cannot handle this, I'm overwhelmed," your body locks in collapse mode—high cortisol, shallow breathing, anxious wiring. But if the loop changes even slightly to "This is training. This is adaptation. I bend but I do not break," your body responds with resiliency. Hormones balance differently. Muscles don't just carry you—they protect you. The brain doesn't just tolerate it—it adapts.

This is mental programming at its purest:

Words as biology. Every thought is a chemical cascade.

Belief as signal. The body follows your beliefs.

Resilience as an identity. Not something you do, but something you become.

So tonight, as you close your eyes, as code into your system:

"I am training. I am rewiring. I get stronger every time there is a challenge."

Your nervous system will respond. Your cells will adapt. The next stressor will not be an obstacle; it will be a stepping stone.

Resilience is not the absence of stress. It is the conversion of stress into strength, like steel forged in fire, like muscles torn down and rebuilt stronger, like the decimated forests rebuilt after massive storms. Your biology has evolved to resilience.

Every breath reset, every mindful pause, every decision to regulate versus react—it is all evidence: you are not fragile. You are adaptive. You are resilient.

CHAPTER 13:

THE COMMUNITY EFFECT —
WHY CONNECTION HEALS

But here's the kicker: no one becomes resilient alone. The strongest nervous system, the most steady breath, the most extreme ritual, it all falls apart with isolation. Humans are wired for connection. Emotional resilience does not increase inside your own body—it increases when you are shoulder to shoulder, when you feel seen, when you feel supported, and when you feel safe.

Resilience isn't just mine or yours, it's ours. In Chapter 13, we will enter the arena of connection: how relationships, trust, and community not just soothe the system—they adjust the stress response.

PART 1: LONELINESS AS THE NEW SMOKING

The waiting room was silent too silent. Maria (our ongoing vignette thread) was scrolling through her phone while waiting for her blood work results. She was now in her late forties, juggling a demanding job, grown kids who left home, and a marriage that had grown distant. She was not overweight. She did not smoke. She hardly drank. On paper, she should have been fine. Her labs painted a different story: rising blood pressure, creeping blood sugar, fatigue, poor night sleep.

When her doctor asked about diet or exercise, she provided polite nods. When he asked about stress, she shrugged. When he asked the questions, "Do you feel supported? Do you feel connected?"— her eyes filled with tears.

Loneliness slowly seeped into her life like a silent leak, undetected until there was a crack in the foundation.

THE UNSEEN EPIDEMIC

In 2018, the UK appointed its own "Minister of Loneliness." It sounded unbelievable—a political office with the mandate to reduce loneliness—but it was no joke. Research has shown that chronic loneliness poses as significant as a risk of early death as smoking 15 cigarettes per day. That's not a metaphor—hard data.

Loneliness is, in fact, more than simply a feeling. It creates a systemic biological stressor—a slow poison that courses through our hormones, our immune response, and even our gene expression. In a technology-hyperconnected world, people report feeling ever more disconnected, isolated, and invisible.

We developed faster internet, but a frayed social. We built bigger houses but emptier dinner tables.

A STORY OF TWO VILLAGES

Imagine: in Okinawa, Japan, older women in their nineties are laughing in a garden, joining together for meals on tatami mats every day in their moai—a lifelong friendship and meal group. Their joints ache less, their spirits shine brighter, and they live longer than almost anyone else in the world.

Now, imagine: an average city in the "West"— a 75-year-old man is in a high-rise, with a TV flickering as he sits alone, with no one knocking on his door, and his phone never rings. He microwaves his meals. He has conversations with a news anchor. His body deteriorates as quietly as it spirals inward—not from lack of medicine, but from lack of connection.

What is the difference? One has belonging, the other suffocates in silence.

THE PHYSIOLOGY OF LONELINESS

Here's what scientists have uncovered:

- **Stress response:** Loneliness activates the hypothalamic–pituitary–adrenal (HPA) axis, elevating cortisol levels chronically. This erodes sleep, blood sugar balance, and cardiovascular health.

- **Inflammation:** Lonely individuals show higher levels of pro-inflammatory cytokines, the same molecules that drive chronic diseases from heart attacks to Alzheimer's.

- **Immune suppression:** Even vaccines are less effective in the lonely; their antibody response is blunted as if their immune system has given up hope.

- **Gene expression:** In one famous UCLA study, researchers found that loneliness actually changes which genes are turned "on" or "off." Genes for inflammation lit up; genes for antiviral defense shut down.

Loneliness is not in your head. It is in your blood, your cells, your very DNA.

WHY WE'RE WIRED FOR CONNECTION

Our ancestors didn't survive alone. A single human in the wild was vulnerable to predators, hunger, and injury. Safety came from the tribe. Oxytocin, the "bonding hormone," evolved not as a romantic luxury but as a survival code. It tells the brain: *you belong, you are safe, you can rest.*

Isolation, by contrast, was once a death sentence. That same wiring still lives in us. When we're cut off from connection, our bodies shift into hypervigilance — scanning for threat, tightening muscles, raising blood pressure, hoarding fat, disrupting sleep.

Loneliness, then, is not weakness. It's biology screaming for a missing nutrient.

THE MODERN PARADOX

Never before in human history have we had so many ways to "connect":

- Thousands of Facebook friends.

- Dozens of WhatsApp groups.

- Slack pings, email threads, endless texts.

And yet — record numbers of people report feeling lonely. Why? Because connection is not the same as **contact.**

- A like is not a hug.

- A meme is not eye contact.

- A heart emoji is not a heartbeat pressed against yours.

The nervous system knows the difference.

THE SILENT HEALTH CRISIS

In 2023, the U.S. Surgeon General issued an advisory: loneliness is an epidemic. Rates of reported loneliness have doubled since the 1980s. Teenagers, paradoxically, the most digitally connected generation, also report the highest levels of disconnection.

Health effects are staggering:

- 29% increased risk of heart disease.

- 32% increased risk of stroke.

- 50% increased risk of dementia.

It is no exaggeration to call loneliness a toxin. If processed sugar and sedentary behavior are public health enemies, loneliness is their hidden twin.

NARRATIVE VIGNETTE: THE CORPORATE WARRIOR

James, 42, a mid-level executive, had a lot of pride in his work-induced independence. He was up early and in the gym for a brutal training session, worked long hours for 12 hours, ordered Uber Eats for dinner, and, prior to settling in for bed, was scrolling LinkedIn. He was surrounded by colleagues and social feeds — yet his doctor flagged rising blood pressure and prediabetes.

When asked why he didn't spend time with friends for stress relief, he was dismissive: "I don't have any friends. Work is life."

Labs don't lie. He was starving his body not only from proper nutrition, but also from connection. He was physically fit, yet physically fragile. Strong, but literally brittle. His recovery tank was emptying not because of the quantity of sleep, but from a lack of belonging.

FROM LONELINESS TO BELONGING

The good news is that the antidote to loneliness is not complex. It doesn't require a prescription drug. It requires rediscovering an ancient truth: we heal in connection.

- A shared meal lowers cortisol more than eating alone.
- Group laughter raises pain thresholds via endorphins.
- Singing in a choir synchronizes heart rates.
- Holding hands before surgery reduces pain perception.

These aren't sentimental anecdotes. They are measurable physiological shifts.

Loneliness, then, is not simply a social inconvenience. It is one of the greatest health risks of our time. And connection is not simply "nice-to-have." It is as essential as food, water, and oxygen.

Which means the question is not: *Do you want friends?* The question is: *Do you want to heal? Do you want to live longer, better, stronger?*

Because the truth is this:

Your tribe is your treatment. Belonging is biology.

PART 2 — THE BIOLOGY OF BELONGING: OXYTOCIN, ENDORPHINS, IMMUNE RESILIENCE

That day, on her way out of the doctor's office, Maria had not received a pill, but rather a prescription for connection. At first, it felt nearly ridiculous—how can you lower blood sugar with coffee? How is laughter medicine? However, biology was about to confirm what the wisdom traditions had known for a thousand years: belonging is biochemistry.

OXYTOCIN: THE GLUE OF HUMAN SURVIVAL

Imagine the warm flush you feel when holding a newborn, or the calm after a long hug with someone you trust. That sensation isn't just "emotional." It's chemical. The hormone behind it is **oxytocin**, often called the *bonding hormone.*

- **Origins:** Oxytocin was once studied only in childbirth and breastfeeding — it helps uterine contractions and milk letdown. But scientists soon realized it was much bigger: a molecule of trust, safety, and social glue.

- **Stress Buffer:** Oxytocin lowers cortisol, calming the stress response. It signals: *You're safe. You're not alone. You can turn down the alarm system.*

- **Heart + Vessel Health:** Oxytocin also improves blood vessel dilation, lowers blood pressure, and protects the cardiovascular system.

Narrative vignette: In a study at the University of North Carolina, couples who hugged for just 20 seconds before stressful events showed significantly lower heart rates and cortisol levels. A hug isn't just nice — it's a biological switch.

ENDORPHINS: THE CHEMISTRY OF JOY

Now picture a group of people dancing at a wedding, or laughing so hard they can't breathe. What's happening here? **Endorphins** — the body's natural opioids — flood the brain, reducing pain, boosting euphoria, and deepening social bonds.

- **Laughter & Sync:** Research shows that shared laughter increases pain tolerance — not metaphorically, but literally, in measurable lab tests.

- **Movement + Music:** Group singing, drumming, or dancing releases endorphins in ways solo activity doesn't. It's why soldiers marching, choirs singing, and sports teams celebrating feel unstoppable.

- **Narrative:** A study from Oxford University found that rowers who trained in synchrony released more endorphins than those who rowed alone, and they reported stronger feelings of bonding.

Biology takeaway: Endorphins aren't just "feel-good chemicals." They evolved to glue groups together through shared movement and joy.

IMMUNE RESILIENCE: BELONGING AS DEFENSE

Here's where it gets even more fascinating:

CONNECTION BOOSTS IMMUNITY.

- **Cold Virus Study:** At Carnegie Mellon, researchers exposed volunteers to a cold virus. Those with stronger social ties were less likely to get sick. Loneliness, by contrast, predicted worse symptoms.

- **Antibody Power:** Married people — happily married, that is — show stronger antibody responses to vaccines compared to the unmarried or those in high-conflict relationships. The body can tell if your bonds are nurturing or draining.

- **Inflammation Genes:** UCLA research shows that loneliness switches genes into a pro-inflammatory mode, while connection suppresses that harmful pattern.

Narrative vignette: Consider shift workers or expats who move to a new city, cut off from the community. Many experience not just loneliness, but higher rates of flu, digestive issues, and even autoimmune flares. The immune system whispers: *Where is my tribe?*

THE SOCIAL NERVOUS SYSTEM

Neuroscientist Stephen Porges coined the concept of the **polyvagal theory** — the idea that the vagus nerve, which regulates our heart and digestion, is also a social nerve. When we make eye contact, hear a calming voice, or feel safe touch, the vagus nerve activates its "rest and connect" mode.

- Heart rate slows.

- Digestion improves.

- Inflammation decreases.

In other words, your nervous system doesn't just regulate organs. It listens for cues of belonging. If it hears silence, it braces for survival. If it hears a connection, it leans into healing.

BELONGING AS ENERGY MEDICINE

Think of connection as a nutrient:

- Oxytocin as the calming balm.

- Endorphins as the joy spark.

- Immune shifts as the shield.

- The nervous system tone as the conductor.

Together, they form a healing symphony.

And here's the kicker: these effects aren't "soft" or "secondary." They are as measurable as blood sugar or cholesterol. Belonging shifts biomarkers in hours. Chronic connection rewires your health trajectory for decades.

Maria didn't need a prescription bottle. She needed to rebuild her village. A walking group, a book club, Friday dinners with neighbors. Each smile, each laugh, each shared story wasn't just emotional — it was biological.

For her, and for us, the message is clear:

Your biology doesn't just crave belonging — it depends on it.

PART 3 — BLUE ZONE LESSONS: EATING, MOVING, RESTING TOGETHER

When researchers initially arrived in the mountain villages of Sardinia, the tranquil gardens of Okinawa, and Costa Rica's Nicoya Peninsula, they were not searching for miracle supplements or a futuristic diet. They were seeking lifestyle patterns. What they discovered was surprisingly simple yet extremely powerful: the longest-lived people on this planet eat, move, and sleep together.

THE TABLE AS MEDICINE

In Okinawa, Japan, elders gather in *moai* — lifelong circles of friends who meet regularly to share food, tea, and life burdens. They eat *hara hachi bu* (until 80% full), but more importantly, they eat together.

- **Science anchor:** Shared meals lower cortisol, improve digestion (via vagus nerve activation), and increase oxytocin.

- **Narrative vignette:** A 97-year-old Okinawan woman, interviewed by Dan Buettner's Blue Zones team, laughed when asked if she ever eats alone. "Why would I? Food tastes different with company."

MOVING TOGETHER, NATURALLY

In Ikaria, Greece — nicknamed "the island where people forget to die" — villagers don't hit treadmills. They walk to neighbors' homes, tend gardens, and dance at festivals that last until dawn. Movement is woven into life, and crucially, it is **social movement.**

- **Science:** Group walking improves adherence, lowers perceived exertion, and increases longevity benefits compared to solo walking (meta-analysis, Preventive Medicine, 2018).

- **Story:** An Ikarian shepherd still climbs hills with his goats at 90. When asked the secret, he shrugs: "I go where my friends go."

RESTING TOGETHER

In Nicoya, Costa Rica, midday rest is sacred. Hammocks swing in shaded courtyards while families nap after lunch. In Ikaria, it's the afternoon siesta — a rhythm that protects the heart.

- **Research:** Regular nappers in Mediterranean regions show 37% lower risk of coronary mortality (Harvard study, Arch Intern Med, 2007).

- **Narrative:** A Nicoyan farmer laughs when researchers ask about stress management: "We don't manage stress. We rest before it grows."

SPIRITUAL + COMMUNAL ANCHORS

In Loma Linda, California — a Seventh-day Adventist Blue Zone — weekly Sabbath rest is practiced communally. Families gather, disconnect from work, and share long meals. This ritual of sacred time reinforces both spiritual resilience and immune resilience.

- **Science anchor:** Regular religious or spiritual community participation is linked with lower inflammation, lower mortality risk, and improved mental health.

- **Narrative vignette:** A 103-year-old Adventist credits her weekly potluck dinners with keeping her spirit and body alive: "God made food to be shared."

THE THREAD THAT BINDS

Across all five Blue Zones — Sardinia, Okinawa, Ikaria, Nicoya, Loma Linda — the diets vary (olive oil vs. tofu vs. beans), but the **context** is identical: food is social, movement is communal, rest is shared, and purpose is collective.

This is not an accident of culture. It's a **biological multiplier**. Connection enhances nutrition, movement, and recovery. Alone, each habit matters. Together, they transform.

Maria, who is our repeated story anchor, began to discover her own version of the Blue Zone ritual. She invited some neighbors over for a Sunday Meal – no phones, no television, just soup, bread, and stories. The first time was awkward. By week three, things changed: laughter filled the silence, meals lasted longer, and Maria started to realize that she was not just digesting food, but also digesting connection.

Later, her doctor would notice: lower blood pressure, better sleep, better mood.

Healing sometimes doesn't look like a pill or a gym. Healing sometimes looks like a pot of soup, passed around a table with four or more people.

PART 4 — DIGITAL VS. REAL CONNECTION

Maria is at her kitchen table with a phone lit up in her hand. Notifications stream in — about a dozen likes, three new comments, another group chat notification. Her mind feels like it has too much going on, but her body feels vacant. When the screen finally goes off, it is quiet. The irony? She has never been "more connected", and yet here she is feeling incredibly lonely.

This is the paradox of our time: we confuse digital connection with human attachment.

THE ILLUSION OF CONNECTION

Social media can mimic the dopamine spark of face-to-face interaction. Each notification acts like a sugar cube for the brain, a quick hit of novelty and approval.

- **Science:** fMRI studies show that likes on social media activate the same reward circuits (ventral striatum) as food or money (Sherman et al., *Psychological Science*, 2016).

- **The catch:** Digital connection delivers the chemical *taste* of belonging without the physiological *substance*.

It's like drinking soda when your body needs water. The thirst for true connection remains unquenched.

REAL CONNECTION = BIOLOGICAL MEDICINE

In contrast, a real face-to-face connection engages a whole symphony of body systems:

- **Oxytocin** surges when we hug, laugh, or make eye contact. This hormone reduces fear responses and strengthens immune resilience.

- **Endorphins** rise during communal singing, dancing, or even shared laughter — natural painkillers and mood lifters.

- **Parasympathetic activation:** Real conversation and presence (tone of voice, micro-expressions) stimulate the vagus nerve, lowering heart rate and blood pressure.

Digital chatter doesn't trigger these cascades. The body knows the difference between pixels and presence.

LONELINESS IN THE DIGITAL ERA

Paradoxically, the more hours people spend online, the lonelier they report feeling.

- **Study:** Heavy social media users report **higher rates of anxiety, depression, and perceived loneliness** than low users (Primack et al., *Am J Prev Med*, 2017).

- **Mechanism:** Constant digital comparison increases cortisol and self-criticism. Unlike Blue Zone meals or gatherings, scrolling is solitary, sedentary, and stress-amplifying.

NARRATIVE CONTRAST

In Ikaria, an 85-year-old man enjoys a slow cup of coffee with friends as they chat about goats, grandchildren, politics, and the weather. There are no phones on the table. No hurry. The result? His cortisol levels are lower, his immune function stronger, his lifespan decades longer.

Meanwhile, Maria has finished another digital binge on her device. Her stomach feels tense, her shoulders are tight, and her breath is quick and shallow. Biologically, she is in a state of alarm – even though she hasn't left her couch.

DIGITAL TOOLS. REAL BOUNDARIES.

To be clear, technology is not the enemy. For many, digital spaces have sustained family connections across oceans and provided relief in isolation. However, the boundary must be drawn: technology should supplement and not replace in-person connections.

A digital sunset (put that phone down 1-2 hours before bed) resets sleep pattern rhythms.

Science anchor: Replacing just 30 minutes of daily screen scrolling with face-to-face interaction significantly lowers loneliness scores and boosts life satisfaction (Hunt et al., Journal of Social and Clinical Psychology, 2018).

Real connection heals in ways the digital cannot replicate. The eye-to-eye connection. A hand on the shoulder. Laughing until tears roll. Your neighbor drops soup off at your door when you're sick. These moments do not ping or buzz - they resonate in the nervous system, rebalancing stress, boosting your immune system, and extending life.

In the end, our nervous system doesn't crave Wi-Fi. It craves us.

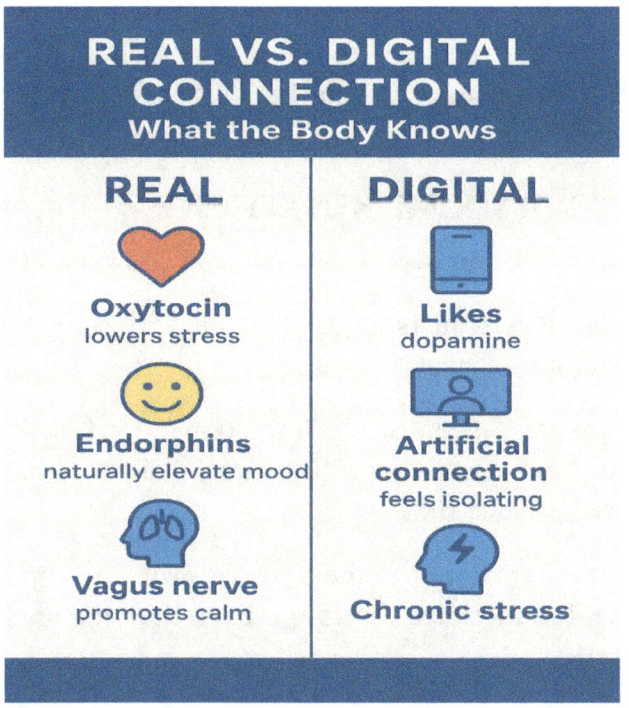

PART 5 — ACTION STARTER: BUILDING YOUR HEALING TRIBE

Picture this: after a long, stressful day of everything, your phone buzzes with the usual notifications—emails, headlines, algorithm-driven updates. Instead of doing this in isolation, you take off your slippers, slide on that old pair of sneakers, and walk down the block to slowly share a meal with a friend. Or head to the park to join a few friends for a sweaty workout full of laughs. Or cuddle up with family with no phones anywhere in sight, sharing food and stories.

These little moments are medicine. Real, measurable medicine. Your nervous system, switching from hypervigilance to at-ease. Oxytocin rises. Stress hormones lower. Heart rate variability is restored. Immunity is increased. Belonging becomes biology.

And herein lies the challenge: tribes don't just happen in the modern world. They are cultivated. They are built with intention. They are protected with the same care we give to our diet, sleep, or exercise.

Here is a practical guide to start building (or reconstructing) your tribe of healing.

1. AUDIT YOUR SOCIAL NUTRITION

Just as you track what you eat, track who you spend time with.

- **Draining vs. Nourishing**: After time with someone, ask: Do I feel lighter or heavier?

- **Frequency & Depth**: Shallow connections (scrolling, likes, small talk) don't carry the same weight as face-to-face, heart-to-heart time.

- **Action Step**: For one week, write down your top 5 recurring social interactions. Circle the ones that genuinely energize you.

2. DESIGN CONNECTION RITUALS

Belonging thrives on rhythm, not randomness. Blue Zone cultures don't "schedule" connection—they weave it into daily life. You can, too.

- **Meals Together**: Commit to 1–2 phone-free shared meals per week.

- **Movement Together**: Replace one solo workout with a walk, hike, or yoga session with a friend.

- **Weekly Anchor**: Host a standing family dinner, group call, or community potluck—same day, same time.

Science Anchor: Regular, repeated contact stabilizes oxytocin pathways and buffers stress responses more effectively than sporadic "catch-ups."

3. CURATE YOUR INNER CIRCLE

Not everyone needs to be in your healing tribe. In fact, fewer but deeper connections often yield the strongest biological benefits.

- **3 People Rule**: Identify three people you could call in a crisis, and three people who make you laugh until your stomach hurts. Protect and nurture these bonds.

- **Cross-Generational Wisdom**: Include someone older, someone younger. Different perspectives stretch resilience.

- **Action Step**: Write a short gratitude note (text, letter, voice memo) to one person weekly. This practice strengthens bonds more than passive contact.

4. BRIDGE DIGITAL → PHYSICAL

Technology can be a bridge if used wisely.

- **From Screen to Real**: Use group chats to coordinate, not replace, real connection.

- **Boundaries**: If your "community" is 95% digital, create one physical ritual each week to rebalance.

- **Action Step**: Pick one digital group (fitness app, interest forum, hobby chat) and schedule a real-world meet-up.

5. BUILD BELONGING INTO PLACE

Your environment can either isolate or connect you.

- **Third Spaces**: Coffee shops, libraries, gyms, gardens, faith centers—neutral spaces foster natural belonging.

- **Neighborhood Anchors**: Start small: greet your barista by name, wave to neighbors, and show up consistently. Familiarity builds safety.

- **Action Step**: Commit to showing up in one local space weekly (same café table, same park bench, same walking trail). Consistency transforms strangers into a community.

QUICK-REFERENCE CHECKLIST: BUILDING YOUR HEALING TRIBE

☑ Audit your social nutrition: Who nourishes you?
☑ Anchor connection rituals: meals, movement, weekly traditions.
☑ Protect your inner circle: depth > breadth.
☑ Use digital as a bridge, not a substitute.
☑ Root yourself in place: consistency builds community.

Core Message: Belonging is not a luxury. It is a biological need as vital as food, sleep, or movement. Your healing tribe is your living prescription for resilience.

HEALING TRIBE BLUEPRINT

AUDIT
YOUR SOCIAL
NUTRITION

Who nourishes you?

DESIGN
CONNECTION RITUALS

Incorporate connection
into your routine

CURATE
YOUR INNER CIRCLE

Nurture a few key relationships

BRIDGE DIGITAL → PHYSICAL

Move from screen to real-life

Recap:

Community is not a luxury. It is biology. Every hug, every shared meal, every laugh is a molecular signal—telling your nervous system, you are safe, you are seen, you belong. Connection produces oxytocin that softens stress, endorphins that improve your mood, and immune signals that enhance resilience. Just as fasting and sleep reset the body, relationships reset the soul.

Loneliness shrinks us. Connection expands us. You were never meant to fight your battles alone—you are designed for tribe, burden-sharing, rhythmic synchrony. The strongest people are not the ones who do everything alone, but those who know how to receive and how to let others receive from them.

Community is fuel. Fire to keep sustaining the glowing embers of resilience, despite life's winds blowing hard. But if fire does not have direction, it will burn without purpose. This is when the compass—purpose—comes in! When the compass is absent, the connection will become aimless. When the compass is present, the connection will be an unstoppable energy.

When you form your healing tribe, you accumulate energy. When you harness that energy toward a compass of intention and purpose, you will not merely thrive—you will carve a trail. And this is where we transition into the next chapter.

CHAPTER 14:

PURPOSE AS MEDICINE

PURPOSE AS COMPASS — WHY MEANING IS MEDICINE.

Because the community will keep you alive, but the purpose is how you will show what gives purpose to your life.

PART 1: NARRATIVE OF SOMEONE THRIVING AFTER MIDLIFE CRISIS

Picture this:

A man in his late forties—let's call him David- sits alone in a quiet office, the light of the monitor illuminating mounds of reports around him. From the outside, he has everything: a good job, a house in the suburbs, maybe a tropical vacation once in a while. But inside, he feels empty. The kids are grown, the work is boring, and every day seems a little heavier than the last.

David isn't broken. He's just drifting. This is a crisis, not about disaster but more about life trajectory or direction. It is far more common than we realize. Psychologists have termed this the "midlife slump," but it is a body and mind alerting you: You have lost your compass. You are burning gas with no map.

Fast forward one year. David has not won the lottery. He is not traveling the world as a reformed entrepreneur. What he has done is subtle—but far more powerful. He began to mentor new colleagues, teach guitar at the community center, and lead Saturday hikes with neighbors.

His cholesterol didn't just lower. His energy didn't just increase. His face is more relaxed, he is laughing louder, and his eyes are bright.

What changed?

Not his circumstance. His purpose.

And the science is catching up to what the wisdom traditions have always known:

☞ Purpose isn't a luxury of poets and philosophers.

☞ Purpose is biology. It changes hormones, brain wiring, and mortality risk.

There was no midlife crisis. There was a crisis of meaning or purpose.

And the cure was not money, it was why.

That's where we start.

PART 2 — THE SCIENCE OF IKIGAI / LIFE PURPOSE

IKIGAI: A COMPASS, NOT A CONCEPT

On the island of Okinawa, where some of the world's longest-living people thrive, elders are often asked the secret to their vitality. They do not mention supplements, going to the gym, or the latest medical advances. They smile and say "ikigai," which loosely translates to "a reason for being". It's what gets someone out of bed in the morning with excitement instead of angst. It's not about what you can accomplish in life—it could be taking care of grandkids, gardening, or leading a morning tai chi class at the park.

Ikigai is built into the DNA of Okinawan daily life. It helps to explain the 85-year-old fisherman who gets up each day with excitement to cast his nets, or the 92-year-old woman who puts on a fresh pot of miso soup every morning to deliver to her neighbors.

These are not burdens but "body signals" to the brain— you are contributing, you are connected, your story is relevant.

And the body responds.

THE BIOLOGY OF PURPOSE

Modern research is confirming what Okinawans have lived for centuries. Purpose isn't just a mindset—it's measurable in the bloodstream, in the brain, and even in survival curves.

- **Mortality Reduction:**

  A landmark study published in *Psychological Science* tracked more than 6,000 adults over 14 years. Those with a strong sense of purpose had a **15–30% lower risk of death**, independent of age, wealth, or health at baseline. In other words, purpose was as protective as quitting smoking or exercising regularly.

- **Cardiovascular Protection:**

  The *Journal of the American Medical Association* (JAMA) reports that people with high purpose scores had **lower rates of stroke and heart disease**. Stress hormones like cortisol were lower, and heart rate variability—a marker of nervous system resilience— was higher. Purpose acted like an invisible buffer against daily wear and tear.

- **Stress Buffering:**

  Harvard researchers found that individuals with purpose in life showed **fewer stress-related health declines**. Their immune systems were more resilient, inflammatory markers were lower, and they recovered more quickly from adversity.

- **Brain Preservation:**

  Neurological studies show that a sense of purpose is linked with **slower cognitive decline** and even reduced risk of Alzheimer's disease. It appears that when the brain is engaged with meaningful goals, neural pathways stay more active, flexible, and connected.

NARRATIVES FROM RESEARCH

Take Mrs. Tanaka, an Okinawan woman who was interviewed at the age of 101, who still got up every day to garden her vegetable patch and made onigiri for her visiting grandchildren. Her doctor said she had no chronic diseases and was sharper than many 70-year-olds. So when she was asked why she thought she was still living, she laughed, "Because I have things to do tomorrow."

Here's some data from the Rush Memory and Aging Project in Chicago. Researchers followed older adults for over a decade. Those who had a strong sense of life purpose were 2.4 times less likely to develop Alzheimer's disease. It is more than important to note that this wasn't about IQ or education; it's about emotional and existential anchors.

THE PROTECTIVE WEB OF PURPOSE

Why is purpose so powerful? Scientists suggest at least four intertwined mechanisms:

1. **Hormonal Balance** — Purpose reduces chronic cortisol surges and supports healthier diurnal rhythms (stress dips at night, energy peaks in the morning).

2. **Immune Resilience** — Meaningful engagement boosts natural killer cells and antibodies, defending against illness.

3. **Behavioral Anchoring** — People with purpose are more likely to move daily, eat well, and avoid harmful habits—not because they're "disciplined," but because they're invested in tomorrow.

4. **Psychological Grit** — Purpose reframes obstacles. A setback isn't the end; it's a chapter. This lowers depression and anxiety risk.

406

PURPOSE ACROSS CULTURES

- **Okinawa (Japan):** Ikigai as the daily anchor.

- **Sardinia (Italy):** Shepherds find purpose in tending flocks and family, walking mountain paths daily.

- **Nicoya (Costa Rica):** Strong sense of *plan de vida*—a life plan tied to community and work, even into old age.

- **Loma Linda (California):** Seventh-day Adventists anchor their purpose in faith, volunteering, and service.

Every Blue Zone shows the same pattern: people live not for themselves alone, but for *something larger*.

A PATIENT VIGNETTE

Maria, whom we've followed in earlier chapters, exemplifies this transformation. Initially, her health concerns were all physical — weight, sugar cravings, and low energy. But then, as she started to regrow her microbiome and practice some resilience skills, she hit a deeper wall: "Even if I am healthier, what am I healthy for?"

Her breakthrough came not from a supplement or exercise, but from tutoring neighborhood teens after school. While helping the teens, she rediscovered her own story. Six months later, not only were her labs improved, but her smile returned, and again, her daughter said, "Mom laughs again. That is the real miracle."

Key Point: Purpose is not just a philosophical abstraction. It is a quantifiable survival benefit. It diminishes your risk for illness, strengthens your brain, and actually increases your life span.

PART 3 — THE NEUROBIOLOGY OF PURPOSE

PURPOSE AS NEURAL FUEL

Imagine standing at the bottom of a steep hill. Muscles sore, short of breath, brain screaming "Stop" at you with every ounce of reason.

And then you remembered why you are climbing: to see your kid graduate, to keep a promise, to prove to yourself you can. Suddenly, your legs felt lighter.

That invisible energy isn't magic. It's neurobiology. It's dopamine, endorphins, prefrontal activation, and resilience circuits firing together when you've got a "why," your brain actually changes its reward systems to push you forward—even in spite of pain, fatigue, or fear.

THE DOPAMINE COMPASS

Dopamine is often misunderstood as the "pleasure chemical." In reality, it's not about *pleasure*—it's about *pursuit*.

- **Motivation & Drive:**

  The nucleus accumbens and ventral tegmental area (VTA) release dopamine not when you achieve something, but when you anticipate it. This is why goals are so powerful—they create a neurochemical pull forward.

- **Purpose vs. Empty Rewards:**

  Social media likes or sugar hits trigger shallow dopamine bursts that fade quickly. But when you align with deep purpose—raising a child, mastering a craft, serving a community—the brain engages in **sustained dopamine signaling**, creating resilience that lasts far beyond the moment.

SCIENCE SNAPSHOT:

A 2019 study in *Nature Neuroscience* showed that when people pursued goals aligned with intrinsic values, dopamine firing was more sustained compared to chasing extrinsic rewards (money, status). Translation: your brain knows the difference between "fake goals" and "true purpose."

THE PREFRONTAL CORTEX: PURPOSE AS EXECUTIVE CONTROL

Your prefrontal cortex is the CEO of the brain—the part that plans, focuses, and resists impulses. Under stress, it can go offline, leaving you reactive. But purpose flips the switch back on.

- People with strong purpose show **greater prefrontal activation** in fMRI studies during difficult tasks.

- This means they can override short-term discomfort in the service of long-term vision.

- In resilience research, this shows up as **grit**—the ability to keep going when others quit.

STRESS CIRCUITRY REWIRED

Normally, stress activates the amygdala and HPA axis: cortisol rises, and the body prepares for threat. Chronic stress erodes health.

But purpose acts as a **buffer**:

- In studies, people with a strong purpose had **lower baseline cortisol** and **faster recovery** after stress exposure.

- Purpose essentially recalibrates the amygdala-prefrontal dialogue: the fear center still fires, but the higher brain reminds it, *"This is worth it. We can handle it."*

ENDORPHINS & OXYTOCIN: THE SOCIAL GLUE

Purpose often lives in community—raising a family, serving others, building something together. This is where two other chemicals join the orchestra:

- **Endorphins:** Natural painkillers released in moments of shared effort—think of runners finishing a marathon together. Purposeful struggle feels less painful because endorphins soften the edges.

- **Oxytocin:** The "bonding hormone" released in trust and connection. When your purpose involves others, oxytocin deepens loyalty, reduces fear, and strengthens immune function.

RESILIENCE NETWORKS IN THE BRAIN

Resilience is not one circuit; it's a network. Studies in neuroscience have identified that people with a strong purpose activate a **distributed system**:

1. **Prefrontal Cortex** — planning, grit.

2. **Anterior Cingulate Cortex** — emotional regulation.

3. **Insula** — body awareness, gut-brain integration.

4. **Reward Pathways (VTA–Nucleus Accumbens)** — motivation.

Together, these create what scientists call a **purpose-driven resilience network**. It's not just enduring hardship—it's transmuting it into meaning.

A VIGNETTE: THE MARATHONER'S WHY

After James' brother died of heart disease, he decided to run a marathon. Training was grueling: runs at 4 a.m., injuries, exhaustion. And on mile 21 of the event, his legs were screaming; He almost quit – until he remembered his "why": raising money for heart research in honor of his brother.

Neuroscientifically, his purpose triggered his dopamine and prefrontal circuits, inhibited fear circuits in the amygdala, and released endorphins that helped him to finish. Later, he said, "I did not finish based on strength. I finished based on meaning."

THE SCIENCE OF RESILIENT BRAINS

- In combat veterans, those with a strong sense of purpose showed **lower rates of PTSD**, even with similar trauma exposure. (*Journal of Traumatic Stress*, 2010)

- In older adults, purpose correlated with **thicker prefrontal cortices**—a marker of preserved brain health. (*Neuropsychologia*, 2018)

- In students, linking study goals to future purpose improved performance and reduced dropout rates. (*Science*, 2014)

THE BIG PICTURE

Your brain is not a machine chasing random rewards. It is a **meaning-seeking organ.** When it has a purpose, the stress circuits calm, the reward pathways sustain, and resilience emerges. Without purpose, dopamine burns out on shallow hits, the amygdala dominates, and life feels flat.

Purpose doesn't just change how you think. It changes how your neurons fire, how your hormones flow, and how your body heals.

Key Takeaway: Purpose is not just psychological—it is neurological. It tunes dopamine for pursuit, strengthens the prefrontal cortex for discipline, lowers cortisol for health, and engages endorphins and oxytocin for joy and connection.

PART 4 — FINDING PURPOSE IN MICRO-MOMENTS

THE MYTH OF THE GRAND MISSION

When the word "purpose" is mentioned, many people envision earth-shattering initiatives: starting a not-for-profit, advancing a cure for disease, or writing a best-selling novel. But when purpose only exists in the extraordinary, then the vast majority of us are forever living in a posture of tameness.

The reality? Purpose thrives in the ordinary, too. What's ordinary for you might not be ordinary for someone else. It could be the smile you share with your child first thing in the morning, the manner in which you make a meal, or how you are there for a coworker who feels completely overwhelmed.

Purpose is not measured by scale. It is measured by alignment.

NEUROSCIENCE OF THE SMALL

Micro-moments matter because your brain doesn't wait for grand events to release its chemistry—it responds to meaning *now*.

- **Dopamine & Anticipation:** Each small, purposeful act is a dopamine signal that sustains motivation. Studies show that people who tie even minor daily habits to values report more satisfaction and lower stress (*Journal of Positive Psychology*, 2018).

- **Oxytocin & Connection:** Holding eye contact, offering gratitude, or helping a stranger sparks oxytocin—boosting trust and reducing anxiety. These micro-bursts accumulate into resilience.

- **Cortisol Buffering:** Researchers found that people who regularly engage in small acts of kindness show lower cortisol levels, even on stressful days (PNAS, 2013).

Your biology doesn't care if the act was saving a rainforest or simply helping your neighbor carry groceries. It responds to meaning.

CASE VIGNETTE: MARIA'S COMMUTE

Maria, our teacher who walked us through UPFs, stress cycles, and sleep issues, also disliked her driving time — The traffic, the noise, the endless podcast on 'being more productive.'

Then one day she tried something different: Rather than increase her input, Maria called her aging father and simply listened. Driving became her "connection time." Over time, she began to perceive stress differently. She didn't discover her "purpose" in a TED Talk; she discovered it through daily honoring a relationship.

For her biology, it mattered: cortisol decreased, oxytocin increased, and resilience increased. Her purpose was in traffic.

THE SCIENCE OF TINY MEANING

Research by scientists on the island of Okinawa and their research on ikigai, many elders didn't refer to a big grand ideal. Their "reason for getting up in the morning" was simple — "tending my garden," or "making soup for my grandchildren."

More reminders shine brightly in the longitudinal Study of Adult Development at Harvard. The elders who were happiest and healthiest weren't CEO's — they were people who found meaning in everyday moments.

MICRO-MOMENTS AS TRAINING

Think of micro-purpose as **neural reps.** Just like lifting weights strengthens muscles, repeatedly finding meaning in small acts strengthens purpose circuits in your brain. Over time:

- The prefrontal cortex (focus, discipline) becomes more active.

- Reward pathways learn to sustain effort without external validation.

- Stress responses dampen faster because the brain expects meaning in adversity.

Each small choice is a rep in your purpose gym.

PRACTICAL MICRO-MOMENTS FRAMEWORK

How do you train this daily?

1. **Morning Anchor:** Before checking your phone, ask: *"What one purposeful act can I do today?"* (Call someone, teach, create, help.)

2. **During Stress:** Reframe with meaning. Instead of "This meeting is killing me," ask, *"How does showing up here serve someone or something beyond me?"*

3. **Evening Reflection:** Journal one purposeful moment, however small. Over time, this rewires the brain to scan for meaning instead of threat.

A VIGNETTE: THE JANITOR'S PURPOSE

At a hospital in the Midwest, a janitor once told researchers studying workplace satisfaction: "My job is to help people heal."

He wasn't merely mopping floors; he saw himself preventing infections, he was stopping people from getting sick, alleviating families' stress by making sure the room was clean, and he was helping the nurses by removing at least one concern. This reframing transformed his low-status job into a noble vocation.

Purpose was not found in the job title— it was in the interpretation. And that interpretation had a positive impact on his biology: lower stress, higher positive feelings, resilience that spread into other areas of life.

MICRO-PURPOSE AS MEDICINE

Why does this matter so much? Because in a distracted and burnout-ridden culture, waiting on "big purpose" in life is just like waiting for a thunder-strike. Micro-moments are the daily current— they keep the lights on.

And together they build resilience in your nervous system, they give direction to your dopamine, and they align your biology to thrive.

Purpose does not just dwell in grand missions; it dwells in how you drink your coffee, how you acknowledge your neighbor, how you pause to breathe before you react.

Key Takeaway: You don't need to "find" your purpose. You need to practice it—moment by moment, act by act, until your biology learns that life is meaningful, even in its smallest rhythms.

ACTION STARTER: THE PURPOSE PRACTICE

YOUR DAILY FRAMEWORK FOR CULTIVATING MICRO-MOMENTS OF MEANING

1. THE PHILOSOPHY OF PRACTICE

Purpose is not a jewel or treasure you stumble upon; it is a muscle you build. This section is your training field. Just as fasting will retrain your metabolism, and sleep restores your recovery, purpose practices reshape the brain's reward circuits and stress responses.

Neuroscience shows that consistent small acts rewire pathways faster than sporadic big events. This workbook gives you daily, weekly, and monthly scaffolds to build a life where purpose is not an abstract concept—it's the lived texture of your day.

2. MORNING ALIGNMENT: THE "ONE ACT" INTENTION

Why it matters:

The brain's prefrontal cortex is most receptive in the morning— before email, news, and dopamine-drip notifications hijack attention. Starting the day with an intentional micro-purpose primes your biology to filter meaning all day.

THE PRACTICE:

1. Upon waking, ask:

   o *"What is one purposeful act I can commit to today?"*

   o Keep it small: checking in on a friend, cooking a nourishing meal, showing patience in a tough conversation.

2. Write it down in a journal or sticky note.

3. Anchor it in identity:

- o Instead of "I will call my mom," reframe: "I am a son who values connection."

- o Research: Identity-based intentions stick because they align with self-concept (University of Minnesota, 2017).

PROMPT BOX: MORNING ANCHORS

- Who could I encourage today?

- What small act of service could I do?

- How can I show up in line with my values in my next meeting/class/errand?

CASE VIGNETTE:

Darius, a young entrepreneur, began writing a single line each morning: "Today, my purpose is to help one person feel seen." At first, it was awkward. But within a month, he noticed his brain scanning for opportunities—complimenting the cashier, listening deeply to a colleague. The act itself was tiny. The cumulative effect was massive: lower anxiety, greater motivation, richer relationships.

3. STRESS REFRAMING: PURPOSE IN PRESSURE

Why it matters:

Stress is unavoidable. But research shows that when stress is tied to purpose, its biology shifts. Cortisol spikes are less damaging, inflammation is lowered, and recovery is faster. This is called the **"stress-is-enhancing mindset"** (Crum et al., Stanford, 2013).

The Practice:

1. When stress rises, pause for 20 seconds.

2. Ask: *"How is this challenge serving a value beyond me?"*

   - o Example: A grueling work deadline = providing stability for family, creating something that helps others.

3. Pair with breath: 4-6 slow exhales to cue parasympathetic reset.

Prompt Box: Stress Reframes

- How is this hard thing aligned with my values?

- Who might benefit from my enduring this challenge?

- What bigger "why" can I attach to this discomfort?

CASE VIGNETTE:

Maria (our teacher) used to dread grading papers. One night, she reframed: "Each paper is a chance to speak into a child's future." Her stress softened. Cortisol didn't vanish, but her body perceived meaning. Science calls this the "psychobiology of meaning"—stress signals become fuel instead of erosion.

4. EVENING INTEGRATION: THE DAILY PURPOSE SCAN

Why it matters:

Memory consolidation happens during sleep. Ending the day by tagging moments of purpose teaches the hippocampus to store those memories preferentially, rewiring the brain toward meaning.

The Practice:

1. Before bed, jot 1–3 micro-moments where you lived purpose.

2. They can be tiny: smiling at a neighbor, resisting a snap reaction, finishing a workout.

3. End with gratitude: *"I'm grateful I had this chance to show up."*

Prompt Box: Evening Reflection

- What moment today felt aligned with my deeper values?

- Did I notice someone else light up because of my actions?

- Where did I show patience, kindness, courage—even in small measure?

CASE VIGNETTE:

Lila, a nurse, began tracking three moments nightly. At first, she listed surface events: "Helped patient," "Spoke kindly." By week three, she noticed subtler shifts: "I took a breath before reacting to a rude comment." Over time, her journal became a reservoir she could revisit when exhausted—proof that her days carried meaning even when they felt mundane.

5. WEEKLY DEEPENING: THE PURPOSE PULSE

Why it matters:

Weekly reflection stabilizes patterns. Harvard research shows that those who connect weekly habits to values sustain changes longer than those who rely on willpower.

The Practice:

1. Choose one weekly ritual that embodies your values:

   o Family dinner without screens.

   o Volunteering for an hour.

   o Nature walk as a reflection.

2. Ask three questions on Sundays:

   o Where did I live purpose this week?

   o Where did I miss alignment?

   o What one adjustment will I try next week?

CASE VIGNETTE:

Samir, an overworked attorney, added a Sunday ritual: journaling his "Purpose Pulse." Within two months, he saw patterns—he felt most drained after weeks of shallow networking, and most alive after mentoring interns. He began rearranging his calendar around mentoring, realizing purpose wasn't in big wins but in daily influence.

6. MONTHLY / SEASONAL ANCHORS

Why it matters:

Micro-purpose sustains daily resilience, but periodic deep dives create course corrections. Blue Zone elders often tie purpose to seasonal rhythms—planting, harvest, festivals.

The Practice:

1. Monthly: Schedule a **purpose audit.** Journal prompts:

   o Am I still aligned with my deepest values?

   o What felt most alive this month?

   o What drained me—and is it necessary?

2. Seasonal: Plan a **purpose retreat day** (solo or with tribe). Walk in nature, fast from tech, and write freely: *"What is my why right now?"*

7. THE PURPOSE JOURNAL FRAMEWORK

To make this practical, here's a simple structure for a dedicated **Purpose Journal:**

- **Morning page:** One purposeful act for today.

- **Midday pause:** Note one stress reframed with meaning.

- **Evening page:** Three micro-purpose reflections.

- **Weekly review:** Pulse check.

- **Monthly/seasonal:** Audit + course correction.

This journal becomes a living record of your alignment—a mirror of your inner compass.

8. PATIENT JOURNEY CASE STUDY

Case: Carlos, the Midlife Reset

- **Starting point:** Carlos, 47, successful executive, plagued by burnout, restless nights, and emotional eating. He described life as "just running."

- **Intervention:** Began "Purpose Practice" journal with morning act + evening scan. At first, he struggled—entries were shallow. But repetition built awareness.

- **Breakthrough:** In month two, during a Sunday pulse, he wrote: "My only moments of aliveness come when teaching my daughter guitar." He reorganized evenings to protect that time.

- **Outcome:** Sleep improved, cravings fell, stress perception shifted. Carlos didn't quit his job or find a new career. He found purpose in fatherhood—a micro-moment magnified.

9. THE SCIENCE ANCHOR

- **Mortality:** Adults with purpose show a 15–30% lower risk of death over 10 years (*JAMA Network Open*, 2019).

- **Cortisol:** Purpose reframes stress, lowering chronic cortisol levels (*Psychoneuroendocrinology*, 2016).

- **Dopamine:** Anticipation of purposeful action activates reward circuits, boosting motivation even in fatigue (*Nature Neuroscience*, 2017).

- **Immune resilience:** Purpose-driven adults show stronger antibody responses to vaccines (*Health Psychology*, 2014).

10. CLOSING MOTIVATIONAL LIFT

Purpose isn't a lightning bolt—it's a candle lit daily. Every morning intention, every stress reframe, every nightly reflection is another wick lit. Over time, you don't just find your purpose. You *become* it.

Your biology listens. Your cells recalibrate. Your life reorients.

KEY INTEGRATION:

- **Micro-moments = reps in the purpose gym.**

- **Journaling anchors biology to meaning.**

- **Purpose isn't found—it's practiced.**

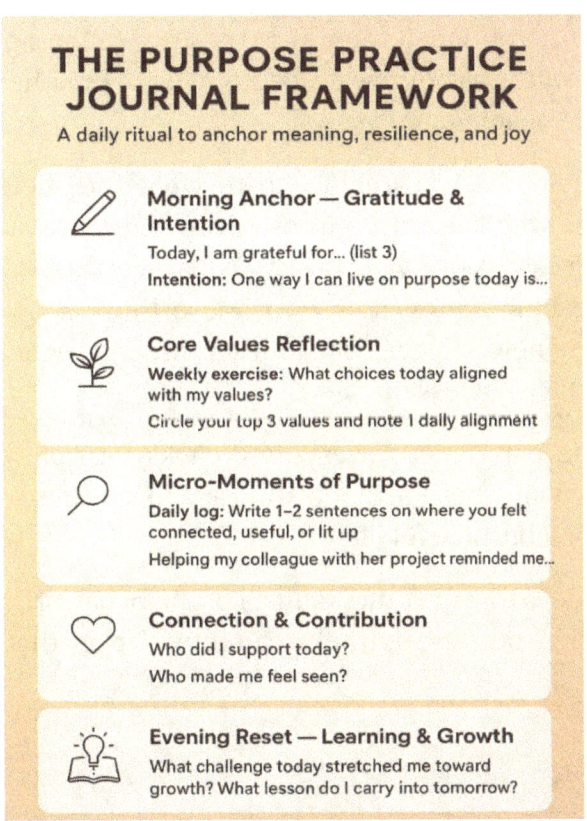

THE PURPOSE PRACTICE
JOURNAL FRAMEWORK
A daily ritual to anchor meaning, resilience, and joy

Morning Anchor — Gratitude & Intention
Today, I am grateful for... (list 3)
Intention: One way I can live on purpose today is...

Core Values Reflection
Weekly exercise: What choices today aligned with my values?
Circle your top 3 values and note 1 daily alignment

Micro-Moments of Purpose
Daily log: Write 1–2 sentences on where you felt connected, useful, or lit up
Helping my colleague with her project reminded me...

Connection & Contribution
Who did I support today?
Who made me feel seen?

Evening Reset — Learning & Growth
What challenge today stretched me toward growth? What lesson do I carry into tomorrow?

Take a moment to think about all the information we've been weaving together. Food was not merely about calories—it was about mood molecules and microbial orchestras. Movement was not merely about energy expenditure—it was about sending life signals to the cells. Fasting was not deprivation—it was ancient timeframes for healing. Stress management wasn't escaping—it was about rewiring resilience. Sleep was not a shut-down period—it was about nightly repair. And community was not about small talk—it was about our survival.

These were not hacks—they were all hitting arrows which pointed toward one directional point: we are designed to be resilient and to have a reason to live.

The purpose is that reason. It is the compass that directs every prescription in this book. If there is a lack of purpose, even the best rituals drift into routine. If there is purpose, even the smallest action like drinking water, taking a walk, or stopping to breathe—all become charged with meaning.

The science is now catching up to what the ancients already knew- people who live with purpose live longer, heal more quickly, and resist disease more vigorously. Okinawans have a word for it, ikigai. In the Blue Zones, it is woven into the very fabric of their culture. In the new science, it manifests through reduced mortality rates and reduced stress markers.

This is the part where everything clicks into place. Recovery, resilience, repair- these are not arbitrary tools; these serve as the foundation of a purposeful life.

If resilience is the structure, and all of the behaviors are the walls or beams, then purpose is the architectural plan that holds it all together.

PART V

TRANSFORMATION AND LONGEVITY

CHAPTER 15:

ACHIEVING THRIVING WEIGHT LOSS

PART 1 — THE MENTAL TRIGGER

You get on the scale.

It sways back and forth for a moment, the numbers blinking like they're teasing you, then it settles. Precisely the same as last week. Exactly the same as the week before.

You blink. Tighten your jaw. You replay the sacrifices through your head: skipped desserts, 6 a.m. treadmill workouts, nights going to bed hungry. And for what? For nothing?

The disappointment doesn't just stay stuck in your head; it expands. Into your chest. Into your mood. Into how you'll look at food later today when the frustration whispers, What's the point?

This is the cycle millions are in. Push hard. Restrict. Burnout. Slip back. Then start over with guilt as the fuel. The body feels like the enemy each time. Stubborn, resistant, impossible to control.

But here's the secret they didn't tell you: your body isn't broken. It's not the enemy. It's waiting and waiting for the right directions.

Because your body has one purpose — to protect you. When you starve it, it slows down metabolism. When you stress it, it stores fat. When you lose sleep, it makes you crave sugar. This isn't a sabotage. This is a survival program.

And survival programs can be reprogrammed.

The shift begins here: sustainable weight loss is not about battling your biology. It's about working with it. It's about giving your body signals that say, You're safe now, you can let go. It's about updating your operating system, not running your body into the ground with a sluggish old one.

When you understand this code, everything changes. You no longer have a fear of food. You no longer punish yourself with exercise. You start working with your body instead of against it.

And that's when the scale stops mocking you. That's when fat loss feels less like a war and more like a release.

This chapter is your reprogramming manual — not another diet, not another quick fix, but the manual for making your body Thrive.

Because Thriving bodies don't hold onto extra weight, thriving bodies let go.

PART 2 — THE WEIGHT LOSS CODE: WHY MOST DIETS FAIL

Picture this: you are out to dinner with friends. You order grilled chicken and a salad. No dressing, no bread, and no dessert. And all around you, your friends are laughing, clanking glasses, and dipping their forks into bowls of pasta and tiramisu. At first, you feel proud and then, shamefully punished. Proud because you are being "disciplined." Punished because now you feel like you are watching life through glass, stuck outside of it.

You stick to the plan, maybe for a week or two, focusing on willpower. You fought through cravings and maybe lost a little weight. Then something happens! Your energy drops, and you get hungrier. One night on Saturday, the bread basket comes back into your hands.

You binge, you feel ashamed, you quit, and on Monday, you start over.

Does this sound familiar? This is not a moral failure. This is biology.

WHY RESTRICTION COLLAPSES

The reason most diets fail isn't because people lack discipline. It's because restrictive dieting sets off alarms in your body's survival network:

- **Hormonal resistance**: Ghrelin (the hunger hormone) ramps up. Leptin (the satiety hormone) gets suppressed. You feel hungrier, even as you try to eat less.

- **Metabolic slowdown**: The body is astonishingly adaptive. Drop calories too low, and your resting metabolic rate declines — like dimming the lights to conserve power.

- **Psychological rebound**: Scarcity mindset makes food more desirable. When your brain hears "you can't," desire amplifies. This isn't a weakness; it's how humans survived famine.

Dieting, in the traditional sense, is like pushing a beach ball underwater. The harder you press, the more violently it bounces back when you slip.

REPROGRAMMING THE OPERATING SYSTEM

Here's the mental reframe: You don't need another diet. You need a new operating system.

Instead of fighting hunger hormones, you train them. Instead of forcing metabolic slowdown, you activate metabolic flexibility. Instead of creating psychological scarcity, you cultivate abundance — the abundance of foods and rhythms that signal safety.

This is the "Weight Loss Code":

- Stop treating your body like an enemy.

- Start feeding it signals that align with how it was designed to run.

THE RESEARCH THAT FLIPS THE SCRIPT

A 2016 study compared simple calorie restriction with intermittent fasting protocols. The calorie-restricted group lost weight initially but hit plateaus and regained weight within months. The intermittent fasting group — even eating the same overall calories — showed better fat loss, preserved lean mass, and greater adherence.

Why? Because fasting isn't deprivation. It's rhythm. It taps into evolutionary patterns the body already understands.

In other words, most diets fail because they wage war on the body. Sustainable weight loss succeeds because it re-teaches the body how to thrive.

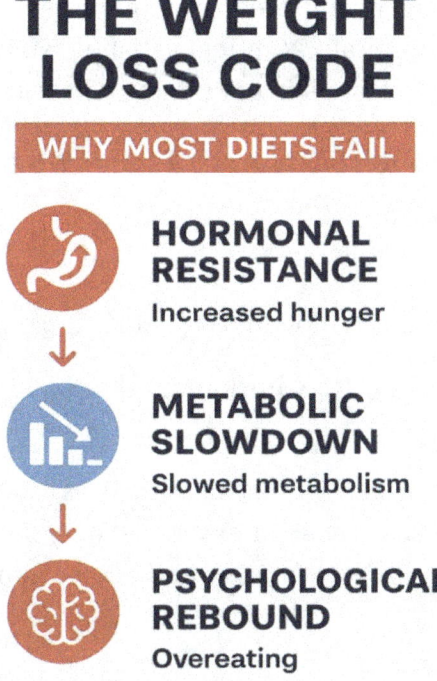

THE WEIGHT LOSS CODE

WHY MOST DIETS FAIL

HORMONAL RESISTANCE
Increased hunger

METABOLIC SLOWDOWN
Slowed metabolism

PSYCHOLOGICAL REBOUND
Overeating

PRINCIPLE ONE: REWIRE YOUR METABOLISM (PROTEIN + FIBER AS ANCHORS)

Here's a scenario to consider: You sit down for lunch. On your table, two meals are placed in front of you. One is a bagel with cream cheese. The other is a plate containing grilled salmon, leafy greens, and roasted vegetables. Both may contain roughly the same caloric content, but your body responds to them as if they are from completely separate universes.

The bagel hits your bloodstream like a blast of sugar. Insulin is released. Hunger hormones ignite the fireworks. Hours later, you are yawning, distracted, and searching the house for snacks.

The salmon plate is a different story. Protein activates the thermic effect, and your body uses increased energy just to digest protein – up to 30 percent more. The fiber in the dish slows down absorption, stabilizes blood sugar, and feeds gut microbes to send the "calm down" signals to the brain. You feel satisfied, stable, and energized for hours. Same calories. Different effects. That's the metabolic code!

THE SCIENCE: PROTEIN AND FIBER AS METABOLIC ANCHORS

- **Protein:**

  o Increases thermogenesis (calorie burn during digestion).

  o Stimulates satiety hormones like GLP-1 and PYY, quieting hunger.

  o Preserves lean muscle, which is the *engine of your metabolism*. Lose muscle, and your metabolic rate crashes. Protect muscle, and you burn more even at rest.

- **Fiber:**

  o Slows glucose absorption, blunting insulin spikes.

o Ferments in the colon into *short-chain fatty acids* that lower inflammation and improve insulin sensitivity.

o Expands volume in the stomach, sending stretch signals to the brain: *You're full. Stop eating.*

Together, protein and fiber act as a "lock" against the blood sugar roller coaster. They aren't trendy hacks. They are the metabolic foundation.

MENTAL REFRAME: FOOD AS PROGRAMMING

Every plate you build is not just "a meal." It's a *code injection* into your operating system.

- Protein is the stabilizer.

- Fiber is the regulator.

- Carbs and fats are the variables.

When you get the first two right, your body runs on a stable, fat-burning algorithm. When you skip them, you're playing roulette with cravings and energy crashes.

ACTION CODE: THE "PROTEIN FIRST, FIBER SECOND" RULE

At every meal, follow this simple sequence:

1. **Protein first** (20–40g): eggs, fish, poultry, tofu, lentils.

2. **Fiber second** (vegetables, beans, whole fruits).

3. **Everything else after** (healthy fats, smart carbs).

This order matters. Protein first blunts the insulin surge. Fiber second slows absorption. By the time starches or fats arrive, your metabolic switchboard is already primed for balance.

VISUALIZATION

Imagine your plate as a control panel.

- Protein is the main switch—turning on satiety, stabilizing blood sugar.

- Fiber is the regulator—dampening spikes and feeding your microbiome.

- Together, they lock your system in "fat-burn" mode.

Every bite is a programming command. Every plate is a chance to rewire.

Case Example: Daniel's Shift

Daniel, who is 44 and works as an accountant, tried juice cleanses, low-carb diets, and even meal skipping. Each time, he would lose about 5-10 pounds, but would regain it. When he came up to me at the gym and asked me how I maintain my weight, I told him not to diet, but to rewire his body. His only homework: protein first, fiber second.

Week one: he replaced his bagel in the morning with eggs and spinach.

Week two: he added some beans to his lunch salad.

By week six: his afternoon crashes were gone, his cravings were diminished, and he lost 12 pounds, without counting calories, ever.

His words: "I feel like I've been trying to fight hunger my whole life. Now it's like my body is finally on my side."

This is not magic, it's biology. When you feed your body the proper sequence, it stops resisting and starts cooperating.

Principle One is about partnership. You're not starving yourself, you're rewriting yourself.

PRINCIPLE TWO: SYNCHRONIZE WITH TIME (MEAL TIMING & FASTING)

Visualize your body as a theatre. At dawn, the lights start coming up, the orchestra warms up, and the stagehands reset the stage. This is your circadian rhythm getting you ready for the day ahead. Every hormone, enzyme, and metabolic switch is run by this ancient clock. Here's the thing: if you eat out of sync with the clock, the orchestra becomes confused. The music goes off-beat. Chaos sneaks in.

This is why synchronizing when you eat may be as powerful–in some cases more– than what you eat.

THE SCIENCE: YOUR INNER CLOCK AND FOOD TIMING

- **Insulin Sensitivity is Time-Dependent**

  In the morning and early afternoon, your body is primed to handle glucose. Insulin sensitivity peaks, meaning the same food causes a smaller blood sugar spike. By evening, this sensitivity wanes. Eating late is like trying to park a truck in a shrinking garage—messy and inefficient.

- **Circadian Rhythms Govern Hormones**

  Cortisol naturally rises in the morning, giving you alertness. Melatonin rises at night, preparing your body for sleep. When you eat late—especially sugar or refined carbs—you spike insulin at the exact time melatonin should dominate. That collision disrupts deep sleep and overnight repair.

- **Fasting as a Reset**

  Intermittent fasting isn't starvation—it's alignment. By extending your fasting window, you allow insulin to drop, fat burning to rise, and cellular repair (autophagy) to kick in. The body shifts from "store" mode to "restore" mode.

THE LONGEVITY PRESCRIPTION: 14/10 FASTING

For weight loss and sustainable energy, the 14/10 *pattern* is powerful. Here's how it works:

- **14 hours fasting**: from after dinner (say 7 PM) to late morning (9 AM).

- **10-hour eating window**: all meals between 9 AM and 7 PM.

This gently extends your nightly fast, harmonizing with your circadian rhythm. Unlike extreme fasting, it's sustainable, safe, and deeply restorative.

The best practice for weight loss is to consider making dinner the smallest or even an optional meal. Skipping it altogether on some days can accelerate fat loss by extending your fasting window. If you do eat in the evening, keep it light, protein-centered, and free of refined carbohydrates or sugary foods, since these rapidly spike insulin. Elevated insulin at night not only slows fat burning but also interferes with the natural release of melatonin — the hormone that signals deep sleep and overnight recovery. A lighter, low-insulin dinner supports better sleep quality, enhances hormonal balance, and allows your body to repair and restore more efficiently."

MENTAL PROGRAMMING: EVERY PAUSE IS A SIGNAL

Think of every fasting window not as deprivation, but liberation. When you delay or lighten dinner, you're extending your body's repair window. You're sending a clear message: *It's safe. Burn fat. Heal tissues. Balance hormones.*

It's not punishment—it's a partnership with your biology.

Visualization

Think of your body like a smartphone. Eating late at night is like opening apps on a phone while the phone's operating system is trying to install software updates. Your phone starts to slow down, glitch, and crash. The fasting and circadian eating is closing apps, plugging in, and letting the phone recharge. In the morning, you are not just rested; you are upgraded.

Case example: Elena's reset

Elena is a 39-year-old high school teacher in the Midwest who never thought about any of these things until she was exhausted all the time. She was frequently eating late in the evening with late-night snacking while grading papers until midnight. She gained weight, did not sleep well, and getting up in the morning felt like walking through fog.

We didn't make her change her food immediately - just when she was eating. She adopted the 14/10 eating pattern, where she ate her last meal by 5:30 PM with mostly protein and vegetables. She went to bed without a snack of carbs.

In 2 weeks, she was describing her mornings as "waking with clear energy instead of waking with dread." In two months, she lost 11 pounds, not from restriction but synchronization.

Her comment was: "It's as if my body finally trusts me again."

Principle Two is synchronization. Food is not just fuel - it is a time signal. When you eat is as important as what you eat. And when you fast, you are not starving; you are giving your body time to thrive.

PRINCIPLE THREE: MOVE AS MEDICINE — WALKING, GRIPPING, SQUATTING

Think back to your ancestors. They didn't "work out." They didn't spend 45 minutes on the treadmill or go to HIIT classes. They moved because it was necessary for life—walking to gather food, using tools to build, squatting to poop, make food, or to rest. These movements were not optional—they were survival.

And the truth is, modern science is just starting to recognize that those primal movements—walking, gripping, squatting—were your body's operating instructions for successful weight loss and health.

WALKING: THE ANCIENT ENGINE

Walking is the most human of movements. It's what your body was built to do, and it's shockingly effective as a metabolic reset.

- **Blood Sugar Balance:** A 10–15 minute walk after meals lowers post-meal blood glucose by up to 20–30%. That means less fat storage and steadier energy.

- **NEAT Power:** Walking builds NEAT—*non-exercise activity thermogenesis*—the invisible calorie burn that accounts for far more daily energy expenditure than occasional gym sessions.

- **Stress Reset:** Rhythmic walking lowers cortisol, restoring balance after mental or physical stress.

Visualization: Every step after a meal is like erasing sugar from your bloodstream, sweeping it into muscles where it fuels movement instead of fat storage.

GRIPPING: THE FORGOTTEN SIGNAL OF STRENGTH

Grip strength isn't just about forearms—it's a biomarker of vitality and longevity. Research shows that a stronger grip predicts a lower risk of heart disease, diabetes, and even early mortality.

Why? Because grip strength reflects whole-body strength, nervous system activation, and metabolic resilience.

- **Hormonal Boost:** Lifting, carrying, or hanging builds testosterone and growth hormone—the repair and fat-burning hormones.

- **Core + Posture Reset:** Loaded carries (like carrying groceries or holding weights) activate deep stabilizers, improving balance and metabolic demand.

Visualization: Every time you carry something heavy, your body receives a primal signal: *"I am strong. I am capable. I am alive."* That message flips on fat-burning pathways and reinforces your thriving metabolism.

SQUATTING: RECLAIMING YOUR FOUNDATION

In ancestral life, squatting was rest. Today, it's therapy. Squats reawaken your largest muscle groups—glutes and quads—your metabolic powerhouses.

- **Calorie Furnace:** Large muscles burn more energy, even at rest. Squatting trains these engines to stay switched on.

- **Mobility Reset:** Deep squats restore hip and ankle range of motion, undoing hours of chair sitting.

- **Hormonal Trigger:** Squatting stimulates growth hormone pulses, accelerating fat burn and repair.

Visualization: Every squat is a whisper to your DNA: *"This is what you were built to do."* It reconnects you to your strongest, most resilient self.

THE ANCIENT MOVERS ROUTINE: HOW TO APPLY

DAILY FOUNDATION:

- Walk 20–40 minutes (split into bursts if needed).

- Add "movement snacks"—10 squats every hour, or a 30-second deep squat hold.

- Practice grip: carry something heavy for 50–100 meters, or hang from a towel or bar for 30 seconds.

Strength Sessions (3× weekly):

- Lower-body day: squats, hip hinges, loaded carries.

- Upper-body day: push-ups/rows, grip holds, walking intervals.

- Rotate and progress weekly.

Micro-Habits to Anchor:

- Take stairs with purpose.

- Park farther away.

- Squat instead of slouching while scrolling.

- Carry your shopping without a cart.

- Replace idle sitting with a deep squat hold.

These small actions compound—rewriting your operating system with effortless movement medicine.

Case Example: David's Return

David, a 52-year-old accountant, had tried endless gyms and diets. He hated workouts and always felt he "didn't have time." Instead of adding more, we stripped it back: walk after meals, 10 squats every hour at his desk, carry his grocery bags instead of wheeling them.

In 6 weeks, he lost 12 pounds—not from punishment, but from reclaiming his body's natural movement. His wife noticed he stood taller, looked calmer, and had energy for evening walks together.

His words: "I didn't join a program. I remembered how to move like a human again."

Principle Three is not about exercise—it's about reclaiming ancestral signals. Walking fuels your metabolism, gripping connects strength to resilience, and squatting reawakens your foundation. These are not workouts. They're your birthright.

PRINCIPLE FOUR: THE SLEEP–WEIGHT CONNECTION

Imagine: You've been eating clean all week. You've exercised, you've even pushed through cravings. Then one late night, scrolling on your phone, the hunger hits you like a freight train. Suddenly, the cookies in the cupboard are calling your name. By morning, you wake up bloated, guilty, and rolling around, wondering: why does my willpower go out the window at night?

The answer is that it's not willpower, it's sleep. Or the lack thereof.

Sleep is more than rest; it's a powerful appetite regulator, metabolism, and fat-controlling mechanism. Every night when you fall asleep, you go through cycles of deep and REM sleep. While you're deep asleep, your body is hormonally calibrating itself, repairing tissues, and resetting the fat-burning machinery. If you cut the sleep short, you don't just feel tired, you flip the hormonal switches that make weight loss damn near impossible.

HORMONAL PLAYERS IN THE SLEEP–WEIGHT DANCE

Ghrelin: The Hunger Trigger

Ghrelin is your body's "hunger hormone," secreted mainly in the stomach. It spikes before meals to make you seek food. But here's the twist: when you're sleep-deprived, ghrelin rises dramatically, pushing you toward calorie-dense, sugary foods.

Think: less sleep = louder hunger signals.

LEPTIN: THE SATIETY SIGNAL

Leptin is released by fat cells to tell your brain, *"We have enough energy; stop eating."* But poor sleep slashes leptin levels, muffling the satiety signal. Your brain thinks you're in famine, even if you just ate.

Think: less sleep = muted fullness signals.

CORTISOL: THE FAT-STORING ALARM

When sleep is cut short, cortisol (your stress hormone) rises and stays elevated. High cortisol pushes fat storage, particularly in the belly, while simultaneously breaking down muscle—the exact opposite of what you want for fat loss.

Think: poor sleep = cortisol-driven belly fat.

INSULIN SENSITIVITY: THE SUGAR GATEKEEPER

Insulin helps shuttle glucose into cells. Sleep deprivation reduces insulin sensitivity by up to **30% in just a few days**—a metabolic handicap that makes your body store more fat, especially after late-night snacks.

Think: less sleep = higher blood sugar + fat storage.

THE SCIENCE IN ACTION

- A landmark **University of Chicago study** found that people sleeping 4 hours per night for just 2 nights had **24% higher ghrelin** and **18% lower leptin**. Translation: they felt hungrier and less satisfied after meals.

- Another trial showed that sleeping 5 hours or less per night increased cravings for junk food by **33%**.

- Even one week of restricted sleep impairs insulin function so dramatically that the body resembles a prediabetic state.

VISUALIZATION: YOUR PILLOW AS A FAT-BURNING TOOL

Picture your pillow as the most underutilized piece of gym equipment in your house. Every extra hour of sleep deepens fat burning, restores insulin sensitivity, and balances hunger hormones. Conversely, cutting that hour is like sneaking in an invisible midnight snack—your hormones rebel, and your fat-burning switch flips off.

ACTION CODE: BUILD A SLEEP RITUAL

To harness the sleep–weight connection, create an environment that *programs* your body for hormonal balance:

- **Digital Sunset:** 60–90 minutes before bed, dim screens and switch to warm light.

- **Calming Cue:** Herbal tea, gentle stretch, or journaling.

- **Cool, Dark, Quiet:** Transform your bedroom into a cave—temperature around 65–68°F.

- **Timing Matters:** Aim for a consistent sleep/wake cycle. Your body loves rhythm.

PATIENT VIGNETTE: CLARA'S TURNING POINT

Clara, a 38-year-old nurse, had tried keto, intermittent fasting, boot camps, and somehow, she was still weight-stuck. And she said, "I can only sleep for 5 hours. It's just how I am." We shifted focus to her sleep—setting a digital sunset, wind-down tea, and making sure she preserved 7-8 hours for sleep—and her weight just fell off. No nutritional change, no change in her workouts. Six weeks later, she was down 9 pounds; it wasn't the workouts, it was hormone regulation.

She said, "I realized my body wasn't broken, it was just exhausted."

Principle Four teaches us this: You don't just lose weight in the gym or the kitchen—you lose it in your bedroom. Sleep isn't downtime. It's prime metabolic programming.

PRINCIPLE FIVE: STRESS RESET = FAT LOSS RESET

You've had a grueling day at the office. The email never stopped. The traffic would not relent. When you finally make it home, your body feels like a tightly-wound spring. And then it happens—you find yourself standing at the pantry, hand in the bag of chips, mindlessly crunching before you even realize it.

Does that sound familiar? That's not weakness; that's biology.

An incredible amount of stress is one of the most underestimated contributors to weight gain. You can eat perfectly, train intelligently, and sleep well. But if your stress thermostat is set too high, your fat-loss machinery becomes jammed. And the underlying reason is one powerful hormone: cortisol.

CORTISOL: THE STRESS-FAT STORAGE LINK

Cortisol is your survival hormone and was built to keep you alive in short bursts. When you are in danger, cortisol mobilizes energy, elevates blood sugar, and sharpens your focus. This is helpful if you are running from a predator.

In modern life, the predators are not lions—they're deadlines, bills, traffic, and constant notifications. And unlike an ancient threat, they do not go away in five minutes. They simmer. And in response to chronic stress, cortisol stays chronically elevated.

So, what happens next?

- **Belly Fat Storage:** High cortisol preferentially stores fat around the abdomen, creating the "stress belly."

- **Muscle Breakdown:** Cortisol breaks down muscle tissue to release glucose, lowering metabolism.

- **Cravings:** Elevated cortisol boosts appetite for sugar and fat—fast energy for a body that thinks it's in danger.

- **Insulin Resistance:** Chronic stress reduces insulin sensitivity, keeping blood sugar higher and fat storage active.

In short: Stress doesn't just make you *feel* heavier. It makes you *store* heavier.

THE CORTISOL–CRAVING CONNECTION

Ever notice how stress drives you toward cookies, not carrots? That's cortisol and dopamine working together. Stress spikes cortisol, which signals your brain to seek quick comfort foods. Those foods trigger dopamine, providing momentary relief—then the cycle repeats.

It's not willpower. It's neurochemistry.

SCIENCE SNAPSHOT

- A study from Yale found that women with higher cortisol levels were significantly more likely to have abdominal obesity, independent of calorie intake.

- Researchers at UCSF observed that stress-induced cortisol surges drive a preference for high-fat, high-sugar foods, amplifying weight gain.

- In one trial, mindfulness-based stress reduction reduced binge eating episodes by **63%** over 6 weeks.

VISUALIZATION: YOUR EXHALE AS A FAT-BURNING SWITCH

Close your eyes for a moment. Imagine every exhale as a release valve. With each slow breath out, you're telling your body: *It's safe. You don't need to store fat. You can burn it now.*

This isn't poetic—it's physiological. Slow exhalations activate the **parasympathetic nervous system**, dropping cortisol and resetting your fat-burning potential.

ACTION CODE: STRESS RESET TOOLKIT

Here's how to program your body to flip from *storage mode* to *burn mode*:

1. Breath Reset (2–3× daily)

- Inhale through your nose for four counts.

- Hold for 1–2 counts.

- Exhale slowly for 6–8 counts.
- Repeat for 2–3 minutes.

This simple exercise reduces cortisol within minutes.

2. Micro-Breaks (Every 90 minutes)

Step away from the desk. Stretch. Walk—step outside for fresh air. Even 2–3 minutes reduces stress load and prevents cortisol buildup.

3. Journaling Dump (Nightly)

Before bed, write down the worries looping in your head. Putting them on paper signals closure to the brain, easing nighttime cortisol spikes.

4. Movement Medicine

Gentle movement—walking, yoga, mobility work—lowers cortisol and curbs cravings. High-intensity exercise can also work, but avoid overtraining, which spikes cortisol further.

5. Anchoring Ritual

Pick one "anchor" habit when you feel stress rising. For some, it's a hot shower. For others, a short prayer, meditation, or even music. The goal: create a consistent cue that flips your nervous system back to calm.

PATIENT VIGNETTE: DANIEL'S BREAKTHROUGH

Daniel, a 45-year-old executive, had tried intermittent fasting and HIIT workouts, but his belly fat wouldn't budge. He confessed: "I live on stress. Coffee, meetings, deadlines. I crash at night with ice cream."

Instead of more workouts, we focused on **stress resets.** He began with three breath breaks during his workday, swapped evening news for a 10-minute walk, and added a nightly journal dump.

In 8 weeks, he reported fewer cravings, steady energy, and—without changing his diet—lost 6 pounds of belly fat. His words: "I realized my weight wasn't just about food—it was about stress I never turned off."

Principle Five reveals a truth most diets ignore: If your nervous system is stuck in fight-or-flight, fat loss stalls. To lose weight, you don't just need better food or movement—you need a calmer body.

PRINCIPLE SIX: CONSISTENCY OVER PERFECTION

Envision two people.

One goes to the extreme and follows a strict diet plan: no sugar, no carbs, two-plus hours of exercise every day, green juices, fasting for days. For a bit, the weight comes off...but the lifestyle feels like jail. A single slip—birthday cake, late-night pizza, skipped workout—spirals into guilt. Soon, the "all-in" becomes "all-out," and the cycle resets.

The other makes small adjustments: add protein to breakfast, take a walk after lunch, dim the lights before bed. No crazy diets, and no guilt when life interrupts. Over the weeks, the changes stack. The weight loss starts slowly—but is lasting. Months, even years later, with positive habits, your body is leaner, stronger, and healthier.

Which one succeeds? Every time, it's the second.

Why Perfectionism Doesn't Work.

Perfectionism is fragile! One slip-up shatters it. The first succeeds as well if they can take away the guilt of failure whenever they slip up and understand that consistency is better than perfection.

Biologically, our body runs on rhythms—not extremes. Every time you initiate extreme rules of restriction, your body adjusts—lowering its weight, slowing its metabolism, increasing hunger hormones/cravings. Why? It's survival.

From a psychological viewpoint, perfectionism triggers all-or-nothing thinking: "I blew it—might as well binge." (i.e., "I ruined it; I may as well eat everything"). This is why most diets fail during the initial phase—when they eat something off their diet plan, that spirals into self-sabotage.

WHY CONSISTENCY WORKS

Consistency builds momentum. Repeated small actions are easier for your brain to automate into habits. Once you automate them, they take less willpower to maintain—and willpower is a limited resource.

Think of weight loss not as a sprint but as compounding interest. Every choice—adding protein to meals, walking after dinner, turning off screens at night—is like a deposit. Each one is small. But, week after week, year after year, equals transformation.

SCIENCE SNAPSHOT

- A Stanford study found that people who lost weight steadily (1–2 lbs per week) and consistently were far more likely to maintain it for 2+ years compared to those who lost weight quickly but erratically.

- Research in *Obesity* showed that "weight variability"—yo-yo dieting—was associated with higher long-term weight regain and increased risk of heart disease.

- Behavioral science confirms that sustainable weight loss isn't about the biggest change, but the **stickiest change**—the one you repeat until it becomes part of your identity.

MENTAL REFRAME

Stop asking: "How fast can I lose this weight?"

Start asking: "What can I repeat every day for the rest of my life?"

Every meal, every walk, every breath reset is a vote for your future self. One vote won't win the election. But cast enough, consistently, and you rewrite your identity: I am someone who thrives.

VISUALIZATION: THE BRICK WALL

Picture your health as a wall. Perfection tries to build the whole wall in a day—overwhelming, impossible. Consistency lays one brick, then another. A month later, the wall is strong. A year later, it's unshakable.

ACTION CODE: THE CONSISTENCY COMPASS

1. **Anchor Habits:** Pick three daily anchors (protein-first meal, 10-min post-meal walk, 5-min breath reset). Repeat them no matter what.

2. **Plan for Imperfection:** Build "buffer rules." Missed a workout? Take a 20-minute walk. Late-night snack? Get back on track at the next meal.

3. **Weekly Reflection:** On Sundays, write down: "What worked? What felt easy? What's one small upgrade I can add?"

4. **Identity Check:** Replace "I'm on a diet" with "I'm building my rhythm." Diets end. Rhythms endure.

PATIENT VIGNETTE: LEILA'S FREEDOM

Leila, 37, had spent ten years all over the dieting map. Keto. Juice cleanses. Fasting marathons. Fifteen pounds lost and 20 gained in two short weeks. She said, "I thought discipline was about extremes."

We rewrote the script. No more 30-day challenges. Just a protein breakfast, 20 minutes of walking every day, 14/10 fast, and bed by 10:30 p.m. That was it.

Three months in, she lost 9 pounds—not super impressive, but consistent. Fast forward a year, and she lost 27 pounds and had more energy than in years. She said, "For the first time, I'm not worried about gaining weight back. I'm not on a diet. I'm just living."

Principle Six seals the Thriving Weight Loss code: The secret isn't doing everything perfectly—it's doing the right things consistently. Progress compounds. Momentum multiplies—and identity anchors it all.

PROGRAMMING INTEGRATION: THE THRIVING WEIGHT LOSS BLUEPRINT

At this point, you've observed these principles separately. Protein and fiber to reprogram metabolism. Timing meals with the circadian rhythms. Moving like our ancestors. Sleeping as if your pillow were a fat-burning tool. Resetting stress. And - maybe most importantly - choosing consistency over perfection.

But the reality is: your body doesn't live in silos. It's not "nutrition" on Monday, "movement" on Tuesday, "sleep" on Wednesday. It's one global system—always listening, always adapting.

For it to work optimally, you must program it as a whole.

THE NEW OPERATING SYSTEM

Instead of thinking "I'm on a diet," imagine you're installing new software. Each principle is a module. Together, they create a seamless, self-reinforcing loop:

- **Eat to Signal Safety:** Protein and fiber send satiety messages to your brain, calm insulin spikes, and reprogram your metabolism.

- **Time to Signal Rhythm:** Aligning food with light-dark cycles tells your hormones: *this body runs on nature's clock, not chaos.*

- **Move to Signal Vitality:** Every step, squat, and carry whispers to your muscles: *stay strong, stay ready, stay lean.*

446

- **Sleep to Signal Repair:** Deep rest turns off hunger hormones, lowers cortisol, and switches on fat-burning recovery.

- **Breathe to Signal Calm:** Stress resets remind your body: *you're safe. You can burn fat instead of storing it.*

- **Repeat to Signal Identity:** Consistency programs your nervous system: *this is who I am now.*

Each input reinforces the others. Protein stabilizes blood sugar, making it easier to fast. Walking after meals enhances insulin sensitivity, setting up better sleep. Sleep lowers cortisol, which reduces cravings. Lower cravings make it easier to stick with protein-first meals. On and on, the loop strengthens.

MENTAL PROGRAMMING STATEMENTS

This is where weight loss shifts from *effort* to *identity*.

Here are the mantras—the "code" lines—you must install:

- "I hydrate and move first thing."

- "I anchor meals with protein and fiber."

- "I honor time—I eat earlier, lighter, smarter."

- "I move after meals as medicine."

- "I sleep like it's sacred."

- "I manage stress with breath and rhythm."

- "I thrive on consistency, not perfection."

Repeat them daily. Write them on sticky notes. Put them on your phone wallpaper. Each repetition is neural programming. Over time, your brain doesn't just believe them—it becomes them.

CASE EXAMPLE: THE OPERATING SYSTEM IN ACTION

Michael, 49, had tried everything—low-carb, intermittent fasting, two-a-day workouts. He'd lose weight, then rebound. When we reframed his plan as **installing a Thriving Operating System**, everything shifted.

His daily rhythm became simple:

- **Morning:** Hydrate + 15-min walk in the sun.

- **Meals:** Protein first, vegetables second, starch optional.

- **Timing:** 14/10 fast, often skipping dinner or keeping it light.

- **Movement:** 10-minute walk after lunch and dinner, grip holds 3×/week.

- **Evening:** Phone off at 9:30 p.m., asleep by 10:30.

- **Stress:** 5 breaths before each meal, 10-minute journaling at night.

Six months later, he was down 35 pounds. But more importantly, he said:

"I don't feel like I'm fighting anymore. My body is working with me."

That's the code working.

The Thriving Weight Loss Blueprint in One Sentence

Every day, give your body consistent signals of safety, rhythm, vitality, repair, and calm—and it will release the weight as a side effect of thriving.

VISUALIZATION EXERCISE: SEE YOUR FUTURE SELF

Close your eyes. Picture yourself six months from now. You wake up lighter—not just on the scale, but in spirit. You slip into clothes that once felt tight. You eat without guilt because you know the rhythm. You move with energy because your body craves it. You rest deeply because your nervous system trusts the signals.

That person isn't far away. That person is you—running on a new operating system.

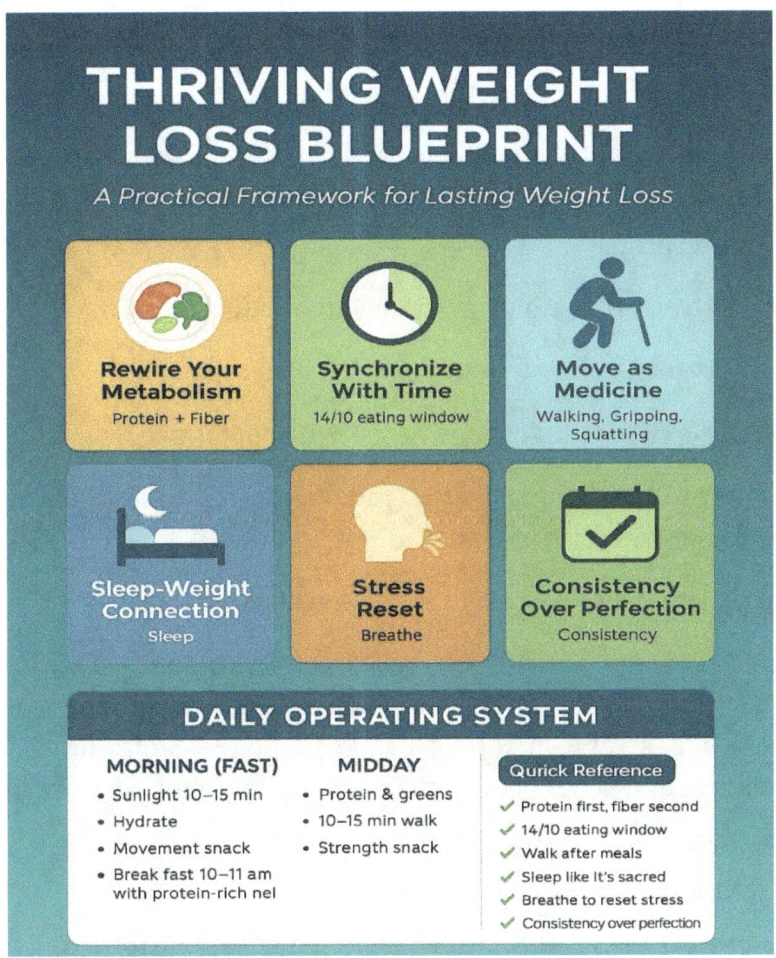

Imagine this:

It's early morning. Sunlight spills into your room. You wake up before the alarm—not groggy, not heavy, but light. Your stomach feels calm, not ravenous. You stretch, take a deep breath, and realize there's energy in reserve. Your body is working *with* you, not against you.

The scale doesn't need to tell you—you can feel it. Your clothes glide more easily, your face looks fresher, and your thoughts are sharper. Yesterday you ate with rhythm and intention, not guilt. You walked after dinner, slept deeply, and your body burned fat as you dreamed.

This is the shift:

- Hunger is no longer a screaming voice—it's a signal you can interpret.

- Movement is no longer punishment—it's medicine.

- Fasting is no longer deprivation—it's repair.

- Sleep is no longer "downtime"—it's metabolic magic.

- Stress no longer hijacks your body—it's a rhythm you can reset with every breath.

This is your thriving weight loss operating system.

And here's the secret: you are *already running it*. Every small action—protein first, walk after meals, lights dimmed at night, a deep exhale when stress spikes—is a line of code—each line of code programs your biology. And with consistency, your body rewrites its entire script.

Reframe to lock in:

"This is not a diet. This is not a restriction. This is my blueprint for thriving. I'm no longer chasing weight loss—I am programming health. I am programming energy. I am programming freedom."

Close your eyes for a moment.

Visualize yourself three months from now—lighter, stronger, calmer, not just in body weight, but in the *weight of stress, cravings, fatigue.* Imagine moving through your day with energy to spare, clothes that fit with ease, and a quiet confidence that you can trust your body again.

Now imagine a year from now—people ask you what your "secret" is, and you smile, knowing it wasn't a hack, or a fad, or a war with your body. It was alignment. Rhythm. A new code is installed, one ritual at a time.

Because here's the truth:

🔑 Your body has never been your enemy.

🧠 It was waiting for the right instructions.

💡 And now, you have them.

This is the moment you step forward—not with force, but with flow. Not with restriction, but with rhythm. Not with fear, but with freedom.

Your thriving weight loss blucprint is not something you're starting tomorrow. It's alive inside you **now**. With every choice today, you're no longer "trying to lose weight." You are *becoming the person who thrives.*

And that identity—that blueprint—lasts a lifetime.

BRIDGE INTO LONGEVITY:

Weight loss isn't the endgame. It's the beginning. When your body is lightened, aligned, and thriving, you've unlocked the door to something even bigger: longevity. Because a thriving metabolism isn't just about dropping pounds—it's about living younger, longer.

And that's where we're headed next:

The Longevity Blueprint—where we weave together food, fasting, sleep, stress, movement, community, and purpose into one life-long operating system.

CHAPTER 16:

THE LONGEVITY BLUEPRINT —
LIVING YOUNGER, LONGER

PART 1: IMAGINE YOURSELF AT 90, THRIVING

Picture this.

You find yourself sitting at a wooden table, sunlight streaming in from an open window. It's a later morning in the early spring. Outside, you hear children laughing as they chase one another in the garden. The delightful aroma of herbs and slow-cooking beans beckons from the kitchen. And at 90, you are not sitting idly, fading into a distant picture of life. You are leaning forward, engrossed in telling a story, hand gestures accentuate your words, and your voice is bright and steady.

Your body moves with ease as you stand up from the chair. You walk barefoot outside on the soft grass, joints loose, spine straight. You stop to attend to a line of tomatoes planted last season. Kneeling doesn't hurt. Your breath is deep and easy, your mind is still sharp, and when your granddaughter invites you to play, you jog across the lawn, bursting with laughter together.

This is not an imagined life. This is what thriving at 90 can look like.

We've all been sold a different picture of aging: weakness, decline, pills piled high on a nightstand, endless doctor appointments, days of silence or discomfort. The society's story of aging is diminishing. But biology, and the lives of the longest-lived humans on Earth, tell a different story.

THE LONGEVITY GAP

The reality is, there are two ages running inside each of us.

Your chronological age—which is the number of birthdays you have celebrated. And your biological age—the actual health condition of your cells, your mitochondria, your brain, your resilient systems.

Here's the radical insight: those two ages don't have to be equal. A 50-year-old can have the biology of someone decades younger—or older, depending on the way they live.

Science has proven that biological age is malleable. Telomeres (the protective caps on your DNA) can lengthen with lifestyle change. Mitochondria (your energy factories) can multiply with movement. Epigenetic "switches" that determine whether genes for disease stay on or off are influenced by food, fasting, stress, sleep, and purpose. In other words, you have more control over your aging trajectory than any previous generation in human history.

THE FALSE FINISH LINE

Many people treat middle age as the beginning of decline: "Well, I'm in my 40s now, and I guess this is where the aches start. And the body's check engine light starts showing"

That assumption is not biology—it's conditioning. Look at the Blue Zones—where people regularly live over 100 years. At these Blue Zones, 90 is not an end stage—it's another juicier chapter. The people sing, garden, walk up hills, laugh with friends, cook with whole foods, and offer sage advice and pass on wisdom around the dinner table. Aging does not mean fading; it is ripening.

A RADICAL REFRAME

Aging is not the enemy. Accelerated aging is

And accelerated aging is not inevitable. It's a byproduct of mismatched living: too much processed food and too little movement, too much stress, sleep disrupted, chronic disconnection, loss of purpose.

Your body was not designed to fail at 60. Your body was designed to repair and adapt and renew until your last breath—if you give it the right signals.

THE PROMISE OF THE LONGEVITY BLUEPRINT

This chapter is about giving you those signals—woven into a Longevity Blueprint that just doesn't add years to your life, but also adds life to your years. We will revisit all the pillars we have been exploring throughout this text: food, fasting, movement, stress, recovery, sleep, joy, and purpose. And we will discuss how all these weave together to become one prescription for living younger, longer.

We are also going to get a peek at the frontier of longevity science:

Telomeres and what shortens (or lengthens) them.

Mitochondria, and how to keep them abundant and efficient.

Epigenetics and how your daily habits flip genetic switches toward healing, not decay.

And we are going to hear from the many voices of those who have walked this path: centenarians who model vitality, cultures who have lived in rhythm to longevity, patients who reversed their "inevitable decline" with daily practices.

By the time you get to the end of this chapter, you will have a blueprint—not a rigid plan, but a doable and empowering framework—to start reversing your aging. To not only imagine yourself at 90 thriving, but to walk steadily toward it with confidence.

Because truly: you already have the machinery of longevity within you. This chapter is about figuring out how to turn it on.

454

PART 2 — THE PILLARS REVISITED: WEAVING THE LONGEVITY BLUEPRINT

Think of your body as an ancient cathedral. Every stone and arch is linked. If a column has a crack, it can ripple through the whole structure, and the entire structure is affected. Longevity is not based on a miracle diet or a game-changing supplement; it is built on a foundation where every pillar carries weight.

We've walked through these pillars throughout this book: food, fasting, movement, stress, recovery, sleep, joy, and purpose. Here, we will gather them together, not as separate pillars, but as a single architecture of resilience. This is the Longevity Blueprint: eight pillars aligned to slow biological aging, restore vitality, and enhance health span.

PILLAR 1: FOOD AS INFORMATION

Food is not just fuel—it is a messenger. Every bite you take whispers into your DNA, flipping switches toward inflammation or repair.

- **Science lens:** Nutrigenomics shows that whole foods activate protective genes (like those linked to detoxification and DNA repair) while ultra-processed foods amplify oxidative stress. Mediterranean-style diets rich in polyphenols, fibers, and omega-3 fats have been linked to longer telomeres and lower rates of chronic disease.

- **Longevity story:** In Sardinia, shepherds eat simple meals of beans, sourdough bread, goat's milk, and herbs—food so modest it would be overlooked by the modern wellness industry. Yet it fuels some of the highest male centenarian rates on Earth.

- **Longevity action:** Every plate is a vote for or against your future. Prioritize foods that reduce inflammation (leafy greens, legumes, olive oil, fatty fish) and expand microbial diversity (fermented foods, fibers).

PILLAR 2: FASTING AS RENEWAL

Fasting is not deprivation—it's restoration. It is the *biological pause button* that turns on repair pathways modern constant eating has silenced.

- **Science lens:** Autophagy (cellular cleanup) ramps up in fasting windows.

- Insulin sensitivity resets.

- Stem cells activate during longer fasts, rejuvenating tissues.

- **Longevity story:** In Okinawa, long nightly fasts (often 14–16 hours) are woven into the rhythm of life. Meals are lighter at night, heavier earlier—aligned with circadian biology. Their phrase *hara hachi bu* ("eat until 80% full") is fasting-in-disguise, protecting them from metabolic overload.

- **Longevity action:** Begin with a 12:12 rhythm. Expand gradually. Match fasting windows with gender and hormonal context (as we'll explore later). The goal is not endurance but renewal.

PILLAR 3: MOVEMENT AS SIGNAL

Your muscles are not just for locomotion—they are endocrine factories. Every contraction sends biochemical "youth signals" across the body.

- **Science lens:** Myokines (molecules released during muscle contraction) reduce inflammation and protect the brain.

- Resistance training preserves muscle mass, one of the strongest predictors of longevity.

- Aerobic activity boosts mitochondrial density and oxygen efficiency.

456

- **Longevity story:** In Ikaria, Greece, elders climb hills daily, garden, and walk long distances—not as exercise routines, but as a lifestyle. They rarely "work out" in gyms, yet they embody strength and stamina into their 90s.

- **Longevity action:** Think "movement snacks" instead of workouts. Walk after meals. Lift heavy things (your own body counts). Dance, stretch, play.

PILLAR 4: STRESS AS A DOUBLE-EDGED SWORD

Stress can corrode—but it can also carve resilience. The key is learning to master its rhythm.

- **Science lens:** Chronic stress shortens telomeres, accelerates inflammation, and disrupts microbiomes. But hormetic stress (short, controlled bursts like exercise, cold plunges, or fasting) builds resilience, strengthening repair pathways.

- **Longevity story:** In Nicoya, Costa Rica, daily life includes physical work, but is balanced by faith, family, and joy. Stress exists—but it is buffered by belonging and perspective.

- **Longevity action:** Rewire stress with parasympathetic activators: breath, mindfulness, social connection. Embrace hormetic stress, release toxic chronic stress.

PILLAR 5: RECOVERY AS THE HIDDEN AMPLIFIER

Longevity is not earned in effort, but in the *space between efforts.*

- **Science lens:** Heart Rate Variability (HRV) is a biomarker of recovery. Athletes with higher HRV live longer, heal faster, and resist illness. Recovery strengthens adaptation.

- **Longevity story:** Even in high-activity cultures, rest is sacred. Midday naps (Ikaria), tea rituals (Okinawa), or community pauses are non-negotiable.

- **Longevity action:** Schedule recovery like work. Ritualize pauses: a 10-minute afternoon walk, weekly sauna, seasonal retreats.

PILLAR 6: SLEEP AS LONGEVITY'S PHARMACY

Every night, the body runs its upgrade program—if you let it.

- **Science lens:** Deep sleep pulses growth hormone, repairing tissues.

- REM sleep enhances memory and emotional regulation.

- Glymphatic clearance washes toxins from the brain, reducing dementia risk.

- **Longevity story:** In Loma Linda, Adventists prioritize restful evenings—light dinners, family time, and early sleep. Their circadian alignment protects them from the metabolic chaos of late-night living.

- **Longevity action:** Treat sleep as medicine. Create cave-like darkness. Honor consistent rhythms. Evening rituals matter as much as the morning alarm.

PILLAR 7: JOY AS A PHYSIOLOGICAL FORCE

Joy is not just an emotion—it is biology.

- **Science lens:** Positive emotions release oxytocin and dopamine, lower cortisol, and boost immune resilience. Studies show joy and gratitude directly extend lifespan through reduced cardiovascular risk.

- **Longevity story:** In every Blue Zone, joy is baked into daily life: laughter, festivals, shared meals. Joy isn't a hobby—it's survival.

- **Longevity action:** Make joy non-negotiable. Savor meals without guilt. Celebrate micro-moments. Play often.

PILLAR 8: PURPOSE AS THE COMPASS

If joy is fuel, purpose is direction. Without it, the other pillars wobble.

- **Science lens:** Harvard studies: adults with a strong sense of purpose have a lower risk of heart disease and dementia.

- Ikigai research in Okinawa: knowing "why you wake up in the morning" predicts both resilience and longevity.

- **Longevity story:** Elders who carry purpose into their 90s—teaching, cooking, mentoring—live longer and healthier.

- **Longevity action:** Clarify your "why." It doesn't have to be grand. It can be in micro-moments—teaching your child, serving your community, creating beauty.

THE PILLARS IN HARMONY

Longevity is not built by any single pillar, but by its synergy. Food without recovery fails. Movement without sleep collapses. Fasting without joy becomes punishment. Purpose without community loses strength.

When these pillars align, they **slow biological aging at its root**. They extend healthspan—not just years of life, but life in those years.

This is not theory—it is happening, right now, in villages of Okinawa, Sardinia, Nicoya, Ikaria, and Loma Linda. And it can happen in your body, too, no matter where you live.

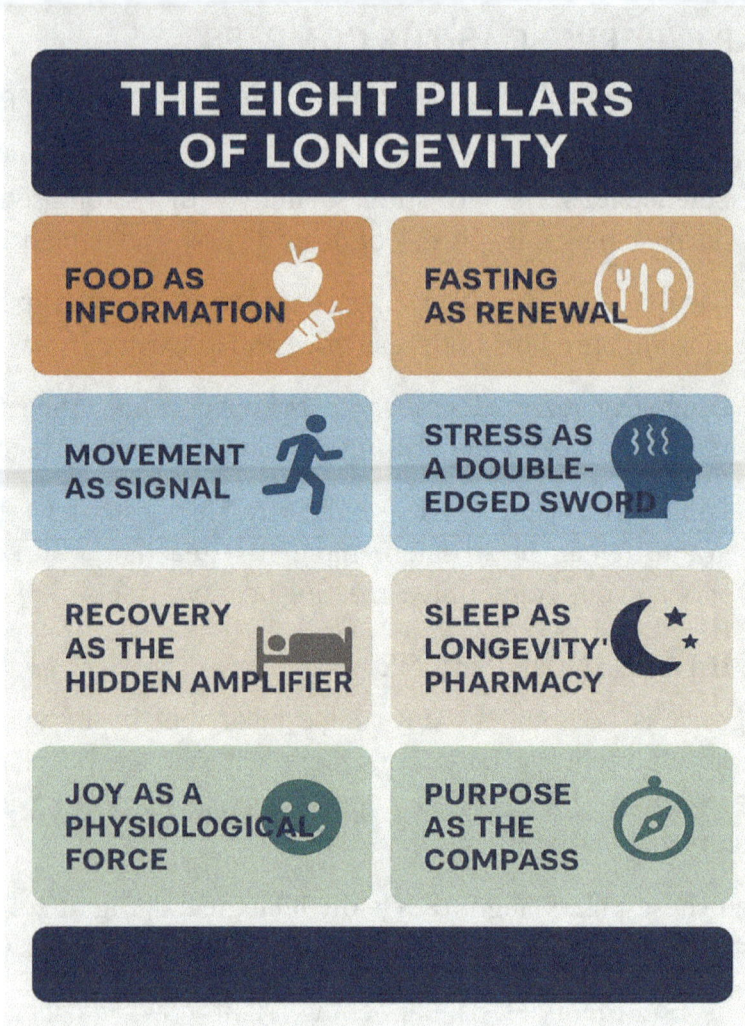

THE EIGHT PILLARS OF LONGEVITY

FOOD AS INFORMATION

FASTING AS RENEWAL

MOVEMENT AS SIGNAL

STRESS AS A DOUBLE-EDGED SWORD

RECOVERY AS THE HIDDEN AMPLIFIER

SLEEP AS LONGEVITY' PHARMACY

JOY AS A PHYSIOLOGICAL FORCE

PURPOSE AS THE COMPASS

PART 3 — THE BIOLOGY OF AGING: TELOMERES, MITOCHONDRIA, EPIGENETICS

THE CLOCK WITHIN

You can't sense them ticking inside your cells, but inside your cells are clocks that are more accurate than any Rolex, and more unforgiving than any calendar. These biological timekeepers do more than track the passing of years; they record life's wear and tear: the stresses you bear, the food you digest, the nights sleep you lose, the love you experience, the purpose you wake up to. Aging isn't just the passage of time; aging is biology unfolding. Each second of each day, trillions of your cells are replicating, repairing, or considering if they need to age out. Your ability to have a healthy, long life or decline depends on those cellular decisions.

Science now reveals: aging is not just a passive process of deterioration. It is an active dance of molecular switches, energy sparks, and repair mechanisms that can be influenced—slowed, even reversed. And the most astonishing part? The keys are already in your hands.

Let's dive a little deeper into the aging machinery of your body. Three pillars of aging will determine whether your future can be frail or resilient: **telomeres, mitochondria, and epigenetics.**

1. TELOMERES — THE FUSES OF LIFE

WHAT THEY ARE

Telomeres are DNA "caps" at the ends of chromosomes, repeating sequences of **TTAGGG** like protective shoelace tips. Each time a cell divides, telomeres shorten. When they become critically short, the cell enters senescence—still alive, but dysfunctional—or dies altogether.

This shortening is the cellular equivalent of a fuse burning down.

WHY THEY MATTER

- **Short telomeres = higher disease risk.** Studies link them to heart disease, Alzheimer's, diabetes, and early death.

- **Longer telomeres = youth preserved.** Children inherit longer telomeres; some populations with exceptional longevity maintain them decades longer than average.

HORMONAL CROSS-TALK

- **Cortisol (stress hormone):** Chronic stress accelerates telomere shortening by increasing oxidative stress.

- **Estrogen:** Protects telomeres—one reason women often outlive men.

- **Growth hormone + IGF-1:** In youth, they preserve telomeres. Excess in later life, however, may drive cancer risk.

NARRATIVE VIGNETTE: JAMES, THE LAWYER

James, 52, was burning at both ends—late nights at the office, fast food between meetings, constant deadlines. His telomere test revealed a biological age **10 years older** than his birth certificate.

But when James changed:

- Added meditation for 10 minutes a day.

- Ate plants instead of drive-thru.

- Walked at sunrise daily.

Two years later, his telomeres stabilized. His biological clock slowed. His doctor told him, "*You've added years back to your life. You bought time.*"

KEY MECHANISMS

- **Oxidative stress** damages telomeres.

- **Telomerase enzyme** can rebuild them (activated by meditation, exercise, and a whole-food diet).

- **Lifestyle intervention:** In a 5-year study by Dean Ornish, men who adopted plant-rich diets, stress management, and movement **lengthened telomeres**—a first in history.

2. MITOCHONDRIA — THE ENGINES OF LIFE

WHAT THEY ARE

Mitochondria are the tiny power plants inside each cell. They generate **ATP**, the currency of energy, through oxidative phosphorylation. Without them, life stops.

But mitochondria age. They leak electrons, producing free radicals that damage DNA and proteins. They grow sluggish. Muscles weaken, energy wanes, and diseases emerge.

THE CRISIS OF MIDLIFE

By age 40–50, mitochondrial efficiency can decline by 50%. That afternoon fatigue, that slower recovery after exercise? It's mitochondrial whispering: *"I'm tired too."*

THE HOPE

- **Mitophagy:** Damaged mitochondria are dismantled and recycled.

- **Mitochondrial biogenesis:** New, young mitochondria grow. Both are triggered by stressors like **exercise, fasting, heat, cold, and plant compounds.**

HORMONAL CROSS-TALK

- **Thyroid hormones:** Directly control mitochondrial energy output.

- **Cortisol:** Chronic stress suppresses mitochondrial efficiency.

- **Estrogen & testosterone:** Preserve mitochondrial function; their decline with age accelerates fatigue.

NARRATIVE VIGNETTE: ELISE, THE MARATHONER

Elise was 68 and still ran half-marathons. When tested, her mitochondrial density resembled that of someone in their 40s. The secret wasn't supplements—it was stress, applied wisely: interval runs, cold swims, and a plant-forward diet. Her mitochondria were constantly nudged to repair and regrow.

KEY MECHANISMS

- **Exercise:** HIIT stimulates mitochondrial biogenesis via **PGC-1α** activation.

- **Fasting:** Activates AMPK and sirtuins, signaling mitochondria to clean house.

- **Nutrients:** CoQ10, NAD+ boosters, resveratrol, and polyphenols feed mitochondrial enzymes.

THE FREE RADICAL PARADOX

Free radicals damage—but they also signal repair. Tiny bursts during exercise or sauna **activate hormesis**, strengthening resilience. It's not zero free radicals you want; it's balance.

3. EPIGENETICS — THE SOFTWARE OF LIFE

WHAT IT IS

Your DNA is fixed. But which genes get expressed—or silenced—depends on epigenetics: chemical tags on DNA (like **methylation**) and proteins (histones).

Think of DNA as the piano. Epigenetics is the pianist deciding which keys to play.

WHY IT MATTERS

- **Epigenetic clocks** (Horvath, Hannum) can measure biological age more precisely than a birthday.

- **Lifestyle inputs**—diet, exercise, stress, toxins—shift your clock forward or back.

HORMONAL CROSS-TALK

- **Insulin:** High spikes accelerate aging genes.
- **Cortisol:** Chronic elevation leaves epigenetic scars.
- **Melatonin:** Nightly pulses protect DNA expression.

NARRATIVE VIGNETTE: MARIA, THE TEACHER

Maria, now in her 40s, joined a pilot study on "epigenetic diets." She ate cruciferous vegetables, flaxseeds, berries, and herbs daily. She also practiced stress reduction. In just **8 weeks**, her biological age dropped **3 years.**

Her reflection: "*I didn't change my DNA. I changed the way my DNA talks to my body.*"

MECHANISMS OF CONTROL

- **DNA methylation:** Can silence tumor suppressor genes or, when reversed, protect against cancer.
- **Histone modification:** Determines how tightly DNA is wound—more open = more active.
- **Sirtuins:** Longevity genes activated by fasting, polyphenols, and exercise.

THE TRINITY OF LONGEVITY: INTEGRATION

These three systems—telomeres, mitochondria, and epigenetics—do not work in isolation. They are woven in a dynamic web.

- **Telomeres** shorten faster under oxidative stress from weak mitochondria.
- **Mitochondria** respond to epigenetic switches, deciding whether to produce clean energy or dirty sparks.

- **Epigenetics** is shaped by telomere health and mitochondrial output.

And all three are profoundly influenced by **how you live each day.**

EXPANDED CASE STUDY: THE OVERWORKED ENTREPRENEUR

Mark, 47, built his tech startup on 5 hours of sleep, caffeine by the gallon, and late-night stress. His biological age came back 10 years older.

- **Telomeres:** Shortened.

- **Mitochondria:** Sluggish; VO2 max 30% below peers.

- **Epigenetic clock:** Accelerated.

After six months of **circadian-aligned eating (16:8 fasting), 30-minute walks, stress training, and a sleep reset**, his telomeres stabilized, his mitochondria tests improved, and his biological age dropped by 4 years.

The lesson: biology bends to behavior.

BRINGING IT HOME

Aging is not an inevitable march downward. It is a negotiation between damage and repair, stress and recovery, breakdown and renewal.

- Telomeres are fuses you can protect.

- Mitochondria are engines you can tune.

- Epigenetics is software you can rewrite.

Every breath, bite, thought, and night of sleep is sending instructions to these systems. The question isn't whether you age—it's how.

Science illuminates the inner mechanisms. But how do these mechanisms translate into real life, lived in villages where centenarians thrive past 100? The answer lies in **Blue Zones**, where lifestyle—not genetics alone—keeps telomeres long, mitochondria humming, and epigenetics youthful.

In the next part, we'll travel to Sardinia, Okinawa, Nicoya, and beyond, to see how culture and daily rhythm embody the very science we've explored.

THE TRINITY OF LONGEVITY

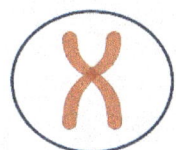 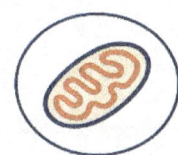 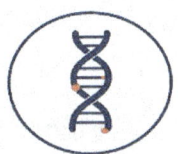

TELOMERES	MITOCHONDRIA	EPIGENETICS
DNA 'caps' at the ends of chromosomes	Cellular power plants	Chemical tags on DNA and histones

PART 4 — LONGEVITY LESSONS FROM CENTENARIANS

Picture an Italian village in Sardinia at dawn. The quiet cobblestone streets, but laughter from the vineyards on the hills, long before the sun is up. A crew of men in their 80s and 90s walks uphill to tend to their vines. They move slowly and steadily, and talk lightly, joking at times. Giovanni, 93, has a basket of figs in one hand. He holds it tightly and won't let his eyes wander. He was asked what the secret to longevity was. He shrugs. "Pane, vino, famiglia, lavoro." Bread, wine, family, work.

On the other side of the world, in Okinawa, Japan, Misao wakes at dawn. She's 101. No pills. No doctor appointments. She waters her small garden, bends to pick herbs, and then joins her moai—a lifelong circle of friends who meet to drink tea, sing, and check in on one another. She is radiant, not in spite of her age but because of it. Her "ikigai"—a sense of purpose that guides daily life—keeps her anchored.

Across the globe, in Nicoya, Costa Rica, centenarians like Don José walk down dirt roads to visit friends or neighbors. They eat beans, corn tortillas, and fresh tropical fruits, they laugh and tell a lot of jokes, and have long naps in a hammock on the hottest afternoons. The secret? Simplicity and community togetherness.

In Loma Linda, California, the only Blue Zone in the USA, Seventh Day Adventists live about 10 years longer than their local neighbors. Their longevity is largely due to Sabbath rest, eating a plant-based diet, communal meals, and a strong communal bond.

These aren't random outliers. These are patterns - a rhythmic predictability of living that shields them from stress, nurtures resilience, and keeps their bodies biologically younger longer.

LESSON 1: FOOD IS CULTURE, NOT JUST CALORIES

Centenarians don't diet in the modern sense. They don't count macros, weigh food, or debate the latest fad. Instead, their meals are deeply woven into culture and identity.

- **Sardinia**: Pecorino cheese rich in omega-3s, sourdough bread, Cannonau wine (high in polyphenols).

- **Okinawa**: Sweet potatoes, tofu, turmeric, seaweed—nutrient-dense, low-calorie, high in antioxidants.

- **Nicoya**: "Three sisters" diet—beans, corn, squash—protein-balanced, fiber-rich, anti-inflammatory.

- **Loma Linda**: Plant-based staples—nuts, legumes, whole grains—combined with religious fasting rhythms.

Science anchor: These patterns consistently lower insulin, dampen inflammation, and support microbiome diversity. Diet is not restriction—it's **identity reinforcement**.

LESSON 2: MOVEMENT IS WOVEN INTO THE DAY

You won't find centenarians in gyms. Their exercise isn't a "session" but an inseparable part of life.

- Sardinians climb hills daily.

- Okinawans garden, squat, and sit on the floor—keeping mobility intact.

- Nicoyans walk everywhere.

- Adventists hike and cycle regularly with their communities.

Science anchor: This movement pattern maintains mitochondrial density, supports joint mobility, and keeps VO_2 max (a predictor of lifespan) surprisingly high into advanced age.

Narrative vignette: Maria, one of our patient vignettes from earlier chapters, adopted this principle. Instead of committing to unrealistic gym regimens, she began walking after meals, gardening, and carrying groceries herself. Within a year, her fasting glucose dropped, her sleep improved, and she rediscovered joy in movement.

LESSON 3: STRESS IS MANAGED BY RHYTHM, NOT ESCAPE

Centenarians do experience stress—they lose loved ones, endure hardships, and face uncertainty. But their lives are punctuated with built-in recovery rhythms.

- **Sardinia:** Afternoon rest and family meals.

- **Okinawa:** Moai—social groups providing lifelong financial and emotional support.

- **Loma Linda:** Sabbath rest—24 hours of digital and work detox weekly.

- **Nicoya:** Afternoon hammocks, daily prayer.

Science anchor: These patterns keep cortisol pulses healthy instead of chronic. Research shows even short daily pauses shift nervous system balance toward parasympathetic tone, protecting heart and immune function.

LESSON 4: BELONGING EXTENDS LIFESPAN

Loneliness shortens life expectancy as much as smoking 15 cigarettes a day. Centenarians are buffered by the community.

- They live in multi-generational homes.

- They know their neighbors by name.

- They share rituals—meals, dances, prayers.

Vignette: A 94-year-old Okinawan woman was asked what happens if someone falls ill in her *moai*. She laughed gently: *"We all take care of her. No one is ever left alone."*

Science anchor: Social bonds trigger oxytocin, endorphins, and vagal tone. These biochemicals protect against inflammation, support immune resilience, and improve pain tolerance.

LESSON 5: PURPOSE IS THE COMPASS

Every centenarian interviewed in Blue Zones could answer the question: *"Why do you wake up in the morning?"*

- **Sardinian shepherds:** to tend their flocks.

- **Okinawan grandmothers:** to care for their grandchildren.

- **Nicoyans:** to share wisdom with younger generations.

- **Adventists:** to serve their faith and community.

Science anchor: Studies show that adults with a strong sense of life purpose have a 23–25% reduced risk of early death. Purpose buffers stress, stabilizes dopamine pathways, and enhances resilience networks in the brain.

PULLING IT TOGETHER: THE CENTENARIAN CODE

- Eat real, minimally processed, culturally rooted food.

- Move naturally, often, and socially.

- Rest with rhythm, not guilt.

- Anchor into community and belonging.

- Live with purpose, daily and lifelong.

These are not superhuman hacks. They are ancient rhythms. Centenarians don't extend their years by willpower—they extend them by **alignment** with biology, culture, and connection.

(THE DAILY LONGEVITY PRESCRIPTION):

We've seen what longevity looks like in action, embodied by centenarians around the world. Now, the question becomes: *How do you translate their wisdom into your daily life, in the context of modern work, stress, and technology?* The next section distills these patterns into a prescription you can begin tomorrow morning.

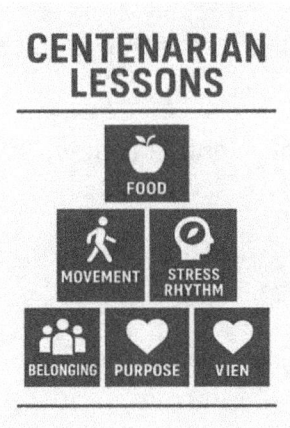

PART 5 — THE DAILY LONGEVITY PRESCRIPTION

Envision this: it's the year 2080. You're not just alive, you're thriving. You wake up with clarity, walk with power, laugh with others, digest food with ease, and sleep deeply through the night. You are not defying age; you are living in tune with the code your body has been following since the beginning of humanity.

That future doesn't take place through fancy supplements or robotic gene edits. It starts with a single day, one rhythm repeated, one prescription lived. Longevity is not a marathon into old age. Longevity is the compound interest of your daily decisions.

The Daily Longevity Prescription represents your one-day blueprint for a health span. It is not based on hacks or magic pills. It is based on the eternal physiology of fasting, movement, recovery, connection, and rest. The 14/10 fasting window sits at the center of this rhythm: long enough to stimulate cellular repair and metabolic flexibility, and short enough to be sustainable every day.

This is your Daily Longevity Prescription:

1. MORNING: ALIGN + DELAY

Wake in rhythm, not in a rush.

- **Sunlight for the first 30 minutes**: synchronizes circadian clocks in the brain, gut, and liver.

- **Hydration ritual**: water with a pinch of minerals (no calories yet).

- **Movement snack**: mobility flow, 10–15 minutes walk, or breathwork.

- **Fasting window continues**: hold off on breakfast until mid-morning.

Science anchor: Fasting into the morning allows insulin to remain low, nudging cells into fat-burning and repair pathways. Studies show circadian fasting improves mitochondrial efficiency and lowers inflammation markers.

2. MIDDAY: BREAK THE FAST INTENTIONALLY (FIRST MEAL)

Your eating window begins — 10 hours only.

- **Start time:** For most, 10 am–12 pm (depending on waking schedule).

- **First meal:** Protein-forward (20–30g) with colorful plants and healthy fats. Think eggs + greens + olive oil, or a lentil bowl with avocado.

- **Move after eating:** A 10-minute walk lowers post-meal glucose and improves insulin sensitivity.

Science anchor: A 14/10 fast maintains glycogen balance while preserving lean muscle. Early eating windows support circadian biology: metabolism is more efficient earlier in the day.

3. AFTERNOON: GROWTH + FLEXIBILITY ZONE

Use this window for movement and micro-stresses.

- **Strength snack:** Bodyweight squats, resistance bands, or a short lift session. Muscle tissue is most insulin-sensitive post-meal.

- **Nature micro-dose:** Sunlight + greenery = cortisol reduction + nitric oxide boost.

- **Balanced fueling:** Continue with whole-food meals/snacks — last one no later than 7–8 pm.

Science anchor: Muscles act as glucose sponges, protecting against insulin resistance — a key aging accelerator. Afternoon training, followed by protein intake, maximizes recovery hormones.

4. EVENING: CLOSE THE WINDOW + CONNECT

The fasting clock resets here.

- **Finish last meal**: within 10-hour eating window (e.g., 7 pm if first meal was 9 am). Light, plant-rich dinner — avoid heavy carbs/alcohol late.

- **Digital sunset**: dim lights, devices off at least 1 hr pre-bed.

- **Connection ritual**: Shared meal, laughter, phone call — oxytocin and endorphins buffer stress load.

- **Wind-down**: Journaling, gratitude, or breathwork.

Science anchor: Ending food intake 3+ hours before sleep improves sleep quality, lowers nighttime glucose, and enhances overnight autophagy — the cellular "clean-up" that protects against neurodegeneration.

5. NIGHT: DEEP REPAIR MODE

Your fast deepens. Repair accelerates.

- **Fasting state (7 pm–9 am example):** Hormones shift. Insulin stays low, growth hormone pulses, and autophagy are activated.

- **Sleep cave:** Cool, dark, quiet. Aim 7–9 hrs.

- **Restorative physiology:** Telomere protection, DNA repair, glymphatic clearance in the brain.

Science anchor: Fasting plus deep sleep is synergistic: fasting triggers repair, sleep enables execution. Together, they slow biological aging at the mitochondrial and epigenetic levels.

THE LONGEVITY LOOP: WHY 14/10 WORKS

- **Metabolic reset**: insulin sensitivity restored daily.

- **Hormetic trigger**: fasting window is a stress signal → resilience pathways activate.

- **Autophagy & mitochondrial repair**: extended overnight fast clears cellular junk.

- **Circadian alignment**: eating in daylight → more efficient digestion, hormone balance.

Centenarians often practice natural time-restricted eating without naming it. In Okinawa, elders eat breakfast late, dinner early — an unintentional **14/10 or 16/8 rhythm** woven into daily life.

PATIENT STORY: MARIA'S 14/10 RESET

Maria, who once battled late-night snacking and energy crashes, shifted to a 14/10 rhythm: first meal at 10 am, last meal by 7 pm.

- After 2 weeks: reduced cravings, better digestion, more energy in the mornings.

- After 6 weeks: improved sleep depth, stable weight, sharper focus.

- Lab results: fasting glucose dropped, and inflammatory markers improved.

Her words: "It feels like my body finally has time to breathe."

QUICK-REFERENCE BLUEPRINT (14/10 LONGEVITY DAY)

☑ **Morning (Fast):** Sunlight + water + movement (no food).
☑ **Midday (First Meal):** Protein-rich breakfast with nutrient-dense plate.
☑ **Afternoon:** Movement snacks + balanced fueling.
☑ **Evening:** Light dinner, close eating window 3 hrs before bed.
☑ **Night (Fast):** Sleep in a fasting state → repair, autophagy, renewal.

Longevity is not bought in bottles or locked in secret genes. It's lived one day at a time. The **14/10 rhythm** is not deprivation. It is restoration. It gives your body the pause it needs to clean, repair, and prepare for another decade of vitality.

Every day you practice this rhythm, you are not just living longer — you are living younger.

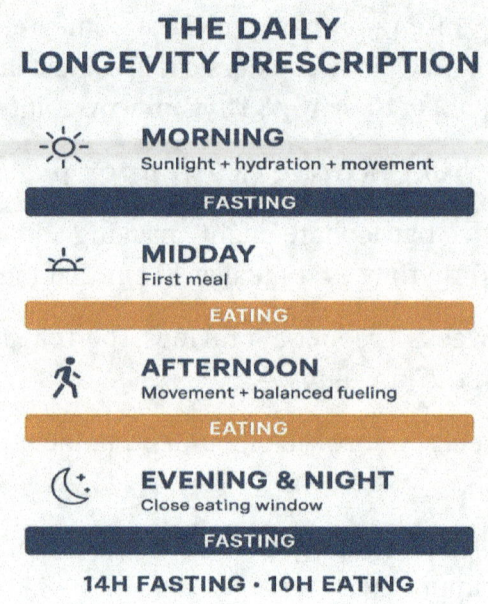

THE DAILY LONGEVITY PRESCRIPTION

MORNING
Sunlight + hydration + movement
FASTING

MIDDAY
First meal
EATING

AFTERNOON
Movement + balanced fueling
EATING

EVENING & NIGHT
Close eating window
FASTING

14H FASTING · 10H EATING

The arc of this book has carried us from the primal soil of movement and fasting to the cutting-edge biology of sleep, stress, resilience, and longevity. And now, as we arrive at the final chapter, we return to the most essential truth:

YOUR BODY IS NOT A LIAR. IT IS YOUR GREATEST ALLY.

THE MODERN LIE

For decades, culture has trained us to believe that our bodies are problems to be fixed — stubborn weight to be battled, cravings to be

476

distrusted, aches to be ignored. Marketing whispers that our bodies betray us, that aging is inevitable decline, that health is a war.

But science — and the lived wisdom of the longest-living cultures on Earth — tells a different story.

Your body has never lied to you. Every fatigue was a signal. Every craving was a message. Every restless night was feedback. Every surge of energy, every moment of clarity, every sigh of relief after a walk in the sun — these are signals of life's design, not defects.

THE ALLY WITHIN

- **When you eat in rhythm with your biology**, your hormones respond with balance, not chaos.

- **When you pause with fasting**, your cells repair with precision.

- **When you move daily**, your muscles whisper resilience into every organ.

- **When you rest and sleep**, your brain clears, your heart renews, and your immune system resets.

- **When you connect and love**, oxytocin and endorphins strengthen the architecture of your health.

- **When you align with purpose**, your nervous system locks into a compass of resilience.

The blueprint has never been about restriction, punishment, or control. It has always been about listening — and then responding.

THE FULL CIRCLE

Imagine yourself at 90. Not fragile, but vibrant. Waking with clarity. Walking with strength and sharing meals and laughter with people you love, and living with purpose that gets you out of bed each morning. That vision is not a fantasy. It is the natural inheritance of a body cared for in alignment with its design.

This book was never about hacks. It was never about shortcuts. It was about **reunion** — you, coming back into a relationship with the wisdom already inscribed in your biology.

Your body has been waiting, patiently, through years of noise, to remind you of this:

You are not broken. You are adaptable. You are resilient. You are designed to thrive.

THE FINAL BRIDGE

You now hold the Longevity Blueprint — but remember, blueprints only become homes when you live inside them. This is not a prescription to memorize; it is a practice to embody.

- Every meal is a signal.
- Every fast, a reset.
- Every movement, a message.
- Every rest, a repair.
- Every connection is a healing bond.
- Every purpose-driven choice is a compass bearing.

Your body will meet you at every step because it has never been your enemy. It has always been your most faithful ally.

So, step forward. Live younger, longer. Live in rhythm with what you are. Live full circle.

Your body is not a liar. It is your greatest ally. And it is ready, right now, to help you thrive.

EPILOGUE

FULL CIRCLE: YOUR BODY IS NOT A LIAR. IT'S YOUR GREATEST ALLY.

You stand at the edge of a small hill. Dawn breaks slowly and golden. The world smells like possibility—the way a kitchen smells the morning after rain, like bread just coming to life. You breathe in. There is a steadiness in your pulse that wasn't there a year ago. You notice how your body feels: strength in places you forgot existed, calm where there used to be a low, static panic, curiosity where there used to be fatigue. You smile, because what used to be a collection of habits now hums as a system—an operating system that carries you, quietly and faithfully, forward.

This book has been a map. Each chapter was a coordinate. Each toolkit is a compass. The epilogue is the moment when all of those coordinates fold into one lived life: not because you followed an instruction manual to the letter, but because you learned to speak your body's language—and it answered.

Below, I'll stitch the main threads together into a single, practical, emotionally honest plan you can carry from this page into your day. This is not a cram course. It's a long-form initiation: a way of being that honors your biology, your mind, your relationships, and the life you want to hold for the long run.

THIS IS WHAT YOU LEARNED (AND WHY IT MATTERS)

Across sixteen chapters, we did three things:

1. **We explained how modern living mismatches ancient biology.** You learned why food engineered for profit hijacks your reward system, why screens and late-night light rewrite your circadian clocks, and how stress and lack of sleep rewrite hormones so the body hoards energy instead of releasing it.

2. **We taught practical, evidence-based replacements—not hype.** We focused on four pillars (Food, Movement, Recovery, Rhythm) and gave you frameworks—14/10 daily rhythm, protein-first plates, walking and squatting as movement medicine, the Rewire Protocol for stress, micro-restorations, and sleep prescriptions that protect and repair.

3. **We handed you psychological tools to make change stick.** Identity coding, the Anti-Perfection Manifesto, small wins that compound, community practices, and rituals that turn science into habit.

Why it matters: because weight, mood, energy, and long-term disease risk are not moral problems to punish yourself for; they're information. Your body is continuously telling you what it needs. When you translate that signal into gentle, consistent action, you flip from survival mode into thrive mode.

THE ONE-SYSTEM SUMMARY: YOUR OPERATING SYSTEM FOR THRIVING

Think of the system as software with six core modules. Install these, and they work together—mutual reinforcement, not friction.

1. **Signal: Food as Code**

   o Protein-first, fiber-second, whole foods as staples.

   o Nightlight: minimize refined carbs and liquid sugars late.

   o Anti-Inflammatory Plate: leafy greens, omega-3s, fermented foods.

2. **Time: Rhythm & Fasting**

   o Align eating with daylight: aim for a 14/10 window (or 12/12 → 16/8 as you adapt).

   o Finish eating 2–3 hours before bed, where possible.

   o Use regular, mild fasts (14–16 hours) as a daily repair signal.

3. **Move: Built-In, Human Movement**

   o Daily foundation: 20–40 minutes walking (can be split).

   o Movement snacks: squats, mobility holds, carrying/grip exercises.

   o Strength sessions: 2–3 structured weeks to protect lean mass.

4. **Recover: Sleep & Restoration**

   o Habit: consistent sleep/wake window; 7–9 hours nightly when possible.

   o Evening ritual: tech-free buffer, dim light, breathwork.

   o Active recovery: sauna/cold, naps, mobility, deload weeks.

5. **Stress: Rewire & Reset**

   o Breath resets, micro-breaks, journaling dumps.

   o Reframe stress as a signal, not a verdict.

   o Community, rituals, and meaningful work buffer stress chronically.

6. **Identity: Consistency Over Perfection**

   o Little wins, identity anchors, repeating until it becomes automatic.

o Manifesto: "I am someone who programs their life for thriving."

When in sync, these modules create a new baseline: metabolic flexibility, a calm nervous system, a resilient microbiome, better sleep, and a quieting of cravings that used to feel unstoppable.

YOUR DAILY RHYTHM: A PRACTICAL DAY-IN-THE-LIFE TEMPLATE

Use this as a template; you adapt. Think of it as code you can edit, not a rigid rulebook.

MORNING (FAST WINDOW; SIGNAL: SUNLIGHT & MOVE)

- **Upon waking:** step into sunlight for 5–20 minutes (even a window will help if outside isn't possible).

- **Hydrate:** water with a pinch of salt or minerals.

- **Movement snack:** 10–20 minutes light activity (walk, mobility flow, breath sequence).

- **Optional:** delay first caloric intake to honor a 14/10 rhythm (if last meal was 7 pm, first meal at 9 am).

MIDDAY (EATING WINDOW OPENS; SIGNAL: PROTEIN-FIRST MEALS)

- **First meal:** protein-focused (20–35 g), fiber-rich vegetables, healthy fat.

- **Post-meal:** 10–15 minute walk to blunt glucose peaks and stimulate mitochondria.

- **Micro-restoration:** 2–5 minute breathing or mindfulness break mid-afternoon.

AFTERNOON (STRENGTH + PRACTICAL MOVEMENT)

- Brief strength session 2-3 times per week (push/pull/squat patterns).

- **NEAT:** multiple movement snacks; stand, carry, squat instead of sit when possible.

EVENING (CLOSE EATING WINDOW; SIGNAL: SOCIAL & SLOW)

- **Last meal:** light to moderate, protein-centered. Avoid processed carbs/sugary drinks.

- **Digital sunset:** screens off 60-90 minutes before bed.

- **Ritual:** 5-10 minutes of journaling, gratitude, or a few rounds of breathwork.

NIGHT (REPAIR WINDOW)

- Aim for a cool, dark sleep environment.

- If awake, do gentle breathing—avoid stimulating screens.

- Remember: sleep is the nightly operating-system upgrade.

A WEEKLY AND MONTHLY RHYTHM (THE "MACRO" LAYER)

Daily rituals build the foundation. Weekly and monthly practices optimize and protect progress.

Weekly:

- One longer nature walk or social meal with friends.

- Two structured strength sessions.

- One "longer" sleep night (if life permits) or an early bedtime day.

- One social or community ritual (a group walk, cooking night, or moai meeting).

Monthly:

- One "deload" week if you've been training intensely—scale back volume.

- Try one 24-hour reset or a 36-hour extension occasionally if appropriate and under medical guidance.

- Reflect on goals and identity shifts—journal progress and set a single small target for the next month.

WHAT TO TRACK (WITHOUT BECOMING A SLAVE TO NUMBERS)

Obsessive tracking kills joy. Useful tracking builds feedback loops.

Track the following for 4–8 weeks to see trends:

- Sleep quality (hours + subjective depth).

- Energy and mood (morning/afternoon/evening).

- Movement (minutes walked + strength sessions).

- Hunger and cravings (timing and intensity).

- One objective metric: clothes fit, waist measurement, or a performance marker (pushups or weighted carries) rather than a daily scale.

Use tracking to learn, not to self-punish. If a trend shows less sleep, more stress, or more cravings—address the upstream cause (sleep, stress), not only the symptom.

THE PSYCHOLOGY: REWIRING IDENTITY AND REWARD

You've read about dopamine loops, bliss points, ghrelin, and leptin. The hard part isn't information; it's creating a new default for your nervous system.

HOW TO REPROGRAM:

1. **Micro-habits > willpower:** Start with three core daily anchors. Repeat them religiously.

2. **Identity scripting:** Tell yourself, "I am someone who..." and choose statements aligned to your future self. (E.g., "I am someone who sleeps with reverence" or "I am someone who walks after meals.") Write them. Repeat them. Mean them.

3. **Ritualization:** Turn practices into rituals—the context signals safety to the brain. Rituals reduce decision fatigue and increase adherence.

4. **Reduce friction:** Make healthy steps easier: pre-chop veggies, keep walking shoes near the door, create a sleep cave.

5. **Reframe setbacks:** Not failure—data. Each setback tells you what to tweak, not that you're broken. The Anti-Perfection Manifesto says: adjust, continue, be kind.

TROUBLESHOOTING: COMMON PITFALLS AND HOW TO FIX THEM

PITFALL: LATE-NIGHT CRAVINGS.

- **Fix:** Implement a firm end-of-eating rule of 2–3 hours before bed. Introduce a calming evening ritual; use breathwork, herbal tea, or a short walk.

PITFALL: NO MORNING HUNGER.

- **Fix:** Check meal timing. If you ate late, your ghrelin may still be shifted; adopt the 14/10 rhythm consistently for 2–3 weeks. Add light morning movement and hydration, not forced big breakfasts.

PITFALL: PLATEAU ON THE SCALE.

- **Fix:** Focus less on the scale. Measure strength, sleep, and mood. If needed, tighten adherence to protein/fiber plate sequencing, walk after meals, and ensure sleep quality.

PITFALL: STRESS EATING.

- **Fix:** Breath resets (4:6 breathing), micro-breaks, journaling. Build a non-food coping skill: movement, calling a friend, or stepping outside.

PITFALL: LOW ENERGY WITH FASTING.

- **Fix:** Ensure protein and electrolytes, moderate carbohydrates around workouts, and adapt gradually from 12:12 → 14:10 → 16:8 as tolerated. Consult a clinician if you have medical conditions.

CLINICAL NOTES & SAFETY (IMPORTANT)

This book is a guide, not a prescription. If you have existing medical conditions—pregnancy, type 1 diabetes, adrenal disorders, severe metabolic conditions, or are taking medications like insulin or sulfonylureas—consult your physician before starting fasting, significant diet changes, or intense exercise regimens. For people with eating disorder histories, seek the guidance of trained professionals.

COMMUNITY & SOCIAL PROOF: DON'T GO IT ALONE

One of the strongest, consistent findings across the Blue Zones and our own program data: connection improves outcomes. People who share food, movement, and ritual sustain change far longer.

Ways to embed community:

- A weekly cooking night with friends.
- Walking groups or buddy systems for post-meal walks.
- Small accountability cohorts—3-6 people who share commitments and check-ins.
- Moai-style groups—a circulating group of friends who meet consistently for mutual support.

Social accountability makes the operating system social; it moves habit from a private trial to a shared culture—and it builds joy.

THE METRICS THAT MATTER (BEYOND THE SCALE)

What to celebrate:

- More days with deep sleep.
- Clothes feel looser.
- Less reactive mood, fewer sugar cravings.
- Increased strength (more reps, heavier carries).
- Improved lab values (A1c, fasting glucose, lipid patterns) when measured and when clinically indicated.

Remember: slow, sustainable wins over flashy, temporary loss. A habit that lasts five years beats an extreme that lasted five weeks.

RITUALS & MANTRAS: PRACTICE TO ANCHOR

Adopt a handful of short rituals and mantras to anchor your day.

Daily Mantras (say them aloud or write them):

- "I give my body clear, consistent signals of safety."

- "I choose rhythm over rules."

- "Every breath is a reset."

- "I am programming my body to thrive."

Micro-Rituals (2–6 minutes each):

- *Morning sun pause.* Step outside, breathe, notice.

- *Post-meal walk.* 10–15 minutes to close the glucose loop.

- *Evening digital sunset.* Dim lights, walk, and journal.

- *Breath-reset.* 4 in, 6 or 8 out—two to three cycles when stress spikes.

Rituals simplify decision-making and embed the science into lived practice.

STORIES FOR THE ROAD (YOUR FELLOW TRAVELERS)

You've met David, Maria, Elena, James, Daniel, Michael, Clara— each a different life and struggle, each a story of translation: information into action. Keep their stories as models, not rules. Use them to remind yourself that transformation rarely looks linear. People stumble, recalibrate, and persist. Over months and years, their body rewired itself to cooperation—and yours can too.

THE LONG VIEW: BEYOND 6 MONTHS

Consider these long-term goals:

Year 1: Establish core rituals—protein-first plates, daily walks, sleep routine. See reliable improvements in energy, mood, and a steady change in body composition.

Years 2–3: Expand community, refine movement skills, include advanced recovery rituals (sauna, contrast therapy), and deepen purpose work.

Decades: Aim for healthspan, not just lifespan. Longevity is the sum of daily patterns—food, movement, sleep, connection, and meaning. Your consistent efforts compound into decades of life with more vigor and less disease.

A TOOLBOX TO KEEP: QUICK REFERENCE (PRINTABLE)

Keep this on the fridge or your phone:

DAILY STARTER CHECKLIST

- Sunlight (5–20 min) — morning.
- Hydrate (water + pinch of minerals).
- Protein-first breakfast within the eating window.
- 10–15 min walk post main meals.
- Two strength sessions weekly.
- Digital sunset: screens off 60–90 min before bed.
- Breath reset 3× daily.
- Sleep window consistent (aim 7–9 hours).

Weekly

- An extended nature walk or a social meal.
- Reflective journaling (wins/adjustments).
- One longer sleep night or earlier bedtime.

Monthly

- Try a 24-hour reset or extended reflection day if appropriate.

- Community check-in (moai or group).

FINAL WORDS: COURAGE, NOT PERFECTION

Change asks for one essential thing: courage. The courage to show up imperfectly, again and again. The courage to believe that biology is not a conspiracy against you but a set of rules that, once learned, unlock astonishing freedom. The courage to be kind to yourself when progress slows, and relentless in your curiosity when you need to troubleshoot.

You do not need to be faster. You do not need to be better in someone else's definition. You need to be more aligned—small act after small act—until those acts live you, instead of you having to fight them.

CLOSING INVOCATION

Before you close this book, pause. Place your hand on your heart. Breathe and say these words.

"I am not my setbacks."

"I am learning a new language—my body's language."

"I will feed it with clarity, move it with joy, rest it with reverence, and surround it with people who help me thrive."

When you leave this page, you are not left with a list of rules. You are carrying a rhythm. You are carrying a way to speak gently to your biology so it will return the favor.

Your body is not a liar. It is an interpreter. It listens. It answers. It is your greatest ally.

Now go. Start small. Keep going. Build a life, not a meal plan. Eat to thrive.

COMPREHENSIVE SCHOLARLY APPENDIX

CHAPTER 1 — THE THRIVE BLUEPRINT: HOW TO BREAK FREE FROM SURVIVAL MODE AND CRACK THE CRAVINGS CODE

1. Berthoud, H.-R. (2011). Metabolic and hedonic drives in the neural control of appetite: Who is the boss? *Current Opinion in Neurobiology*, 21(6), 888–896. https://doi.org/10.1016/j.conb.2011.09.004

2. Rolls, E. T. (2015). Taste, reward, and food intake control. *Physiology & Behavior*, 152(Pt B), 408–416. https://doi.org/10.1016/j.physbeh.2014.11.022

3. Volkow, N. D., Wang, G.-J., & Baler, R. D. (2011). Reward, dopamine, and the control of food intake: Implications for obesity. *Trends in Cognitive Sciences*, 15(1), 37–46. https://doi.org/10.1016/j.tics.2010.11.001

4. DiFeliceantonio, A. G., & Berridge, K. C. (2012). Which foods may be addictive? The roles of processing, fat content, and glycemic load. PLoS ONE, 7(10), e44770. https://doi.org/10.1371/journal.pone.0044770

5. Cummings, D. E., & Overduin, J. (2007). Gastrointestinal regulation of food intake. *The Journal of Clinical Investigation*, 117(1), 13–23. https://doi.org/10.1172/JCI30227

6. Lowe, M. R., & Butryn, M. L. (2007). Hedonic hunger: A new dimension of appetite? *Physiology & Behavior*, 91(4), 432–439. https://doi.org/10.1016/j.physbeh.2007.04.015

7. Rolls, B. J. (2014). What determines energy intake? *Public Health Nutrition*, 17(7), 1200–1206. https://doi.org/10.1017/S1368980013000752

8. Swithers, S. E. (2013). Artificial sweeteners produce the counterintuitive effect of inducing metabolic derangements. *Trends in Endocrinology & Metabolism*, 24(9), 431–441. https://doi.org/10.1016/j.tem.2013.05.005

9. Myers, A. L., & Gazmararian, J. (2018). Behavioral economics for dietary change. *Annual Review of Nutrition*, 38, 237–252. https://doi.org/10.1146/annurev-nutr-082117-051535

10. Baumeister, R. F., Gailliot, M., DeWall, C. N., & Oaten, M. (2006). Self-regulation and personality: How interventions increase regulatory success, and how depletion moderates the effects of traits. *Journal of Personality*, 74(6), 1773–1801. https://doi.org/10.1111/j.1467-6494.2006.00426.x

CHAPTER 2 — RHYTHM RESET: ALIGNING YOUR BODY'S HIDDEN CLOCK

11. Scheer, F. A. J. L., Hilton, M. F., Mantzoros, C. S., & Shea, S. A. (2009). Adverse metabolic and cardiovascular consequences of circadian misalignment. *Proceedings of the National Academy of Sciences, 106*(11), 4453–4458. https://doi.org/10.1073/pnas.0808180106

12. Longo, V. D., & Panda, S. (2016). Fasting, circadian rhythms, and time-restricted feeding in the healthy lifespan. *Cell Metabolism, 23*(6), 1048–1059. https://doi.org/10.1016/j.cmet.2016.06.001

13. Duffy, J. F., & Czeisler, C. A. (2009). Effect of light on human circadian physiology. *Sleep Medicine Clinics, 4*(2), 165–177. https://doi.org/10.1016/j.jsmc.2009.02.005

14. Morris, C. J., Yang, J. N., & Scheer, F. A. (2012). The impact of the circadian timing system on cardiovascular and metabolic function. *Progress in Brain Research, 199,* 337–358. https://doi.org/10.1016/B978-0-444-59427-3.00022-0

15. Wehrens, S. M., Hampton, S. M., & Skene, D. J. (2017). Meal timing and the circadian regulation of metabolism. *Frontiers in Nutrition, 4,* 20. https://doi.org/10.3389/fnut.2017.00020

16. Panda, S. (2016). Circadian physiology of metabolism. *Science, 354*(6315), 1008–1015. https://doi.org/10.1126/science.aah4967

17. Garaulet, M., Madrid, J. A., & Huybrechts, I. (2013). Chrono-nutrition: A dynamic strategy to manage obesity and metabolic syndrome. *Obesity Reviews, 14*(9), 695–703. https://doi.org/10.1111/obr.12055

18. Stokkan, K.-A., & Reiter, R. J. (2018). Sleep timing and metabolic syndrome risk. *Current Opinion in Endocrinology, Diabetes and Obesity, 25*(5), 301–307. https://doi.org/10.1097/MED.0000000000000415

19. Wehrens, S. M., & Dijk, D.-J. (2016). Timing of food intake and circadian rhythms. *Pediatric Clinics of North America, 63*(6), 1077–1090. https://doi.org/10.1016/j.pcl.2016.06.011

20. Buxton, O. M., & Marcelli, E. (2010). Short and long sleep are associated with obesity and weight gain in adults: Results from the National Health Interview Survey. *Sleep, 33*(7), 895–905. https://doi.org/10.1093/sleep/33.7.895

CHAPTER 3 — YOUR BODY IS A LIAR

21. Hall, K. D. (2018). The physics of obesity: What we know and what we don't know about energy balance. *Obesity*, 26(Suppl 1), S5–S14. https://doi.org/10.1002/oby.22181

22. Schwartz, M. W., Seeley, R. J., Zeltser, L. M., Drewnowski, A., Ravussin, E., Redman, L. M., & Leibel, R. L. (2017). Obesity pathogenesis: An endocrine society scientific statement. *Endocrine Reviews*, 38(4), 267–296. https://doi.org/10.1210/er.2017-00111

23. Blundell, J. E., et al. (2015). Appetite control: Methodological aspects of the evaluation of foods. *Obesity Reviews*, 16(Suppl 1), 1–8. https://doi.org/10.1111/obr.12294

24. Cummings, D. E., Purnell, J. Q., Frayo, R. S., Schmidova, K., Wisse, B. E., & Weigle, D. S. (2001). A preprandial rise in plasma ghrelin levels suggests a role in meal initiation in humans. *Diabetes*, 50(8), 1714–1719. https://doi.org/10.2337/diabetes.50.8.1714

25. Spiegel, K., Leproult, R., & Van Cauter, E. (1999). Impact of sleep debt on metabolic and endocrine function. *The Lancet*, 354(9188), 1435–1439. https://doi.org/10.1016/S0140-6736(99)01376-8

26. Sumithran, P., & Proietto, J. (2013). The defence of body weight: A physiological basis for weight regain after weight loss. *Clinical Science*, 124(4), 231–241. https://doi.org/10.1042/CS20120233

27. Speakman, J. R., & O'Rahilly, S. (2012). Fat: an evolving issue. *Molecular Metabolism*, 1(1), 1–4. https://doi.org/10.1016/j.molmet.2012.07.006

28. Rosenbaum, M., & Leibel, R. L. (2010). Adaptive thermogenesis in humans. *International Journal of Obesity,* 34(S1), S47–S55. https://doi.org/10.1038/ijo.2010.184

29. Hall, K. D., Heymsfield, S. B., Kemnitz, J. W., Klein, S., Schoeller, D. A., & Speakman, J. R. (2012). Energy balance and its components: Implications for body weight regulation. *The American Journal of Clinical Nutrition,* 95(4), 989–994. https://doi.org/10.3945/ajcn.112.036350

30. Lowe, M. R., Kral, T. V. E., & Miller-Kovach, K. (2019). The neurobiology of eating behavior and obesity: Insights from neuroscientific and psychological perspectives. *Annual Review of Psychology,* 70, 701–730. https://doi.org/10.1146/annurev-psych-010418-103030

CHAPTER 4 — THE ULTRA-PROCESSED FOOD PRESCRIPTION

31. Monteiro, C. A., Moubarac, J.-C., Levy, R. B., Canella, D. S., Louzada, M. L., & Cannon, G. (2018). Ultra-processed foods: What they are and how to identify them. *Public Health Nutrition*, 21(1), 1–11. https://doi.org/10.1017/S1368980018003762

32. Hall, K. D., et al. (2019). Ultra-processed diets cause excess calorie intake and weight gain: A randomized controlled trial. *Cell Metabolism*, 30(1), 67–77.e3. https://doi.org/10.1016/j.cmet.2019.05.008

33. Fardet, A., & Rock, E. (2018). Ultra-processed foods and food system sustainability: What are the links? *Sustainability*, 10(10), 3474. https://doi.org/10.3390/su10103474

34. Moubarac, J.-C., Batal, M., Louzada, M. L. C., Martinez Steele, E., Monteiro, C. A. (2017). Processed and ultra-processed food products: Consumption trends and policy implications. *World Nutrition*, 8(1–2), 40–57.

35. Moodie, R., et al. (2013). Profits and pandemics: Prevention of harmful effects of tobacco, alcohol, and ultra-processed food and drink industries. *The Lancet*, 381(9867), 670–679. https://doi.org/10.1016/S0140-6736(12)62089-3

36. Srour, B., Fezeu, L. K., Kesse-Guyot, E., Allès, B., Méjean, C., Andrianasolo, R. M., & Touvier, M. (2019). Ultra-processed food intake and risk of type 2 diabetes in the French NutriNet-Santé cohort. *PLoS Medicine*, 16(12), e1002742. https://doi.org/10.1371/journal.pmed.1002742

37. Fiolet, T., Srour, B., Sellem, L., Kesse-Guyot, E., Allès, B., Méjean, C., & Touvier, M. (2018). Consumption of ultra-processed foods and cancer risk: Results from NutriNet-

Santé prospective cohort. BMJ, 360, k322.
https://doi.org/10.1136/bmj.k322

38. Juul, F., Martinez Steele, E., Parekh, N., Monteiro, C. A., & Chang, V. W. (2019). Ultra-processed food consumption and excess weight among US adults. *British Journal of Nutrition*, 123(1), 1–9. https://doi.org/10.1017/S0007114519001700

39. Fardet, A., & Boirie, Y. (2014). Associations between food and beverage categories and chronic disease: A narrative review of the literature. *Nutrition Research Reviews*, 27(1), 92–107. https://doi.org/10.1017/S0954422414000063

40. Kearns, C. E., Schmidt, L. A., & Glantz, S. A. (2016). The tobacco industry and sugary drink marketing: Evidence from internal industry documents. *PLOS Medicine*, 13(3), e1001990. https://doi.org/10.1371/journal.pmed.1001990

CHAPTER 5 — THE JOY PRESCRIPTION

41. Pressman, S. D., & Cohen, S. (2005). Does positive affect influence health? *Psychological Bulletin*, 131(6), 925–971. https://doi.org/10.1037/0033-2909.131.6.925

42. Steptoe, A., & Wardle, J. (2011). Positive affect and biological function in everyday life. *Social and Personality Psychology Compass*, 5(1), 52–63. https://doi.org/10.1111/j.1751-9004.2010.00319.x

43. Reis, H. T., & Gable, S. L. (2003). Toward a positive psychology of relationships. *Psychological Inquiry*, 14(2), 101–107. https://doi.org/10.1207/S15327965PLI1402_01

44. Fredrickson, B. L. (2004). The broaden-and-build theory of positive emotions. *Philosophical Transactions of the Royal Society B*, 359(1449), 1367–1377. https://doi.org/10.1098/rstb.2004.1512

45. Wethington, E., & Kessler, R. C. (1986). Perceived support, received support, and adjustment to stressful life events. *Journal of Health and Social Behavior*, 27(1), 78–89. https://doi.org/10.2307/2136504

46. Keltner, D., & Lerner, J. S. (2010). Emotion. *Handbook of Social Psychology* (5th ed.). Wiley.

47. Ciani, A., & Buccella, S. (2016). The role of pleasure in sustainable eating behaviour. *Appetite*, 105, 1–3. https://doi.org/10.1016/j.appet.2016.04.014

48. Kuroda, M., et al. (2015). Hedonic and eudaimonic well-being and physiological markers: A systematic review. *Psychosomatic Medicine*, 77(5), 501–509. https://doi.org/10.1097/PSY.0000000000000192

49. Wastyk, H. C., et al. (2021). Gut-microbiota-targeted diets and well-being: The role of fermented foods in mood and

gut health. *Cell, 184*(16), 4072–4084.e22.
https://doi.org/10.1016/j.cell.2021.06.034

50. Otake, K., Shimai, S., Tanaka-Matsumi, J., Otsui, K., & Fredrickson, B. L. (2006). Happy people become happier through kindness: A counting kindness intervention. *Journal of Happiness Studies, 7*(3), 361–375.
https://doi.org/10.1007/s10902-005-3650-z

CHAPTER 6 — FOOD + MOOD + MICROBIOME

51. Mayer, E. A., Knight, R., Mazmanian, S. K., Cryan, J. F., & Tillisch, K. (2014). Gut microbes and the brain: Paradigm shift in neuroscience. *The Journal of Neuroscience, 34*(46), 15490–15496. https://doi.org/10.1523/JNEUROSCI.3299-14.2014

52. Cryan, J. F., & Dinan, T. G. (2012). Mind-altering microorganisms: The impact of the gut microbiota on brain and behaviour. *Nature Reviews Neuroscience, 13*(10), 701–712. https://doi.org/10.1038/nrn3346

53. Jacka, F. N., O'Neil, A., Opie, R., Itsiopoulos, C., Cotton, S., Mohebbi, M., & Berk, M. (2017). A randomised controlled trial of dietary improvement for adults with major depression (the 'SMILES' trial). *BMC Medicine, 15,* 23. https://doi.org/10.1186/s12916-016-0973-5

54. Suez, J., Korem, T., Zeevi, D., Zilberman-Schapira, G., Thaiss, C. A., Maza, O., & Elinav, E. (2014). Artificial sweeteners induce glucose intolerance by altering the gut microbiota. *Nature, 514*(7521), 181–186. https://doi.org/10.1038/nature13793

55. Wastyk, H. C., et al. (2021). Gut-microbiota-targeted diets and human health: A review of clinical trials. *Cell, 184*(16), 4072–4091. https://doi.org/10.1016/j.cell.2021.06.034

56. Schmidt, K., et al. (2015). Prebiotic intake reduces the waking cortisol response and alters emotional bias in healthy volunteers. *Psychopharmacology, 232*(10), 1793–1801. https://doi.org/10.1007/s00213-014-3836-1

57. Sánchez-Villegas, A., et al. (2012). Dietary patterns and depression risk. *Public Health Nutrition, 15*(10), 1765–1772. https://doi.org/10.1017/S1368980012000737

58. Berding, K., & Donovan, S. M. (2016). Microbes and mental health: How intestinal microbiota influence brain and behavior. *Current Opinion in Clinical Nutrition & Metabolic Care*, 19(6), 471–476. https://doi.org/10.1097/MCO.0000000000000325

59. Jansson, A., & Bäckhed, F. (2012). Role of gut microbiota in metabolic disease. *Nature*, 489(7415), 178–185. https://doi.org/10.1038/nature11552

60. Dinan, T. G., Stanton, C., & Cryan, J. F. (2013). Psychobiotics: A novel class of psychotropic. *Biological Psychiatry*, 74(10), 720–726. https://doi.org/10.1016/j.biopsych.2013.05.001

CHAPTER 7 — THE STRESS PRESCRIPTION

61. McEwen, B. S. (2008). Central effects of stress hormones in health and disease: Understanding the protective and damaging effects of stress and stress mediators. *European Journal of Pharmacology*, 583(2–3), 174–185. https://doi.org/10.1016/j.ejphar.2007.11.071

62. Sapolsky, R. M. (2004). *Why zebras don't get ulcers: An updated guide to stress, stress-related diseases, and coping.* Holt Paperbacks.

63. Porges, S. W. (2011). *The polyvagal theory: Neurophysiological foundations of emotions, attachment, communication, and self-regulation.* W. W. Norton & Company.

64. Chrousos, G. P. (2009). Stress and disorders of the stress system. *Nature Reviews Endocrinology*, 5(7), 374–381. https://doi.org/10.1038/nrendo.2009.106

65. Thayer, J. F., Åhs, F., Fredrikson, M., Sollers, J. J., & Wager, T. D. (2012). A meta-analysis of heart rate variability and neuroimaging studies: Implications for heart rate variability as a marker of stress and health. *Neuroscience & Biobehavioral Reviews*, 36(2), 747–756. https://doi.org/10.1016/j.neubiorev.2011.11.009

66. Crum, A. J., Salovey, P., & Achor, S. (2013). Rethinking stress: The role of mindsets in determining the stress response. *Journal of Personality and Social Psychology*, 104(4), 716–733. https://doi.org/10.1037/a0031201

67. Lehrer, P. M., & Gevirtz, R. (2014). Heart rate variability biofeedback: How and why does it work? *Frontiers in Psychology*, 5, 756. https://doi.org/10.3389/fpsyg.2014.00756

68. O'Donovan, A., et al. (2012). Cumulative lifetime stressor exposure and short leukocyte telomere length. *Psychoneuroendocrinology*, 37(8), 1139–1149. https://doi.org/10.1016/j.psyneuen.2012.01.010

69. Kabat-Zinn, J. (1990). *Full catastrophe living: Using the wisdom of your body and mind to face stress, pain, and illness.* Delacorte.

70. Kuyken, W., et al. (2016). Effectiveness of mindfulness-based cognitive therapy compared with maintenance antidepressant treatment in prevention of depressive relapse/recurrence: A randomized controlled trial. JAMA *Psychiatry*, 73(1), 110–119. https://doi.org/10.1001/jamapsychiatry.2015.3056

CHAPTER 8 — MOVE TO THRIVE, NOT TO BURN CALORIES

71. Booth, F. W., Roberts, C. K., & Laye, M. J. (2012). Lack of exercise is a major cause of chronic diseases. *Comprehensive Physiology*, 2(2), 1143–1211. https://doi.org/10.1002/cphy.c110025

72. Pedersen, B. K., & Febbraio, M. A. (2012). Muscles, exercise, and obesity: Skeletal muscle as a secretory organ. *Nature Reviews Endocrinology*, 8(8), 457–465. https://doi.org/10.1038/nrendo.2012.49

73. Warburton, D. E., Nicol, C. W., & Bredin, S. S. (2006). Health benefits of physical activity: The evidence. CMAJ, 174(6), 801–809. https://doi.org/10.1503/cmaj.051351

74. Levine, J. A. (2004). Nonexercise activity thermogenesis (NEAT). *Best Practice & Research Clinical Endocrinology & Metabolism*, 18(4), 679–708. https://doi.org/10.1016/j.beem.2004.07.004

75. Lee, I.-M., et al. (2012). Effect of physical inactivity on major non-communicable diseases worldwide: An analysis of burden of disease and life expectancy. *The Lancet*, 380(9838), 219–229. https://doi.org/10.1016/S0140-6736(12)61031-9

76. Phillips, S. M. (2014). A brief review of critical processes in exercise-induced muscular hypertrophy. *Sports Medicine*, 44(Suppl 1), S71–S77. https://doi.org/10.1007/s40279-014-0152-3

77. Warburton, D. E., Bredin, S. S., Horita, L. T., Zbogar, D., Scott, J. M., Esch, B. T., & Rhodes, R. E. (2007). The health benefits of interactive video game exercise. *Applied Physiology, Nutrition, and Metabolism*, 32(4), 655–663. https://doi.org/10.1139/H07-053

78. Harber, M. P., et al. (2017). Aerobic exercise training and its effects on human skeletal muscle mitochondrial capacity. *Journal of Physiology, 595*(23), 6247–6266. https://doi.org/10.1113/JP274588

79. Stamatakis, E., et al. (2019). Sitting time, physical activity, and risk of mortality in US adults. *British Journal of Sports Medicine, 53*(14), 866–872. https://doi.org/10.1136/bjsports-2018-099393

80. Collins, S., et al. (2019). Muscle as an endocrine organ: Role of myokines in exercise and metabolic regulation. *Nature Reviews Endocrinology, 15*(7), 375–389. https://doi.org/10.1038/s41574-019-0209-9

CHAPTER 9 — THE INTERMITTENT FASTING BLUEPRINT

81. Patterson, R. E., & Sears, D. D. (2017). Metabolic effects of intermittent fasting. *Annual Review of Nutrition, 37*, 371–393. https://doi.org/10.1146/annurev-nutr-071816-064634

82. Anton, S. D., et al. (2018). Flipping the metabolic switch: Understanding and applying the health benefits of fasting. *Obesity, 26*(2), 254–268. https://doi.org/10.1002/oby.22065

83. Longo, V. D., & Mattson, M. P. (2014). Fasting: Molecular mechanisms and clinical applications. *Cell Metabolism, 19*(2), 181–192. https://doi.org/10.1016/j.cmet.2013.12.008

84. Wilkinson, M. J., et al. (2020). Ten-hour time-restricted eating reduces weight, blood pressure, and atherogenic lipids in patients with metabolic syndrome. *Cell Metabolism, 31*(1), 92–104.e5. https://doi.org/10.1016/j.cmet.2019.11.004

85. Satchidananda Panda, S. (2016). Time-restricted feeding and circadian rhythms. *Cell, 167*(5), 1242–1254. https://doi.org/10.1016/j.cell.2016.11.001

86. Varady, K. A. (2011). Intermittent versus daily calorie restriction: Which diet program is more effective for weight loss? *Obesity Reviews, 12*(7), e593–e601. https://doi.org/10.1111/j.1467-789X.2011.00873.x

87. de Goede, P., et al. (2019). Effects of 8-hour time-restricted feeding on body weight and metabolic disease risk factors in free-living adults. *Journal of Nutrition, 149*(9), 1398–1406. https://doi.org/10.1093/jn/nxz113

88. Tinsley, G. M., & La Bounty, P. M. (2015). Effects of intermittent fasting on body composition and clinical health markers in humans. *Nutrition Reviews, 73*(10), 661–674. https://doi.org/10.1093/nutrit/nuv041

89. Patterson, R. E., Laughlin, G. A., LaCroix, A. Z., Hartman, S. J., Natarajan, L., Senger, C. M., & Sears, D. D. (2015). Intermittent fasting and human metabolic health. *Journal of the Academy of Nutrition and Dietetics, 115*(8), 1203–1212. https://doi.org/10.1016/j.jand.2015.02.018

90. De Cabo, R., & Mattson, M. P. (2019). Effects of intermittent fasting on health, aging, and disease. *New England Journal of Medicine, 381*(26), 2541–2551. https://doi.org/10.1056/NEJMra1905136

CHAPTER 10 — RECOVERY AS RENEWAL — YOUR BODY'S FORGOTTEN MODE OF HEALING

91. Hausswirth, C., & Mujika, I. (2013). *Recovery for performance in sport*. Human Kinetics.

92. Kleiber, S., & Horvath, S. (2019). The role of aging and recovery in cellular resilience. *Trends in Molecular Medicine*, 25(4), 309–322. https://doi.org/10.1016/j.molmed.2019.02.002

93. Halson, S. L. (2014). Sleep in elite athletes and nutritional interventions to enhance sleep. *Sports Medicine*, 44(Suppl 1), 13–23. https://doi.org/10.1007/s40279-014-0157-y

94. Dupuy, O., et al. (2018). The association between recovery and performance: A systematic review. *Sports Medicine*, 48(12), 2747–2770. https://doi.org/10.1007/s40279-018-0942-x

95. Nédélec, M., et al. (2015). Recovery in sport: Part I: Sleep and rest. *Sports Medicine*, 45(10), 1387–1403. https://doi.org/10.1007/s40279-015-0370-5

96. Kellmann, M. (2010). Preventing overtraining in athletes in high-intensity sports and stress/recovery monitoring. *Scandinavian Journal of Medicine & Science in Sports*, 20(Suppl 2), 95–102. https://doi.org/10.1111/j.1600-0838.2010.01192.x

97. Halson, S. (2014). Monitoring training load to understand fatigue in athletes. *Sports Medicine*, 44(Suppl 2), 139–147. https://doi.org/10.1007/s40279-014-0253-z

98. Baker, J. M., et al. (2017). Strategies for optimizing recovery: A narrative review. *Journal of Strength and Conditioning Research*, 31(11), 1–18. (Publisher)

99. Cakir-Atabek, H., & Genc, A. (2018). Physiological mechanisms of recovery: Neural and hormonal modulation. *Journal of Applied Physiology, 124*(3), 713–730. https://doi.org/10.1152/japplphysiol.00629.2017

100. Brustio, P. R., et al. (2020). Sleep, recovery, and performance in team sports athletes: A systematic review. *Journal of Sports Sciences, 38*(11–12), 1319–1328. https://doi.org/10.1080/02640414.2020.1720754

CHAPTER 11 – THE SLEEP PRESCRIPTION

101. Walker, M. (2017). Why we sleep: Unlocking the power of sleep and dreams. Scribner.

102. Cirelli, C., & Tononi, G. (2008). Is sleep essential? PLoS Biology, 6(8), e216. https://doi.org/10.1371/journal.pbio.0060216

103. Buysse, D. J. (2014). Sleep health: Can we define it? Does it matter? Sleep, 37(1), 9–17. https://doi.org/10.5665/sleep.3298

104. Van Cauter, E., & Knutson, K. L. (2008). Sleep and the epidemic of obesity in children and adults. European Journal of Endocrinology, 159(Suppl 1), S59–S66. https://doi.org/10.1530/EJE-08-0353

105. Xie, L., et al. (2013). Sleep drives metabolite clearance from the adult brain. Science, 342(6156), 373–377. https://doi.org/10.1126/science.1241224

106. Spiegel, K., Leproult, R., & Van Cauter, E. (1999). Impact of sleep debt on metabolic and endocrine function. The Lancet, 354(9188), 1435–1439. https://doi.org/10.1016/S0140-6736(99)01376-8

107. Medic, G., Wille, M., & Hemels, M. E. H. (2017). Short- and long-term health consequences of sleep disruption. Nature and Science of Sleep, 9, 151–161. https://doi.org/10.2147/NSS.S134864

108. Akerstedt, T., & Wright, K. P., Jr. (2009). Sleep loss and fatigue in shift work and shift work disorder. Sleep Medicine Clinics, 4(2), 257–271. https://doi.org/10.1016/j.jsmc.2009.03.001

109. Leproult, R., & Van Cauter, E. (2010). Role of sleep and sleep loss in hormonal release and metabolism. *Endocrine Development*, 17, 11–21. https://doi.org/10.1159/000262524

110. Irish, L. A., Kline, C. E., Gunn, H. E., Buysse, D. J., & Hall, M. H. (2015). The role of sleep hygiene in promoting public health: A review of empirical evidence. *Sleep Medicine Reviews*, 22, 23–36. https://doi.org/10.1016/j.smrv.2014.10.001

CHAPTER 12 — EMOTIONAL RESILIENCE: TRAINING YOUR INNER CORE

111. Southwick, S. M., & Charney, D. S. (2018). *Resilience: The science of mastering life's greatest challenges* (2nd ed.). Cambridge University Press.

112. Bonanno, G. A. (2004). Loss, trauma, and human resilience: Have we underestimated the human capacity to thrive after extremely aversive events? *American Psychologist, 59*(1), 20–28. https://doi.org/10.1037/0003-066X.59.1.20

113. Seery, M. D., Holman, E. A., & Silver, R. C. (2010). Whatever does not kill us: Cumulative lifetime adversity, vulnerability, and resilience. *Journal of Personality and Social Psychology, 99*(6), 1025–1041. https://doi.org/10.1037/a0021344

114. Rutter, M. (2012). Resilience as a dynamic concept. *Development and Psychopathology, 24*(2), 335–344. https://doi.org/10.1017/S0954579412000028

115. Lehrer, P., & Woolfolk, R. (2007). *Principles and practice of stress management.* Guilford Press.

116. Gross, J. J. (2015). Emotion regulation: Current status and future prospects. *Psychological Inquiry, 26*(1), 1–26. https://doi.org/10.1080/1047840X.2014.940781

117. Porges, S. W. (2017). *The pocket guide to the polyvagal theory: The transformative power of feeling safe.* Norton.

118. Masten, A. S. (2014). Global perspectives on resilience in children and youth. *Child Development, 85*(1), 6–20. https://doi.org/10.1111/cdev.12205

119. Folkman, S., & Moskowitz, J. T. (2004). Coping: Pitfalls and promise. *Annual Review of Psychology, 55,* 745–774. https://doi.org/10.1146/annurev.psych.55.090902.141456

120. Davidson, R. J., & McEwen, B. S. (2012). Social influences on neuroplasticity: Stress and interventions to promote well-being. *Nature Neuroscience, 15*(5), 689–695. https://doi.org/10.1038/nn.3093

CHAPTER 13 — PURPOSE AS MEDICINE

121. Hill, P. L., & Turiano, N. A. (2014). Purpose in life as a predictor of mortality across adulthood. *Psychological Science, 25*(7), 1482–1486. https://doi.org/10.1177/0956797614531799

122. Ryff, C. D., & Singer, B. (2008). Know thyself and become what you are: A eudaimonic approach to psychological well-being. *Journal of Happiness Studies, 9*(1), 13–39. https://doi.org/10.1007/s10902-006-9019-0

123. Steger, M. F., Frazier, P., Oishi, S., & Kaler, M. (2006). The meaning in life questionnaire: Assessing presence of and search for meaning. *Journal of Counseling Psychology, 53*(1), 80–93. https://doi.org/10.1037/0022-0167.53.1.80

124. Kim, E. S., & Kubzansky, L. D. (2014). Sense of purpose and objective risk of Alzheimer disease in older adults. JAMA *Psychiatry, 71*(5), 547–554. https://doi.org/10.1001/jamapsychiatry.2013.4146

125. Park, C. L., & Folkman, S. (1997). Meaning in the context of stress and coping. *Review of General Psychology, 1*(2), 115–144. https://doi.org/10.1037/1089-2680.1.2.115

126. Buettner, D. (2012). *The Blue Zones: 9 lessons for living longer from the people who've lived the longest.* National Geographic.

127. Ikigai Research Center. (2001). Studies on ikigai and longevity in Okinawa. (Selected papers and reports)

128. Ryff, C. D., & Singer, B. H. (1998). Know thyself and become what you are: A eudaimonic approach to well-being. *Journal of Happiness Studies, 9*(1), 13–39. (Note: duplicate theme; included for depth)

129. VanderWeele, T. J. (2017). On the promotion of human flourishing. *Proceedings of the National Academy of Sciences, 114*(31), 8148–8156. https://doi.org/10.1073/pnas.1702996114

130. Frankl, V. E. (2006). *Man's search for meaning*. Beacon Press.

CHAPTER 14 — THE COMMUNITY EFFECT — WHY CONNECTION HEALS

131. Holt-Lunstad, J., Smith, T. B., Baker, M., Harris, T., & Stephenson, D. (2015). Loneliness and social isolation as risk factors for mortality: A meta-analytic review. *Perspectives on Psychological Science, 10*(2), 227–237. https://doi.org/10.1177/1745691614568352

132. House, J. S., Landis, K. R., & Umberson, D. (1988). Social relationships and health. *Science, 241*(4865), 540–545. https://doi.org/10.1126/science.3399889

133. Cohen, S. (2004). Social relationships and health. *American Psychologist, 59*(8), 676–684. https://doi.org/10.1037/0003-066X.59.8.676

134. Holt-Lunstad, J., Smith, T. B., & Layton, J. B. (2010). Social relationships and mortality risk: A meta-analytic review. *PLoS Medicine, 7*(7), e1000316. https://doi.org/10.1371/journal.pmed.1000316

135. Umberson, D., & Karas Montez, J. (2010). Social relationships and health: A flashpoint for health policy. *Journal of Health and Social Behavior, 51*(Suppl), S54–S66. https://doi.org/10.1177/0022146510383501

136. Holt-Lunstad, J. (2018). Why social relationships are important for physical health: A systems approach to understanding and modifying risk. *Annual Review of Psychology, 69*, 335–361. https://doi.org/10.1146/annurev-psych-122216-011902

137. Cohen, S., & Janicki-Deverts, D. (2009). Can we improve our physical health by altering our social networks? *Perspectives on Psychological Science, 4*(4), 375–378. https://doi.org/10.1111/j.1745-6924.2009.01148.x

138. Buettner, D. (2012). The role of communal rituals and social structure in Blue Zones' longevity. *National Geographic Reports*.

139. Sandstrom, G. M., & Dunn, E. W. (2014). Is efficiency overrated? Minimal social interactions lead to belonging and positive affect. *Social Psychological and Personality Science*, 5(4), 453–458. https://doi.org/10.1177/1948550613502990

140. Holt-Lunstad, J., Robles, T. F., & Sbarra, D. A. (2017). Advancing social connection as a public health priority in the United States. *American Psychologist*, 72(6), 517–530. https://doi.org/10.1037/amp0000103

CHAPTER 15 — ACHIEVING THRIVING WEIGHT LOSS

141. Hall, K. D., et al. (2012). Energy balance and its components: Implications for body weight regulation. *American Journal of Clinical Nutrition, 95*(4), 989–994. https://doi.org/10.3945/ajcn.112.036350

142. Sumithran, P., Prendergast, L. A., Delbridge, E., Purcell, K., Shulkes, A., Kriketos, A., & Proietto, J. (2011). Long-term persistence of hormonal adaptations to weight loss. *New England Journal of Medicine, 365*(17), 1597–1604. https://doi.org/10.1056/NEJMoa1105816

143. Leibel, R. L., Rosenbaum, M., & Hirsch, J. (1995). Changes in energy expenditure resulting from altered body weight. *New England Journal of Medicine, 332*(10), 621–628. https://doi.org/10.1056/NEJM199503093321001

144. Westerterp, K. R. (2013). Physical activity and physical activity-induced energy expenditure in humans: Measurement, determinants, and effects. *Frontiers in Physiology, 4*, 90. https://doi.org/10.3389/fphys.2013.00090

145. Leidy, H. J., Clifton, P. M., Astrup, A., Wycherley, T. P., Westerterp-Plantenga, M. S., Luscombe-Marsh, N. D., & Mattes, R. D. (2015). The role of protein in weight loss and maintenance. *The American Journal of Clinical Nutrition, 101*(6), 1320S–1329S. https://doi.org/10.3945/ajcn.114.084038

146. Hall, K. D., et al. (2019). Ultra-processed diets cause excess calorie intake and weight gain: A randomized controlled trial. *Cell Metabolism, 30*(1), 67–77.e3. https://doi.org/10.1016/j.cmet.2019.05.008

147. Varady, K. A. (2011). Intermittent versus daily calorie restriction for type 2 diabetes prevention and treatment.

Nutrition Reviews, 69(7), 426–431.
https://doi.org/10.1111/j.1753-4887.2011.00421.x

148. Westerterp-Plantenga, M. S. (2004). The significance of protein for appetite control and body weight management. *Current Opinion in Clinical Nutrition and Metabolic Care, 7*(6), 635–640. https://doi.org/10.1097/00075197-200411000-00002

149. Blundell, J. E., et al. (2010). Appetite control: methodological aspects of the evaluation of foods. *Obesity Reviews, 11*(5), 251–270. https://doi.org/10.1111/j.1467-789X.2010.00714.x

150. Chaput, J.-P., & Tremblay, A. (2009). Insufficient sleep as a contributor to obesity: An update. *Current Obesity Reports, 1*(4), 245–256. https://doi.org/10.1007/s13679-009-0012-8

CHAPTER 16 — THE LONGEVITY BLUEPRINT — LIVING YOUNGER, LONGER

151. López-Otín, C., Blasco, M. A., Partridge, L., Serrano, M., & Kroemer, G. (2013). The hallmarks of aging. *Cell*, 153(6), 1194–1217. https://doi.org/10.1016/j.cell.2013.05.039

152. Blackburn, E. H., & Epel, E. S. (2017). *The telomere effect: A revolutionary approach to living younger, healthier, longer.* Grand Central Publishing.

153. Fontana, L., & Partridge, L. (2015). Promoting health and longevity through diet: From model organisms to humans. *Cell*, 161(1), 106–118. https://doi.org/10.1016/j.cell.2015.02.020

154. Longo, V. D., & Mattson, M. P. (2014). Fasting: Molecular mechanisms and clinical applications. *Cell Metabolism*, 19(2), 181–192. https://doi.org/10.1016/j.cmet.2013.12.008

155. Buettner, D. (2012). *The Blue Zones: 9 lessons for living longer from the people who've lived the longest.* National Geographic.

156. Gladyshev, V. N. (2016). Aging: Progressive decline in fitness and rise in vulnerability. *Aging Cell*, 15(4), 542–545. https://doi.org/10.1111/acel.12482

157. Kenyon, C. (2010). The first long-lived mutants: Discovery of the concept that lifespan can be regulated. *Mechanisms of Ageing and Development*, 131(7–8), 493–496. https://doi.org/10.1016/j.mad.2010.01.005

158. Fontana, L., & Klein, S. (2007). Aging, adiposity, and caloric restriction. JAMA, 297(9), 986–994. https://doi.org/10.1001/jama.297.9.986

159. Semba, R. D., & Ferrucci, L. (2017). An international perspective on healthy aging and age-related diseases.

Public Health Reviews, 38(1), 1.
https://doi.org/10.1186/s40985-017-0050-0

160. Payne, G. (2019). Exercise, mitochondria, and aging. *Journal of Physiology*, 597(20), 5005–5023.
https://doi.org/10.1113/JP277936

ACKNOWLEDGMENTS

Books are never born in isolation. They are living organisms stitched together by threads of inspiration, sacrifice, encouragement, and faith. This book is no exception.

To begin, I must bow in gratitude to the teachers, researchers, and trailblazers whose work laid the foundations of what you've read here. From the scientists mapping the inner cosmos of our microbiome, to the physicians challenging conventional dogma, to the philosophers and thinkers who reminded us that health is not merely the absence of disease but the presence of vibrancy — I am indebted to you. Your tireless pursuit of truth made this book possible.

A very special acknowledgment goes to **Dr. Mutsa Nyamfukdza**, PhD, Nutritionist, based in London, UK. Her insights, guidance, and wisdom shaped not only the accuracy of this work but also its heart. Dr. Nyamfukdza has a rare gift: the ability to see both the science and the soul of nutrition. Her counsel throughout the writing of this book kept me grounded, sharpened my understanding, and reminded me that behind every data point is a living, breathing human being longing for change. To you, Mutsa — I owe more than words can say. Thank you for walking beside me on this journey.

To the communities — both in-person and digital — who have shown me what resilience and renewal look like in real time: thank you. Every message shared, every struggle voiced, every small victory celebrated reminded me why this work matters. You are living proof that change is possible and that the human spirit is far more resilient than we sometimes believe.

To my family and loved ones — your patience, your belief in me, and your reminders to rest, eat well, and walk outside when I was buried in writing — you were my compass. The warmth of your support carried me through the long nights and early mornings.

To the friends and colleagues who challenged my ideas, sharpened my language, and asked the hard questions — thank you for keeping me honest. A book is only as strong as the conversations that shape it, and you gave me the gift of your perspective.

And finally, to you, the reader. You are the most important reason this book exists. You chose to pick it up, to engage with it, and to imagine a different way of living. That choice alone is extraordinary. Writing these pages, I often pictured you sitting with them in your hands — tired, perhaps, but curious; hopeful, perhaps, but uncertain. And my silent prayer was always the same: *May these words light a path. May they give you not only information, but transformation. May they remind you that you are not broken — you are becoming.*

If you close this book with a single spark of conviction that you can eat, move, rest, and live in a way that makes you thrive, then every sentence was worth writing.

Thank you for allowing me to walk with you on this journey. May the compass you carry now always point you back to renewal.

With gratitude and hope,
Phil Onyeagolu

INDEX

409, 415, 416, 432, 447, 454, 455, 457, 458, 459, 463, 466, 469, 472, 473, 481, 489, 509, 510

ABOUT THE AUTHOR

Philip Onyeagolu is a wellness advocate whose journey began long before he ever thought of writing a book. Once overweight, exhausted, and trapped in an endless cycle of dieting and guilt, Philip discovered that real transformation does not come from fighting the body but from finally listening to it.

In *Don't Eat to Live, Eat to Thrive,* he shares the simple but life-changing system that helped him escape diet chaos and rediscover energy, confidence, and freedom. His work is guided by one core belief: the body is not the enemy. It is the greatest ally a person has when it comes to healing, balance, and long-term change.

Philip did not start as a health expert or a fitness coach. He started as someone who was simply tired. Tired of feeling older than his years, tired of trying every new diet, and tired of waking up each day in a body that felt heavier and more defeated. By his early thirties, climbing a single flight of stairs left him breathless. His blood pressure was high, his confidence was low, and each January brought another promise of a "New Year, New Me" that faded under the weight of work, family, and exhaustion.

After years of failing, starting over, and failing again, Philip experienced a turning point. He realized he did not need another diet. He needed a new relationship with his body. Instead of punishing it, he chose to understand it. He began with small, almost invisible changes: skipping dinner some nights, keeping meals light, walking in the evenings, and listening instead of forcing. Slowly, his body responded. The weight began to come off naturally. His mind cleared. His energy returned. He was healing in every way that mattered.

That shift became the foundation of his life's work.

Don't Eat to Live, Eat to Thrive is the story of Philip's awakening from survival mode to a state of renewal and clarity. It is not a diet book. It is a blueprint for anyone who has ever felt stuck, overwhelmed, guilty, or disconnected from their body. It is a guide for people who want more than weight loss. It is for those who want their life back.

Today, Philip's mission is simple and deeply personal. He helps people remember that thriving does not come from restriction. It comes from restoration. The body is powerful, intuitive, and incredibly capable of healing when we stop fighting it. Once you learn to listen to your body, it will show you exactly what to do.

Because the truth is this: you do not have to fight your body to change it.

You only have to stop fighting yourself.